THE WOMAN'S GUIDE TO GOOD HEALTH

THE WOMAN'S GUIDE TO GOOD HEALTH

Mary Jane Gray, M.D./Florence Haseltine, M.D./
Susan Love, M.D./Kathleen Mayzel, M.D./
Artemis P. Simopoulos, M.D./with Beverly Jacobson
and the Editors of Consumer Reports Books

CONSUMER REPORTS BOOKS
A Division of Consumers Union
Yonkers, New York

Library of Congress Cataloging-in-Publication Data:

The Woman's guide to Good Health / Mary Jane Gray . . . [et al.] and the
editors of Consumer Reports Books.
    p.   cm.
    Includes index.
    ISBN 0-89043-382-8
    1. Women—Health and hygiene.   I. Gray, Mary Jane.   II. Consumer
Reports Books.
RA778.W752 1991
613'.04244—dc20   91-27256
                                                                          CIP

Design by GDS / Jeffrey L. Ward
First printing, November 1991
Manufactured in the United States of America

Contents

Introduction

It is more than two decades since the ground-breaking books on women's health and health care focused national attention on the need for women to take greater responsibility for their own health and well-being. Voicing a growing distrust with the medical establishment, these books provided women with crucial information about the prevention, diagnosis, and treatment of "female problems." Popular texts of the 70s encouraged women to administer treatment, perform minor surgical procedures, and sidestep conventional medical advice that had proved to be insensitive and/or inadequate to women's real needs.

As a result of the women's movement and other social, economic, and political changes, health care in America in recent years has become more receptive to the demands of women. Licensed midwives deliver babies in the comfort of a woman's own home, or in birthing centers that provide more intimate care than that of a large municipal hospital. New treatments for breast cancer that minimize disfigurement and psychological damage have replaced routine radical mastectomies. Hysterectomies performed vaginally minimize the risk and discomfort of traditional procedures. More women have entered the medical profession—women now account for over 32 percent of medical school graduates—and many have entered the fields of medical research with a deep commitment to furthering knowledge of women's health issues.

While health care for women has improved since the 1960s, there is still much to be done. In many areas of the country, routine repeat cesareans put women needlessly at risk, while many unnecessary hysterectomies continue to be performed. Because of an uneven allocation of public funds for research that favors male problems, much still remains to be learned about women and heart disease; premenstrual syndrome; safe, dependable birth control; the interaction of hormones; osteoporosis; and many other women's health issues.

Nevertheless, the Editors of Consumer Reports Books believe the do-it-yourself medicine of the past is no longer necessary or recommended. Enough women have joined and influenced the medical establishment to ensure that women's issues will not be overlooked. The recent explosion of technical knowledge and advances in medicine, the confusing claims and counterclaims of miracle drugs and procedures, make it particularly important to seek out the best professional advice. On the other hand, the best defense against inadequate or risky treatment is knowledge and skepticism. The more a woman knows about her own body, the better she will be able to evaluate the medical advice she receives. As the practice of medicine has become increasingly complex and specialized, it is crucial that women know what questions to ask their health-care professional, when to seek a second opinion, and how to decide between alternative treatment plans.

Conceived and developed by the Editors of Consumer Reports Books, and written by a team of women doctors who are experts in their field, *The Woman's Guide to Good Health* combines sensitivity to women's needs and issues with mainstream medical expertise. Here is the most up-to-date information on prevention, diagnosis, and treatment of disease, with special attention to such controversial areas as cancer treatment, breast reconstruction techniques, hormone-replacement therapy, and alternatives to hysterectomy. Frank discussions about the role of heredity in breast cancer, the growing threat of sexually transmitted diseases, and the newest technologies for artificial insemination address women's most intimate concerns in clear, easy-to-understand language. A book of knowledge for women of all ages, *The Woman's Guide to Good Health* will help provide the information women need to make intelligent decisions about health care for themselves and their families.

The Editors of Consumer Reports Books

1

Medical Politics and Medical Personnel

Mary Jane Gray, M.D.

WOMEN AND THE HEALTH-CARE SYSTEM

It is no accident that American women have taken such a major role over the past few decades in health-care advocacy. Research on women's health has been neglected, with only 13 percent of the National Institutes of Health (NIH) budget devoted to women's diseases. In fact, it was not until 1990 that the NIH established the first women's health bureau. There is, therefore, a severely inadequate research base for normal female physiological functions such as menstruation, childbirth, and menopause, and far too little information is available about such "female" diseases as osteoporosis and breast cancer. We have only one treatment for the discomforts of menopause, and that one, estrogen-replacement therapy (ERT), while effective, has not been proved to be totally safe. Moreover, practically nothing is known about cardiovascular disease in women because all the studies have been done on men; this is true despite the fact that 247,000 women die annually of heart attacks, compared with about 40,000 deaths from breast cancer and an equal number from lung cancer; in fact, cardiovascular disease is the leading cause of death for older women.

1

The power structure in medicine is still heavily dominated by males. Despite the surge of women in medical schools, only 16.7 percent of the nation's doctors are female, and only a handful of women serve as full professors, medical school deans, and directors of research institutes. On the other hand, females dominate the lower end of the health-care spectrum, providing 97 percent of all practical and registered nurses, 86 percent of health aides, and 71 percent of health technicians.

The women's movement has produced some national organizations that have lobbied successfully for improvements in women's health, including better care for DES daughters (those whose mothers during pregnancy were given the synthetic estrogen hormone diethylstilbestrol, which was later found to cause cancer), removing hazardous contraceptives from the market, and creating family-centered birthing arrangements within American hospitals. But even they have not been able to bring to the United States the more effective contraceptive methods in use abroad, among them male contraceptives researched in China and RU-486, the postconception abortion pill developed in France. And millions of women and their children have no health insurance at all, either because they work for companies that do not provide it to their employees, are part-time workers not covered by their company's health-care plan, or earn too much money to qualify for Medicaid but not enough to buy their own health insurance policy.

Research on women's experiences with the health-care system in the United States has shown that although they seek medical care more frequently than men, they are often treated with less respect, particularly by male doctors. Two studies showed that nurses, too, display more regard for male than female patients. Women also receive far more psychotherapeutic medications, although there are no valid studies that contend they are any less emotionally stable than men.

Women are also subjected to more surgical procedures than they need, specifically hysterectomy and cesarean section, particularly if they have health insurance. Many observers of the health-care scene believe that women have been victims of overtreatment in the area of cancer surgery as well. For example, a number of surgeons still perform radical mastectomies without considering other possibilities, even though studies have established that lumpectomy and radiation—which are far less disfiguring—are often viable alternatives. One reason for this overtreatment, and its companion overtesting, is the large number of lawsuits being brought against doctors today, leading them to practice "defensive medicine" without enough regard for the consequences to the patient. The best safeguard against inadequate or unnecessary treatment is, therefore, knowledge and caution.

PHYSICIANS AND SPECIALISTS

Medicine has become so specialized in the United States that even if your health is excellent, you probably will have a variety of health-care providers in your lifetime. These may range from your primary-care physician to highly trained specialists who treat specific medical or surgical problems to the technicians who handle routine or sophisticated testing procedures. The proliferating number of categories and medical services supplied today require both your attention and your understanding if you are to be an enlightened health-care consumer.

A physician is a person who has graduated from medical school; a specialist is a physician who has received postgraduate training. Most women have a primary-care physician who is either a general practitioner (GP), a specialist in family practice, or an internist, whom they consult for general checkups and specific problems. Some GPs and family doctors still deliver babies and care for infants and children as well, but if your primary-care physician is an internist, you will probably consult an obstetrician-gynecologist (OB-GYN) when you become pregnant and later select a pediatrician to look after the baby. In practice, the obstetrician-gynecologist often becomes the primary-care physician for many women from puberty to menopause. Certain sections of the country suffer from a shortage of adequately trained physicians who attend births because a growing number are understandably reluctant to risk the threat of malpractice lawsuits and the consequently prohibitive costs of malpractice insurance.

A general practitioner, a dying breed and therefore difficult to find as medicine becomes more sophisticated, has had one year of internship training beyond medical school before going into practice. A family practitioner trains for three postgraduate years, while internists, obstetrician-gynecologists, and pediatricians complete internship and residency programs that vary in length from three to five years.

The organizations that test and certify doctors in their specialties after completion of their residencies are the American boards of these specialties. Being board-eligible means only that the physician has had enough postgraduate training to be allowed to take the board examination. When a physician is board-certified, it means that he or she has taken and passed a written, and often an oral, examination in a particular specialty.

You can tell how much training a doctor has by the category of specialization, which is indicated by the initials that appear after his or her name in listings and diplomas. F.A.C. means Fellow of the American College and is followed by the specialty designation, so that F.A.C.P. indicates that the doctor is a Fellow of the American College of Pediatrics, and F.A.C.O.G. specifies a Fellow of the American College of Obstetricians and Gynecologists. These organizations have standards of training, and all applicants are carefully screened before they are allowed to use their designation.

In addition to these most commonly consulted physicians, many other specialists exist should you need them, including surgeons (general, vascular, cancer, neurological), anesthesiologists, cardiologists, dermatologists, radiologists, and psychiatrists. There are hematologists (specialists in blood diseases), oncologists (cancer specialists), urologists (doctors who treat diseases of the urinary system), jnephrologists (doctors who look after the kidneys), rheumatologists (those who treat arthritis and other diseases of the joints and connective tissue), neurologists (whose expertise is the brain and nervous system), orthopedists (who treat bone problems), gastroenterologists (who look after the digestive tract), otolaryngologists (specialists in ear, nose, and throat diseases), ophthalmologists (eye problems), and gerontologists (doctors who specialize in the treatment of the elderly). Your primary-care physician will refer you to a specialist should you need one, but you should always ask about the specialist's qualifications and experience in performing the procedures in question, and make it a point to participate in the choice.

OTHER PRACTITIONERS

Some health-care providers have not been to medical school but have taken alternative training. Nurse practitioners, physician assistants, and midwives, for example, variously offer care in clinics, hospitals, and sometimes in private medical practices.

NURSE PRACTITIONERS (NPs)

The University of Colorado established the first nurse practitioner training program in 1960, and today there are 25,000 NPs in the United States. These registered nurses, who have completed courses in advanced nursing education, have clinical experience in family health, caring for adults, children, adolescents, and the elderly. Some have special training in women's health, psychiatric conditions, and occupational health. They work for physicians in private practice and in clinics, health departments, home health-care agencies, health-maintenance organizations, nursing homes, and correctional facilities. Some nurse practitioners have independent practices, but you are most likely to encounter an NP either in your doctor's office or in a women's health clinic, where she or he may serve as a gynecologic nurse practitioner. These specialized NPs take patients' histories, perform physical exams—including pelvic exams and Pap smears—and treat typical gynecologic problems—including sexually transmitted diseases (STDs), abnormal bleeding, vaginitis, and urinary tract infections.

Nurse practitioners emphasize the value of health education and counseling in allaying medical problems, which includes giving advice on nutrition, exercise, and beneficial changes in life-style and advising about the management of stress and family problems. NPs diagnose and treat common conditions, such as sprains, infections, and rashes; manage chronic illnesses—including high blood pressure, diabetes, and arthritis—under the supervision of a physician; perform physical examinations and order laboratory work and X rays; and put on casts and perform minor office surgery. In some states they can prescribe medication. By and large, NPs work under protocols developed by physicians that spell out the specific mode of treatment for various medical conditions. If the patient has vaginitis, for example, the protocol will specify which tests the NP should order—cultures for gonorrhea, wet preparations, and so on. It will also define what action the nurse practitioner is to take upon receiving the test results. In most medical practices that include an NP, the physician reviews and signs the chart of each patient the NP treats.

PHYSICIAN ASSISTANTS (PAs)

When four ex–navy medical corpsmen enrolled in Duke University's new program for physician assistants in 1965, they became the forerunners of the 20,000 PAs who practice today, largely in American hospitals. PAs train for 24 months, covering a curriculum that is roughly equivalent to the middle two years of medical school. They take a certification exam upon graduation. PAs do not practice privately; they are trained by physicians to help them as needed. Many assist with surgery, while some work for internists and others are employed by corporate health programs, where they cut costs for their employers because their salaries are far lower than those of doctors. PAs also make a significant contribution to the staffs of nursing homes.

In your doctor's office, the physician assistant may be the person who spends time with you explaining test results, going over your prescribed treatment, or getting you started in an exercise or weight-loss program. As with NPs, most supervising doctors sign the chart of a patient seen by a physician assistant.

MIDWIVES

A midwife ("with woman" in Middle English) is the person who stays with a woman throughout her labor and delivery. He or she may also deliver babies in a hospital, a free-standing birth center, or the woman's home.

Midwifery in the United States predates the Republic, with the first one arriving on the *Mayflower*. During the colonial period and into the nineteenth century, midwives assisted most women at childbirth. As early as 1722, six Louisiana physicians administered qualifying examinations to three French midwives who had diplomas from European universities, allowing two to practice without supervision and deeming the qualifications of the third inadequate. In 1760, New York State began licensing midwives, and other states soon followed. Yet many experienced midwives continued to practice outside the licensing system.

Until well into the twentieth century, childbirth among all social classes took place at home. The death knell of American midwifery began in 1855, when Dr. J. Marion Sims, the "father" of obstetrics and gynecology, began his specialty practice at Women's Hospital in New York City. By 1876, there were enough physicians specializing in gynecology to organize the American Gynecologic Society. Although female midwives continued to work among the poor and still delivered half of the nation's babies at the beginning of the twentieth century, and despite the fact that studies comparing physician- and midwife-attended births showed little difference in fetal outcome and the rate of infection, the stereotype of the dirty, drunken midwife persisted. By 1912, the trend toward improving the training of doctors was in full force, and by 1920 the move to hospital births, where women were attended by male obstetricians, had begun in earnest. Home births declined rapidly; today, 98 percent of all babies are born in the hospital.

Midwifery began its renaissance in the 1960s, spurred by women who wanted natural childbirth and objected to the obstetrical technology and anesthesia that accompanied hospital birth.

If you are at low risk of developing complications during pregnancy and birth, you may want to consider being cared for by a midwife. Women attended by midwives usually see a doctor once during the pregnancy to evaluate their health and make sure they have no chronic conditions that need medical care. If you have a complicating condition, such as toxemia, kidney or heart disease, severe anemia, a serious infection, hypertension, diabetes, or Rh sensitization; if the fetus or placenta is in an abnormal position, lying across the birth canal; or if the baby is in the breech position with the buttocks or legs rather than the head presenting at the birth canal; if you are carrying twins; or if you are addicted to drugs, you are not a candidate for midwifery care.

Nurse-Midwives

Nurse-midwives are registered nurses who have taken additional training in midwifery. There are 29 midwifery schools in the United States, 9 certificate programs, 8 that award a master's degree, and 2 precertification programs that serve as refresher courses for midwives returning to practice after an absence. These programs differ in the length of the course and level of training.

The American College of Nurse-Midwives (ACNM) has established training standards and certifies nurse-midwives; in fact, 45 states either recognize or require this certification. Nurse-midwives are trained to manage all aspects of pregnancy, birth, and post-partum care; take medical histories; give nutritional advice; assess problems; and make referrals to medical specialists when specialized treatment is needed. In some states they can prescribe medication. Nurse-midwives usually practice in hospitals or free-standing birth centers as part of a team and have an obstetrician available for consultation or in case of emergency. Some have private practices. Reimbursement by private and government insurers varies; 16 states mandate private insurance reimbursement for nurse-midwifery services, and 32 states have regulations covering Medicaid reimbursement. If you intend to choose a midwife as your birth attendant, check your health insurance policy to see if it covers midwifery services.

Independent Midwives

Independent midwives learn their skills by apprenticing with experienced midwives or by attending one of several schools around the country that teach midwifery. At least 24 states regulate practice by midwives who are not certified by ACNM, and some, such as New Hampshire and New Mexico, have developed requirements for state certification that include oral and written examinations and clinical observation. The Midwives Alliance of North America (MANA) is the professional organization that represents independent midwives, and it is currently working to develop national certification guidelines. Most independent midwives are in private practice and attend some births, although some work in staff clinics, such as the Maternity Center in El Paso, Texas.

The requirements—and the availability—of physician backup for lay-midwives varies, but in any case it is important to determine if your midwife has a doctor she can call on if there is an emergency. Many independent midwives have doctors who not only assist them if needed but also see each of the midwife's clients at least once during her pregnancy. Insurance reimbursement varies; check your health insurance policy to see if it covers the services of an independent midwife and home birth. If you plan to give birth at home, you and your midwife should know the location of the nearest hospital and have transportation available to it should the need arise.

DIETITIANS

If you intend to make significant changes in your eating habits and believe you need professional help and advice, you may want to consult a dietitian. Registered dietitians have been trained to provide a comprehensive analysis of your current diet and eating habits and to recommend—and supervise—changes that will improve your health and your general well-being. If your doctor refers you to a dietitian, the services may be covered by your health insurance policy.

MEDICAL SOCIAL WORKERS

You may also consult with a medical social worker if you need assistance with a problem—for example, you might have an elderly hospitalized parent who needs either home care or long- or short-term nursing-home care once he or she leaves the hospital. These practitioners are most commonly employed by hospitals, but there are many in private practice. Given the bureaucratic maze that characterizes our Medicare and Medicaid programs, some medical social workers have specialized in providing advice on how to negotiate these systems effectively while securing the best medical care available.

FINDING COMPETENT CARE

It may be more difficult to find a general or family practitioner than it is to find an internist, OB-GYN specialist, or pediatrician because more American doctors tend to specialize. If there is a health maintenance organization (HMO) in your area, you may want to visit it and interview the doctors and other medical personnel who work there. At an HMO, you pay an annual fee for medical care that is provided by member-doctors; this arrangement is usually less costly than buying health insurance to cover care by private practitioners and hospitals. The larger HMOs have a number of doctors and a variety of other medical personnel on staff; while they do not have specialists available in all areas, your HMO primary-care physician can usually refer you to one if needed. Be sure to check on the HMO's referral policy, as some narrow your choice by limiting referrals to certain specialists in the community. The choice between an HMO and health insurance is an important one that will be affected, among other matters, by the quality of the HMOs in your area. It is well worth researching the kind of care available before you decide which to choose. Of course, your employer may have made the choice for you, but many large employers now offer a variety of health plans.

Once you decide what kind of doctor you are looking for, it's a good idea to collect information from several sources. Friends who are doctors or nurses or who otherwise work in the medical field are a good place to start. You might also check with medical professional organizations that recommend physicians; call your local hospital or medical society for the names of doctors on the hospital's staff who also see private patients; or call the nearest medical school for a list of professors with a private practice. Or you might consult community-based groups such as Planned Parenthood or a women's health clinic if there is one in your community.

After you have collected a few names, a credential check is in order. You can do this easily by contacting the hospital with which the doctor is affiliated. Before granting a physician privileges to admit patients, a hospital committee checks the doctor's credentials, including medical school attendance, specialty training, board certification, and state licensure. If the physician actually practices at the hospital, you can usually be assured that those basic requirements have been met. Although it is true that medical communities sometimes protect incompetent doctors—those who abuse alcohol or drugs, or have become otherwise dangerous or unable to function properly—from public attention, it is not a common occurrence and is therefore a minor consideration in your accepting a recommendation from such sources.

When checking the credentials of nonphysician medical practitioners, you can contact their employers, who will have verified their education, training, and certification. If you plan to consult a midwife or a nurse practitioner in private practice, you can ask her or him directly about training and certification from either

ACNM or the particular state health board that certifies credentials in your locality. The same is true of dietitians, nutritionists, and medical social workers who maintain private practices. Check credentials with the licensing organization.

The final step is an interview. This allows you to meet the clinician and to evaluate his or her office. This is the time to tell your prospective doctor what is important to you and what you expect from your medical care—for example, your desire to be as fully informed as possible and to participate in all decision making about your treatment. This informs the practitioner that you expect honest and accurate information about the purpose and necessity for any testing that may be ordered, about any medical condition you may develop, a clear explanation of what is wrong, and an explanation of the various treatment options that are available. Use this initial contact to determine if you can talk to the practitioner easily and find out about his or her basic approach to patients. Will the doctor encourage you to participate in decisions about your own treatment? How does the doctor feel about obtaining second opinions? Will the doctor take time to talk with you about your treatment? Is there someone else in the office—a nurse, PA, or NP—who will be available to answer your questions? What procedure should you follow in case of an emergency, especially at night or on weekends?

How long is the average waiting time for office appointments, and how long can you expect to wait to see the doctor when you arrive? Waiting can be a real problem, particularly in large cities or when dealing with doctors who think a waiting room full of patients impresses newcomers—if possible, you will want to avoid the latter. Are the facilities clean and up-to-date? Is the secretarial or auxiliary staff pleasant and helpful?

You might also want to use this time to find out what the doctor expects from you. Giving an accurate medical history and presenting your symptoms clearly and early in the visit are indispensable if the doctor is to provide the best care. Come prepared with a good sense of your own priorities so you can communicate your concerns about symptoms, treatment, and the nature of the relationship you would like to have with the doctor.

If you also use this initial appointment for a routine physical, or to seek care for a specific problem, you will be able to judge the clinician's skill, sensitivity, and knowledge. A recent survey evaluating women's reactions to their first pelvic exam found that despite the fact that 40 percent of the study population rated their gynecologic care as excellent, 14 percent reported that they were "extremely terrified" by their first pelvic, while 26 percent rated the experience as frightening, 33 percent as embarrassing, and 28 percent as anxiety-provoking. One-fifth of these women felt their physicians were overly abrupt when conducting a pelvic exam, and one-third said the contact between themselves and the doctor was too brief.

If you are seeking maternity care, find out during this visit what the clinician's philosophy is and whether it meshes with your own. Does the doctor lean toward natural or technological childbirth, or somewhere in between? How much prenatal testing does the doctor recommend? How often does the doctor find episiotomies and cesarean sections necessary? Does the doctor use fetal monitors during labor, or check the fetal heartbeat with a stethoscope? What about your having family members with you during labor? If the doctor cannot provide you with comprehensive information about nutrition during pregnancy, smoking cessation, exercise, and childbirth education, is there someone else in the practice prepared to do so? Try to determine if the physician really enjoys delivering babies or instead is overly concerned with testing to protect himself from potential lawsuits. Bring your partner or a friend with you, because even if you take notes during your conversation, another person's impressions and perspective will be helpful, both during the interview and later.

Whether the medical care you're seeking is general or specialized, be sure to discuss fees. Many people, including physicians, are uncomfortable addressing this subject, but it is particularly important as costs skyrocket. Ask the doctor or the office supervisor what the charges are for various services, including office visits and tests, then check your health insurance policy to see how much of the cost is covered. Some policies don't reimburse for preventive care, while others require that you be responsible for paying a high deductible before they begin to cover any costs. In either case, unless you are a member of an HMO, you will be paying some fees out of your own pocket; make certain you know what to expect. It's sometimes possible to negotiate the period of time over which your payments are made, or the fees themselves.

If you become dissatisfied with your physician, you should find another. Patients leave doctors for many reasons: a breakdown in communication, a conflict of personalities, another physician was consulted for a second opinion and he or she was liked better, a move to a different area, a loss of confidence as the result of something the doctor said or did. You can explain your decision to the practitioner or not, as you see fit. If you decide to do so, either by phone, letter, or in person, it might help the doctor understand what went wrong. For example, some older physicians think of women primarily as people who need protecting, and they may not understand that this attitude is condescending, patronizing, or otherwise offensive. Sometimes talking it over can save a doctor-patient relationship and prevent bitterness on either side. In any case, if your reason for leaving is a serious breach of medical ethics, such as alcohol or drug abuse or the practitioner's making sexual advances, you should report it by letter to the local county medical society to protect other patients.

PATIENTS' RIGHTS

Most physicians and other medical workers try to give patients the best available care when they are hospitalized, and to make them as comfortable as possible. (See Chapter 14.) Nevertheless, many problems can arise. If you need treatment in a hospital, your rights include the following:

- If your life is in danger, you must be admitted to an emergency room and receive immediate medical care regardless of your race, color, sex, religion, type of illness, or how your bill will be paid. However, hospitals in major cities may reach a saturation point and close their emergency rooms. If this happens, you will have to go elsewhere. If your life is not threatened, the emergency room staff will determine what your condition is and either treat you or refer you elsewhere.
- When you enter a hospital voluntarily, you have the right to know the rules and regulations that will apply to you. Don't sign anything unless you read and understand it. If you object to something in a hospital form, cross it out before signing.
- After admission, you have the right to proper medical care;

if you are transferred to another hospital, you should know why and what your other choices are. Be sure the second hospital has agreed to accept you and has the treatment facilities and/or staff that were unavailable at the first hospital.

- If the hospital intends to include you in any research or medical teaching, it must gain your consent and apprise you of your rights as a patient. You have the right to know the purpose of the research or teaching, how it will benefit you or others, and what possible negative effect it can have on you and your recovery. You have the right to refuse these activities, and you should not be intimidated by the fear of antagonizing medical workers if you decide to refuse. This may take courage at the time you need it most.
- You have the right to an explanation, in language you can understand, of your condition, proposed treatment, and chances of recovery. You have the right to know what will happen if you decide against the proposed treatment. If you consent to treatment, you or the friend or advocate you enlist to do so should ask what the procedure entails, what the possible side effects are, whether and to what extent the treatment will cause you pain, who will perform the procedure, how much it will cost, how long you will be hospitalized, and what kind of care you will need when you go home.
- You have the right to refuse treatment and leave the hospital at any time. (There are exceptions for psychiatric patients who are considered dangerous to themselves and others, and these vary from state to state.) However, you should find out all the possible consequences you might experience if you leave. If you depart without being discharged by your doctor, you will have to sign a form absolving the doctor and the hospital of liability if your condition worsens.
- You have the right to be treated with dignity.
- You have the right to privacy and confidentiality.
- You have the right to have your bill explained. If you think your rights have been violated, tell the person involved. If that does not correct the situation, speak to the person's supervisor. If that doesn't work, ask for the hospital's patient representative (a staff person who is available at some, but not all, hospitals) or a social worker. You or your advocates

should try to resolve the situation by directing attention to the problem itself rather than to the person involved, as physicians and supervisors will then be freer to resolve the matter without their feeling threatened by having to choose sides between the staff they depend on and you.

• You have the right to an explanation of the tests the doctor recommends: how they will be performed, if they will be painful, what they will show, and how much they will cost.

The best way to avoid problems is for you or your advocate to keep in touch with the supervising nurse to determine what procedures—tests, medication, surgery—are scheduled for you. Here your relationship with your doctor will be crucial in terms of your being protected—as much as possible—against the risk of being overtested and overtreated.

TRENDS FOR THE FUTURE

Both women's health needs and the care women receive from doctors will undergo considerable change in this last decade of the twentieth century, as well as in the decades to come. U.S. demographics predict fewer women between the ages of 15 and 44, fewer births, and many more women in the older age groups. Consequently, women will need less obstetrical care, but because the number of older mothers will increase, the care they need may require more testing, counseling, and supervision than younger women need during pregnancy.

Women's health care in the future will focus on how women are affected by cardiovascular disease, hypertension, obesity, diabetes, cigarette smoking, hormone therapy, and osteoporosis. As researchers discover new ways of controlling uterine bleeding, halting and reversing tumor growth, and treating infection, the justification for surgery will greatly decrease. Screening will become an increasingly important part of medical practice as doctors try to catch diseases early, when they have the best chance of curing them.

Prevention and education will be increasingly stressed, and the doctor's office may become the place to go to learn how to change negative behaviors, encourage a healthy life-style, and achieve the benefits of good nutrition and exercise. For this to happen, however, insurers will have to begin paying for preventive treatment. If the Women's Research Bureau at NIH is successful, research studies in the future will at last include women, and far greater emphasis will be placed on accumulating data about the normal physiological parameters of women's biology. Much greater attention will be devoted to the natural process of aging and to the diseases that occur with aging, and some of that information will provide data on what women can do in their younger years to prevent problems later in life. This has already begun to happen with the study of osteoporosis; we now know, for example, that adequate calcium intake up to age 25 can build stronger bones and delay or prevent the onset of this crippling disease after menopause.

Women will continue to educate themselves so they can participate responsibly in their own health care, and also will need to go on educating themselves about the diseases to which they are particularly vulnerable. At present, each woman should be the preeminent member of her health-care team, enabling her to receive the best quality medical experience.

2

The Reproductive System

Florence Haseltine, M.D.

Because you will want to develop the best possible partnership with the health-care providers in your life, including a good understanding about when and whether to consult them at all, it's wise to be equipped with a basic understanding of just how your body works.

THE ANATOMY OF THE REPRODUCTIVE SYSTEM

The female reproductive tract is a complex system that contains a variety of components. These include the direct reproductive organs, such as the external genitalia that we can see and feel; the internal organs, such as the cervix and uterus, some of which we can feel and others that the doctor examines during a routine medical checkup; and certain glands, such as the adrenal, pituitary, and hypothalamus glands within the brain, which powerfully affect our reproductive abilities.

It is important to know the names of the organs that make up your reproductive system so that you can accurately report to your doctor any problems that occur. It is also vital to recognize how structures you can see and touch, such as the breasts and the vagina, look and feel when normal; in this way you can spot any changes that might indicate an infection or a disease process is starting. This familiarity will allow you to conduct the self-examinations of your breasts and vulva that are so vital if you are to prevent minor problems from becoming major ones and to see your doctor for an early diagnosis of adverse conditions that do occur.

THE EXTERNAL ORGANS

THE BREASTS

The breasts are the most obvious part of a woman's reproductive physiology, and the beginning of their development signals the onset of puberty. Breasts are symmetrical, with a round circle of darker skin in the middle containing the areola and the nipple. The nipples usually point outward, but they can also lie flat or turn inward. Nipples are highly sensitive and responsive to touch because they are made of erectile tissue; they play an important role in sexual responsiveness. During sexual arousal and orgasm, they are usually erect. (See Chapter 4, Fig. 4.1.)

The areola is also sensitive to touch. Oil glands within the areola, which can appear as tiny bumps on the surface, secrete a lubricant to protect the nipple during nursing.

One breast is usually slightly larger than the other; folklore says it is often the left breast, but there is no real evidence to support this. The breasts change with age and childbearing. Young women have firm breasts, and the tissue appears taut; the breasts of older women are more relaxed, and some will have stretch marks from childbearing. Breasts come in all sizes and can only be compared to each other, as there is no norm or standard, only averages.

The internal structure of the breast consists of fat, connective tissue, and mammary glands, which contain milk-producing areas and ducts that carry the milk to the nipples so a mother can nurse her infant. Although women generally have approximately the same amount of glandular tissue in their breasts, the amount of fat can vary; this is what accounts for the differences in women's breast size, and it is partially governed by heredity.

Because breast cancer now affects one in every nine women in the United States, you should examine your breasts monthly. (See Chapter 4 for a description of how to do a breast self-exam.) If you find that your nipples change in appearance between these examinations, or you feel a lump that wasn't present at your last medical checkup or monthly breast self-exam, consult your doctor promptly.

THE VULVA

The vulva is the entire genital area visible when you spread your legs, including the mons pubis—the soft tissue that contains the growth of hair that extends over the top of the pelvis, down the outer portion of the vulva, and, in some women, along the inside of the thighs. Sometimes the hair extends up the abdomen as far as the navel. Normal patterns of pubic hair range from generous amounts to scanty, and vary with hereditary and ethnic qualities. Most Caucasian women have curly pubic hair, for example, while that of Asian women is straight and usually far sparser. Changes in those hair patterns can occur if a hormonal abnormality causes the body to produce an excessive amount of male hormones (androgens). (See Chapter 3.)

The best way to see the vulva is to squat in front of a mirror with your legs apart or to lie on your back with a mirror held between your spread legs. Either way allows you to look at the various external structures and to examine them yourself. In a mature woman, the outer lips—labia majora—are covered with pubic hair. In women who have not had children, the outer lips lie close to each other; after childbirth they separate, and it's possible to see the opening of the vagina more readily. Fat, sebaceous glands, and connective tissue are the predominant ingredients that make up the labia majora. The inner lips, or labia minora, lie just inside the outer lips; they are hairless and extremely sensitive when touched. The vestibule, the area within the labia minora and visible if you separate them, joins a soft fold of skin right below the mons. This structure, called the hood of the clitoris, is sexually responsive. The vestibule also contains bundles of erectile tissue called the bulbs of the vestibule. Beneath the vestibule, on either side of the vaginal opening, are the Bartholin's glands, which produce a thin, lubricating mucus. The clitoris, located at the top of the vulva, consists of the shaft, a movable cord of responsive tissue just beneath the skin; the tip, or glans, which is the most sensitive and sexually responsive part of the entire vulva and faces the vagina; and the crura, the suspension ligaments that connect the clitoris to the pelvic bones. The bulbs of the vestibule, the clitoris, and the network of connecting blood vessels and muscle throughout the pelvic area all fill with blood and swell during sexual arousal.

The vulva also contains the urinary opening, located just below the clitoris; the outer portion of the vagina, located beneath the urinary openings; the smooth skin between the vagina and anus, called the perineum, which stretches remarkably during vaginal birth; and the anus itself.

As we develop during the fetal stage, the outer portion of the vagina forms from tissue of the perineum that turns inward; doctors call this process invagination. This perineal tissue grows in to meet the cervix, or the bottom of the uterus, and the upper vagina. Frequently, the vagina does not become a totally open tube, leaving a rim of tissue called the hymen, covered by a lining of flattened, platelike cells. The amount of the hymeneal tissue that remains in each of us varies, and even after childbearing, hymeneal tags or remnants are visible. The perineal body, which is the remaining area of the external organs, is composed of the muscles that surround the anus—the external anal sphincter, the bulbocavernosus muscles, and the superficial transverse perineal muscles.

THE INTERNAL ORGANS

THE VAGINA

Internally, the vagina is not a smooth muscular tube; once puberty begins, vaginal ridges form, with the thickness and folds of these ridges varying from one individual to another. The vagina is about three to five inches long and connects the uterus with the exterior of the body. The top wall of the vagina is usually shorter than the bottom wall, which lies next to the rectum. After menopause, the vaginal ridges diminish.

The vagina sheds its cells along with vaginal secretions, a process that women experience as the normal, everyday discharge. (If the vagina becomes infected, this discharge can become infused with

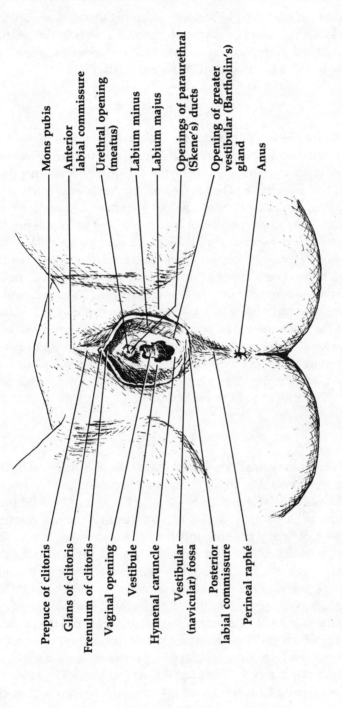

Mons pubis

Anterior
labial commissure

Urethral opening
(meatus)

Labium minus

Labium majus

Openings of paraurethral
(Skene's) ducts

Opening of greater
vestibular (Bartholin's)
gland

Anus

Prepuce of clitoris

Glans of clitoris

Frenulum of clitoris

Vaginal opening

Vestibule

Hymenal caruncle

Vestibular
(navicular) fossa

Posterior
labial commissure

Perineal raphé

Fig. 2.1 Perineum and External Genitalia: Female

pus and emit an odor.) Laboratory examination of these expelled vaginal cells can identify various hormonal events in the ovarian cycle. Vaginal secretions contribute to the vaginal moisture that permits lubrication to occur with sexual arousal.

THE CERVIX

Located at the top of the vagina, the cervix, which is the bottom of the uterus, or womb, varies in structure from woman to woman; its appearance also changes during the course of the monthly cycle and with childbearing. The surface of the cervix is smooth, with an opening, the endocervical canal, in its center. The endocervical canal forms the lower portion of the uterus, and its glands are the source of the cervical mucus that appears in the middle of the monthly menstrual cycle. Menstrual blood passes through the endocervical canal as it exits the uterus each month; vaginally delivered babies also make their way through it during childbirth, which is when tears can occur. In the center of the cervix is the os, the opening into the uterus. It is about the width of a thin straw, and you can feel it with your finger by reaching up through your vagina. The opening of the cervix is circular in some women and a slit in others. Covering the os is a mucous plug that prevents bacteria from penetrating above the cervical level.

THE UTERUS

The uterus contains three basic segments: the cervix with the endocervical canal, the lower uterine segment, and the fundus, or top. Normally the size and shape of a Seckle pear (or a small Bosc pear), the uterus weighs about two ounces in a mature woman. Three sets of ligaments suspend it in the abdominal cavity: the round ligaments, which run from the top of the uterus to the abdominal wall; the broad ligament, which extends from the side wall of the pelvis to the uterus and contains the large vessels that deliver its blood supply; and the utero-sacral ligament, extending back to the sacrum. At the base of the broad ligament is the cardinal ligament, which encloses the major uterine vessels.

Most women have a uterus that flexes forward, toward the bladder, but in about a third of women it is tipped backward, in which case it is referred to as retroverted. The uterus has a thick muscle

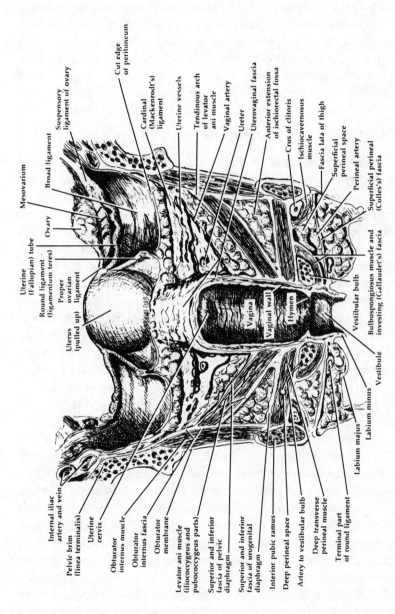

Fig. 2.2 Uterus, Vagina, and Supporting Structures

wall and is lined with tissue called the endometrium, which changes dramatically throughout the menstrual cycle. (See Chapter 3.) The main function of the uterus is to provide a protective environment in which a fetus can grow and develop. By the end of pregnancy, for example, the uterus has increased to 18 times its original weight, resembling a large honeydew melon or a medium-size watermelon. Its ability to return almost to its prepregnancy size is typical of its remarkable flexibility.

THE OVARIES

The ovaries, located on either side of the uterus, are between one and two inches long and one inch wide. During each menstrual cycle, one of them enlarges and forms a small cyst, which can be as big as two inches. The ovaries are complex endocrine organs. During each cycle they produce an egg (also called an oocyte or ovum), which, if fertilized, allows a woman to become pregnant. The ovaries also manufacture a series of endocrine hormones that prepare the uterus and the rest of the body for pregnancy. The eggs reside in follicles, groups of cells that are present in the female infant at birth and are maintained in a resting state until chosen for ovulation. Of the hundreds of thousands of egg-containing follicles in the ovaries at birth, only a small number—under 500— ever develop into mature eggs. The cells that surround the resting egg, called granulosa cells and theca cells, together with the egg, make up the follicle. These cells nurture the egg. The follicle and its supporting tissues also make the hormones estrogen, progesterone, and testosterone.

During the ovarian cycle, the pituitary gland, located at the base of the brain, releases the follicle-stimulating hormone (FSH), which, as the name implies, signals the ovaries to initiate follicle development. Researchers do not understand the mechanism that selects the follicle, but they do know that, while several follicles are recruited each month, usually only one goes on to develop. One theory is that the follicles produce certain substances that are self-regulatory.

The next step occurs at mid-cycle, when the ovaries release large quantities of luteinizing hormone (LH), the hormone that causes the follicle to release its egg. One of the fallopian tubes then picks up the egg and transports it down the tube to the uterus. In addition, the ovaries produce growth factors that regulate the pituitary gland. It is through the role of the pituitary gland that the brain is actually the main reproductive organ in the body, sending signals to the ovaries to start functioning at puberty and regulating the cycles from then on. Damage to the brain, particularly to the pituitary, can have severe adverse effects with respect to fertility.

THE FALLOPIAN TUBES

The fallopian tubes are thin, hollow structures about four to five inches long that lie on either side of the uterus, falling away from the ovary like a pair of inverted animal horns. Attached at their uterine end, the narrow tubes, about the width of an electrical cord, flare out at the ovarian end to become the flowery fimbriae, uneven undulating strands of tissue that, unconnected to the ovaries, hover just above them, surrounding and capturing the egg once it emerges from the ovary. Fertilization usually takes place in the fallopian tube, with the fertilized egg then taking four or five days to make its leisurely way to the uterine lining, where it must implant for a successful pregnancy. The delicate, corrugated lining of the fallopian tube, which contracts rhythmically, may help move the egg toward its destination. An unfertilized egg simply passes through the tube, taking several days to move through the uterus, cervix, and vagina, where the body expels it. (See Chapter 3.)

MEDICAL EXAMINATION OF THE REPRODUCTIVE TRACT

A woman usually makes an appointment with her gynecologist or family doctor for a routine review of her reproductive tract for a variety of reasons: She suspects a problem or has experienced one; she wants contraceptive advice; she is pregnant or thinking of becoming pregnant and needs information; or it's been a year since her last physical and she wants to be sure everything is normal. (We recommend annual gynecologic checkups for all women over 21 and for every woman after she becomes sexually active, to diagnose problems early and treat them promptly.)

A routine medical exam begins once you enter the doctor's office and exchange your street clothes and your underwear for a robe that opens in front. A nurse will record your weight, height, and blood pressure, all indicators of your general health. You will also be given a paper cup for a urine sample.

The doctor begins by feeling the thyroid gland at the base of your neck to see if it is enlarged or if nodular glands are present. While it is not an integral part of the reproductive tract, the thyroid gland influences fertility, and thyroid disease is one of the factors that can cause both premature birth and an irregular menstrual cycle. The clinician will also listen to your heart and lungs to determine if there are any unusual murmurs or breath sounds that need to be evaluated further.

Next, the physician will look at your breasts to see if they appear normal and will feel the breast tissue for any abnormal growths—this is done by rolling the breast tissue between the fingers. The doctor will also examine the tissue in the armpit (the axilla) because breast tissue extends up into it. The lymph nodes that drain the axilla are located there as well, and the doctor will note whether the lymph nodes are enlarged, which may indicate an infection or cancer of the breast tissue. To complete the breast examination, the doctor will ask you to lie down on your back and will then use the chest wall as a firm surface for further palpating the breast tissue.

If the doctor detects a mass in the breast, you may be referred to a specialist for further examination. The presence of such a mass shouldn't alarm you; most lumps are benign, and actual breast cancers are slow-growing. (See Chapter 4.) During the examination, the doctor gently squeezes the nipples to detect any discharge. If your nipples are retracted or inverted, they will be carefully brought out and examined. If a discharge is present, the doctor will take a sample and send the material to the lab for identification and study. A small amount of milky discharge is normal, especially for women who have had children. If you are over 35, the doctor will refer you for a mammogram, a series of X rays that detect possible irregularities in breast tissue. (See Chapter 4.) If the results show tumors with calcification or other X-ray findings that might indicate the presence of breast cancer, then early identification and treatment are possible.

Next, the physician will evaluate your abdomen to make sure the liver is not enlarged and that none of the pelvic organs—uterus, ovaries, and so on—are out of place. When normal, they remain within the confines of the pelvis and are accessible only during pelvic (internal) examination. The abdomen of a woman who has had children is easier for a doctor to examine because it is relatively soft, but if you relax as much as possible, your abdomen can be felt (palpated) easily, regardless of your past reproductive history.

Your physician will then examine your genitals, asking you to spread your legs apart so the vulva is accessible. Doctors perform this procedure differently in various parts of the world. In countries without modern medical examination tables, the health-care provider asks a woman to hold her legs below her knees and manually angle them out. In the United States, thanks to the availability and design of the examination table, you can rest your feet in stirrups and relax your legs to the side. This puts your buttocks at the end of the table so that you and the examiner are both as comfortable as possible under the circumstances. You might want to ask for a hand-held mirror so you can follow the examination and ask questions about the different organs.

During the examination of the vulva, your clinician is looking for cysts or irregularities that occur within or on the surface of the tissues, such as ulcers or warts. Sebaceous cysts and ingrown hairs may also be present. This is the time for you to point out any spots that itch or swell or cause you pain or discomfort, so that the doctor can examine them more closely. One common problem is an infection or blockage of the Bartholin's glands, which may require drainage. These glands can be injured during childbirth or when the obstetrician repairs an episiotomy, the hospital procedure that creates a small cut in the perineum during childbirth to make it easier for the baby's head to emerge. The glands can also become painful if their secretions cannot be discharged when you become sexually aroused. (See Chapter 14.)

The next part of the workup involves inspecting the vaginal wall. To do this, the doctor inserts a speculum into the vagina. Made of metal or plastic, the speculum looks like two shoehorns placed together, with the overall appearance of duck bills. The doctor inserts the speculum in its closed position, opening it once it's within the vagina, thus allowing a view of the vaginal walls. Many advocates for women's health have encouraged women to obtain their own plastic speculums and to familiarize themselves with their bodies by examining themselves at home with the help of a mirror.

An integral part of the examination is obtaining a Pap smear (named for Dr. George Papanicolaou, who devised it). In order to find any incipient problems and treat them early, the doctor takes a sample of cells from the cervix and the cervical canal, a scraping procedure that should be painless. (See Chapter 14.)

After examining the vagina and cervix, the doctor moves on to the internal pelvic exam, inspecting the uterus and ovaries. At this point in the examination many women steel themselves, fearing pain, but the fact is that the more you are able to relax your legs and pelvis, the quicker, easier, and more comfortable the procedure will be. Sometimes, even if you're able to relax well, you will experience feelings of discomfort, pressure, and pain during the pelvic exam; the best way to negotiate this encounter is to focus on breathing deeply and evenly and relaxing your pelvis.

The pelvic exam is a bimanual maneuver. The doctor stands either between your legs or to your side and places two fingers within your vagina and one hand on your abdomen; she or he then lifts your uterus and palpates it with the abdominal hand. In this way the position, size, shape, and possible tenderness of the uterus can be felt and evaluated. The doctor will then examine your ovaries. They can be difficult to feel, and the thinner—and the more relaxed—you are, the easier the examination is. It is not abnormal, for example, for the doctor to be able to feel an ovary with a two-inch cyst on it; if such a cyst is present, it must be followed to determine whether it goes away of its own accord or whether further measures are required. (See Chapters 12 and 14.) The ovaries and the uterus should be mobile on examination; if the doctor is unable to move them it may mean that they have been fixed in place by some disorder. If you have reported having problems, such as pain during intercourse, the doctor will check the uterus further. Tenderness of the uterus can occur if it has become infected from an intrauterine device (IUD) or if a fibroid is present that has outgrown its blood supply and is causing pain. The fallopian tubes are sometimes particularly difficult for an examiner to feel, but if either tube is blocked, it can become swollen and will be palpable.

To explore the back of the uterus and the space between the vagina and the rectum, the area called the cul-de-sac, the examiner must place a finger in the rectum. This gentle probing also has the advantage of detecting rectal pathology and is considered a routine part of the examination, particularly for women over 50. A rectal-vaginal examination permits the doctor to evaluate the back surface of your uterus and to define the ovaries further. If your uterus is tipped backward, for example, it's often easier to examine it this way. This probing also allows the doctor to feel the utero-sacral ligaments, which run from the bottom of the uterus to the sacrum, and to determine if there is damage to the pelvic organs, which might show up as scarring and puckering of this region.

Another indicator that helps the clinician determine the condition of the uterine lining, the endometrium, is the history of your menstrual pattern, including the amount of bleeding during your period and its length. The bleeding you experience at the end of each cycle should be predictable and consistent. If you notice changes, particularly bleeding between periods, it's important to consult the doctor for an evaluation. If the doctor finds abnormalities or notes changes that can indicate a potential for malignancy, she or he can take a sample of endometrial tissue for laboratory testing. At the end of the exam, the doctor puts aside a sample of the stool that was on the examination glove and tests it for evidence of blood.

If the physician has difficulty feeling your uterus or ovaries with either a bimanual or rectal exam, recent technology now makes it possible to obtain a definition of these organs by ultrasound (e.g., sonogram).

Following the examination, be sure you discuss the results with your doctor. Were any abnormalities found? Were there other matters that deserve your attention—the presence of a fibroid to be watched, for example, or any other finding that needs to be followed? This is the time to ask the questions that haven't been covered during the physical examination and to put on the record any medical fact or problem you may not have had the opportunity to mention before.

3

Puberty and Menstruation

Florence Haseltine, M.D.

Puberty marks the beginning of sexual maturity. Although the ovaries and testes are formed before birth, the signaling stations that bring them to life are quiescent until puberty begins. Normally, girls enter puberty between the ages of eight and 14, with the average first menstrual period coming at age 12; boys enter puberty two years later.

While we still do not know all the factors that influence human development, we know that the age of puberty for girls in this country dropped steadily until the 1950s, when it leveled off, probably paralleling the improvement that has taken place over the years in the basic nutrition of children. Another factor that influences when puberty begins is genetic predisposition; some girls begin to menstruate at about the same time as their mothers and older sisters did. The degree of the child's physical activity also plays a role; in general, more active girls menstruate later than their less energetic counterparts.

SIGNS OF PUBERTY

The first signs of normal puberty in girls are an acceleration of linear growth and the onset of breast development. Next, hair appears in the pubic region and under the armpits (axillary hair), followed by the beginning of menstruation. In some girls, axillary and pubic hair emerge before the breasts begin to develop. Boys at puberty produce testosterone, which causes testicular enlargement, the appearance of pubic hair, and the growth of the penis. While boys can see the changes that take place in their testes, girls are unaware that their ovaries are maturing. What girls do notice is that they are growing more rapidly, their figures are changing as they accumulate body fat and take on the relatively rounded shape typical of a mature woman, their breasts are developing, and they are acquiring body hair.

BREAST GROWTH

Breast growth has been measured by a convention called Tanner stages, a classification process first implemented by Dr. J. M. Tanner and now used almost universally as a way of describing breast development. The nipple consists of an inner portion called the papilla and the surrounding tissue called the areola, and it is the reference point for the growth of the breast. The underlying breast tissue enlarges after the nipple develops (see Table 3.1).

Before puberty, the papilla is the only elevated portion of the breast. This is described as Stage 1. With the onset of puberty, Stage 2, the breast bud stage begins; the papilla becomes elevated, some enlargement of the diameter of the areola takes place, and a small amount of tender breast tissue forms under the nipples. Stage 3 brings further development of the breast and areola, but they remain on the same plane and have not yet separated. At Stage 4, the nipple area appears to rise above the breast tissue. Stage 5 represents the mature breast, in which only the papilla projects above the breast tissue and the areola appears as a continuum with the breast tissue. Nipples vary widely in size, shape, and even direction; almost all these variations are normal.

Table 3.1 Age Ranges for Tanner Pubertal Developmental Stages[1]

Stage of Development		Age*	
		Mean (Years)	Range (95% Limits)
Breast growth			
B-1	Preadolescent		
B-2	Breast budding and areolar enlargement	11.2	8.9–13.3
B-3	Breast tissue enlarged beyond areola in a visible mound	12.2	10.0–14.3
B-4	Areola and papilla project beyond contour of breast	13.1	10.8–15.3
B-5	Mature breast with areola recessed to contour of breast	15.3	11.9–18.8
Pubic hair growth			
PH-1	Absence of sex hair		
PH-2	Sparse hair, usually along labia majora	11.7	9.3–14.1
PH-3	Coarse curled hair sparsely over mons veneris	12.4	10.2–14.6
PH-4	Abundant hair limited to mons veneris	13.0	10.8–15.1
PH-5	Adult hair spread to medial aspects of thighs	14.4	12.2–16.7

During adolescence, growth velocity accelerates for the first one to two years, with *peak height velocity* usually occurring about one year after the onset of breast budding and one and a half years before menarche. The mean age of *menarche* in European and North American populations varies from 12.6 to 13.5 years (range 9–16 years). There is a clear tendency for puberty to occur earlier in overweight girls. The secular trend toward earlier menarche that was observed over the last century now appears to have ceased in the industrial nations.

---

*North American standards are approximately six months earlier for each stage.
[1]Data from W. A. Marshall and J. M. Tanner, "Variations in the Pattern of Pubertal Changes in Girls," *Archives of Diseases in Childhood* 44 (1969): 291.

BODY HAIR

Dr. Tanner also described the stages of pubic hair growth, which extend from Stage 1, in which pubic hair is not yet visible, to Stage 5, in which the hair exhibits its adult appearance and is in the inverse triangular shape that is characteristic of the mature woman. Most girls don't notice their pubic hair until they reach Stage 3, when it becomes dark and coarse even though it is still quite sparse; the pubic hair of girls with blond hair is darker than their scalp hair. By Stage 4, a girl has the pubic hair typical of an adult woman. While it covers the pubic area, it has not appeared on the thighs or abdomen, which is typical of Stage 5. These characteristics vary, of course, with genetic and ethnic qualities. For example, women of Asian descent have sparser pubic and axillary hair growth, and the hair is usually straight, not curly. Also, Asian women often display fully mature pubic hair growth at about what would be Tanner's Stage 4 in other groups.

Axillary hair can also be staged, although it is the custom for most American girls to shave leg and underarm hair very early, usually by Stage 4, partly to conform with cosmetic convention and, in the latter case, partly as an effort to reduce the odor that develops from the newly functioning apocrine glands under the arms. This body shaving is a cultural convention, not mandated by standards of either health or cleanliness.

HORMONES

Hormones are the secret ingredient of puberty; we can't see them, but they have profound effects on the body. They are controlled and released by the pituitary-hypothalamic axis.

The hypothalamus is the key to sexual and reproductive development. Located at the base of the brain, this gland controls our basic drives—hunger, thirst, aggression, and sex—as well as our body temperature. (See Chapter 2.) In order for a child to enter and complete puberty, the hypothalamus must send signals in the form of hormones to the nearby pituitary gland. The substance the hypothalamus secretes is called gonadotropin-releasing hormone (GnRH), which causes the pituitary to secrete gonadotropins, the follicle-stimulating hormone (FSH) and the luteinizing hormone

(LH) that will in turn be carried by the blood to the ovaries, where they will stimulate the ovarian follicles there to begin developing until one becomes a mature egg. Researchers do not yet fully understand what triggers this release, but we know it involves a clocklike mechanism in the brain that develops with age and weight gain and, when mature, sends out a signal every 60 to 90 minutes. This signal initiates a pulse of GnRH, which, in turn, makes the pituitary gland secrete the hormones that bring the ovaries to life. Recent research has indicated that body composition may be as important as weight gain in pubertal development, and that girls need a certain percentage of body fat before menstruation and ovulation can occur.

THE ROLE OF ESTROGEN

As the ovaries produce the hormone estrogen, the rest of the reproductive organs start to mature. The uterus begins to grow rapidly, from the size of a sugar cube weighing .04 ounce (a gram) in the young child to the size of a small orange or golf ball weighing a third of an ounce (10 grams). Before menstruation occurs, a pubescent girl's uterus usually weighs about one ounce.

The vagina also develops, and as the lining of the vagina responds to estrogen, girls often notice a white mucus discharge on their underwear. Many youngsters worry about this, but the discharge is normal and simply means that the vagina is producing typical secretions and shedding its mature lining. The fallopian tubes, through which the eggs will pass on their way from the ovaries to the uterus, develop now as well.

Besides contributing to the general growth spurt of adolescence, estrogen accelerates bone growth in adolescent girls and stops the growth of the long bones, particularly those in the arms and legs, when the bones have matured. (In boys, testosterone performs this function.) Estrogen also promotes the distribution of typical female fat and protects against the loss of bone density.

THE ADRENAL GLANDS

Located on either side of the spinal column just above the kidneys, the adrenal glands also mature during puberty. Researchers still do not understand the interaction between the hypothalamic-gonadal axis and the development of the adrenal glands. The ovaries and the female adrenal glands both produce androgens, or male hormones, but obviously, while present in females, the level is not nearly as high as it is in males (the total amount that the ovaries and the adrenal glands in females manufacture is one-tenth of that made by males).

It is these male hormones that produce axillary and pubic hair in females. Androgens also affect female bone growth, contributing to the "growth spurt" of puberty, and cause acne; one of the ways physicians try to treat acne in young girls is to reduce the amount of ovarian androgen by prescribing an estrogenic birth control pill, which suppresses it. Since the acne of puberty can be a serious cosmetic problem that causes a great deal of emotional suffering, particularly when severe, it should not be dismissed as unimportant. A young girl with severe acne should see a gynecologist to have her androgen levels measured and a dermatologist to make sure she receives the best possible skin care. Although acne was considered almost impossible to cure a generation ago, the situation is very different today.

THE MENSTRUAL CYCLE

Once the hypothalamic clock begins sending signals to the pituitary to release GnRH, the system must become regular and rhythmic. Initially, estrogen signals the brain that the ovaries have started their work. (Actually, there is a continuous exchange of information between the ovaries and the brain throughout the human life span.) The ovaries are very sensitive to the level of gonadotropins (FSH and LH), and the brain is equally responsive to the level of estrogen—and later, progesterone—that the ovaries produce. The ovaries send other signals as well in the form of proteins that in some way make the pituitary gland more or less sensitive to the estrogen and progesterone levels in circulation.

Puberty does not happen overnight. The ovaries take about two to four years to mature completely so that one of them will expel an egg each month. This is why many girls find that their periods are not evenly spaced at first. Bleeding can occur twice a month or every two to three months, and the flow can vary from light to heavy and still be normal.

As the hypothalamus matures, the ovaries start to function in a cyclic fashion. Each egg is surrounded by a layer of cells that form a primordial follicle. At first, the pituitary sends out more FSH than LH. With the initial burst of follicle-stimulating hormone, a few of these primordial follicles start to grow. Researchers do not know why only a few follicles react, but the system is a clever one because, if all responded, we would lose all our follicles at the first exposure to FSH, making continuous fertility over many years impossible.

The follicles grow as the egg enlarges until it becomes mature enough to be expelled by the ovary in the process called ovulation. After ovulation, the follicle becomes a much more complicated hormone-secreting entity. Although several follicles begin to mature, only one survives to ovulation; the rest undergo degeneration. Again, no one knows why one follicle becomes active and the others remain dormant, but it is clear that the follicles self-select.

As the follicle grows it becomes multilayered and differentiated; it enlarges so much that, instead of being barely visible to the unaided eye, it eventually measures three-quarters of an inch (two centimeters) across. There are at least three different cell types that nurture the egg and excrete hormones into the blood to signal the uterus that ovulation is approaching and that it should be ready to receive a fertilized egg if fertilization occurs. During this period, called the preovulatory or follicular part of the cycle, the follicle mainly produces estrogen.

Surrounding the enlarged egg is a mass of cells called the cumulus, so named because when we look at a mature egg and the cells encircling it under the microscope, the complex looks like a sparkling galaxy in the night sky. The ovary releases the egg and its cumulus through a small hole in its surface when it receives a signal from the brain in the form of a surge of luteinizing hormone (LH). One of the fallopian tubes picks up the egg along with the cumulus of cells and transports them to the uterus.

During ovulation, which usually takes place 14 days before menstrual bleeding begins, a woman can become pregnant if sperm reaches the fallopian tube and penetrates the egg. The egg lives for 12 to 48 hours, but sperm can survive for two to three days in the tube. Some women experience pain with ovulation when the follicle and the surface of the ovary dissolve and release the egg, causing a kind of minirupture that may produce slight bleeding. This is called *mittelschmerz*, the German term for mid-cycle pain, which may resemble the kind of cramp associated with menstruation.

Even after ovulation, the follicle's function is not complete. It continues to produce estrogen to support the lining of the uterus; once the egg is released, the follicle secretes another hormone, progesterone, which transforms the estrogen-primed lining of the uterus into a state fully receptive to a fertilized egg. If fertilization of the egg does not take place, the follicle will have a short life span, lasting only the 14 days until regular menstrual bleeding occurs, as the uterine lining (endometrium) responds to the changing ovarian hormones.

During the follicular phase of the cycle, the endometrium grows. The thick muscle wall of the uterus is lined with hormonally sensitive tissue; it is this layer of tissue—called the basal layer or basal endometrium—that forms the endometrial lining during each monthly cycle. Responding to the high level of estrogen, this basal layer divides. The new, or cycling, endometrium is composed of tubules of straight glands, supporting tissue or stroma, and blood vessels. The cycling endometrium appears uniform in composition and the glands and blood vessels are lined up in an orderly array. Once ovulation has occurred, however, the cycling layer matures rapidly. The cells of the glands expand and fill with secretions, and the tubules and blood vessels become tortuous in appearance. The stroma swells, and the lining takes on a spongy appearance. The endometrium can stay in this condition only with the support of progesterone and estrogen. As the levels of these hormones drop, which occurs if the egg has not been fertilized, the membranes that hold the blood vessels intact disintegrate, and the support tissue fills with blood. The endometrial structure collapses, and the cycling layer of the uterine lining is shed, down to the basal layer of endometrium. Following this shedding and bleeding—menstruation—the lining of the uterus gets ready for the next monthly cycle as the low levels of estrogen and progesterone signal the hypothalamus that it is time to begin the process all over again.

NORMAL VARIATIONS IN THE MENSTRUAL CYCLE

Menstrual cycles vary enormously from person to person in terms of the timing of the cycle, its length, and its characteristics. A normal cycle can range between 21 and 42 days, or three to six weeks. The difference reflects the length of time of the first, or follicular, part of the cycle. The second phase of the cycle, from ovulation to menstruation, called the luteal phase, lasts more consistently—about 14 days. If the second phase of the monthly cycle does not run its full length of about 14 days, the lining of the uterus may not mature properly to accept the implantation of a fertilized egg, a phenomenon that can be a cause of infertility. Whatever particular pattern of menstrual bleeding a woman develops in the early years of menstruation, it can change with age, childbearing, exposure to oral contraceptives, and other physiological and psychological factors.

The number of days of menstrual bleeding can be as short as half a day or as long as 10 days. The amount of menstrual fluid a woman produces also is not standard, though the average is about two to two and a half ounces of fluid (including cervical mucus and other secretions) and one ounce of blood. Normal menstrual blood is usually reddish or brownish in color, but not bright red. Although the menstrual blood may clot within the uterus, the clots usually dissolve before the uterus expels the blood. If you expel large amounts of clotted blood during your period, it may mean that the bleeding is abnormal, and you should see a physician. (See Chapter 12.)

IF THE EGG IS FERTILIZED

If fertilization takes place and the fertilized egg embeds in the uterine lining, the follicle does not subside after 14 days. Instead, it continues to produce estrogen and progesterone. Fertilization creates a change in the entire hormonal pattern of the body. The fertilized egg releases an early-pregnancy hormone called human chorionic gonadotropin (hCG), which is similar to luteinizing hormone in that both can stimulate the follicle to continue manufacturing estrogen and progesterone. However, hCG is a longer-lived protein, and the early embryo manufactures much more of it than the amount of LH generated. With the production of hCG, the follicle, now called the corpus luteum (yellow body), functions only for the first six to seven weeks of pregnancy. Although it remains throughout the pregnancy, it does not contribute to the development of the fetus—or, indeed, to anything—after the early stages.

PRECOCIOUS PUBERTY

If a child begins puberty before the age of eight, medical evaluation by a specialist is necessary since one possible cause of this condition is an estrogen-producing tumor. Sometimes, however, the cause is less worrisome and can be as simple as a young girl having found and consumed a supply of her mother's birth control pills.

Currently doctors are able to stop precocious puberty in some youngsters by giving them hormones (Nafarelin, Lupron) that act to block the production of gonadotropin. These medications are related to gonadotropin-releasing hormones, and they bind to the same locations in the pituitary as hCG, but instead of stimulating the release of LH, they block it so that the ovaries stop functioning. Physicians usually continue to treat these girls with prescribed drugs until they are eight to 10 years old, following them as long as they are taking medication.

PAINFUL MENSTRUATION (DYSMENORRHEA)

Painful periods are a common phenomenon among women of all ages, varying greatly in degree. Young women often suffer severe enough uterine or abdominal cramps during their periods that they stay home from school. Doctors usually categorize dysmenorrhea as "primary," describing pain that starts within the first few menstrual periods, and "secondary," pain that comes on later in life.

PRIMARY DYSMENORRHEA

Typical primary menstrual pain consists of uterine cramps, often accompanied by backache, headache, and, occasionally, nausea and diarrhea.

One cause of the condition can be the prostaglandin that is released into the bloodstream as the endometrium breaks down.

High levels of prostaglandin make the uterus contract, decreasing the blood flow and the amount of oxygen to the uterine muscle and initiating pain. This substance also makes the smooth muscle in the intestinal tract contract, precipitating abdominal pain, diarrhea, nausea, and vomiting in some women.

In young girls, cramping pain may be produced by blood and tissue passing through the cervix, causing it to stretch slightly as the uterus contracts to force out the blood and other contents of the menstrual flow. Many young women find that menstrual pain disappears as they become older, when they use the birth control pill as a contraceptive (it suppresses ovulation), or after they give birth to a first child. During delivery, the cervix opens (dilates) and, although it closes again afterward, it never becomes as tight as it was before childbirth; as a result, it does not have to stretch to expel the menstrual flow.

Treatment

Aspirin was the first of the antiprostaglandins that was sometimes successful in reducing pain from menstrual cramps. Doctors prescribed it long before they understood how it worked. There are now a number of more effective antiprostaglandins available, with ibuprofen (Motrin, Advil, Nuprin, etc.) the most common and least expensive. When ibuprofen first became available as an over-the-counter (OTC) medication, its manufacturers reduced the strength of this drug to 200 milligrams per pill, but doctors rarely prescribe less than 400 to 600 milligrams at a time. If ibuprofen fails to relieve menstrual pain, it is usually because the dose taken is inadequate—although doses in excess of 400 mg are unwise without medical supervision. Because of slight differences in ingredient levels, often one combination will provide relief when others won't, so it is worth trying two or three brands or generics if you experience painful cramps. There are also more than a dozen prescription drugs available that act as antiprostaglandins (prescription Motrin—which is stronger than OTC Motrin—Anaprox, Naprosyn, Ponstel, Ansaid). All these drugs can cause ulcers if taken in high doses for long periods of time.

Almost immediately after the oral contraceptive pill (OCP) was made available, it became evident that the shorter, artificially induced periods that the women who were using it experienced were also much less painful than their previous naturally occurring periods. The Pill changes the hormonal environment of the uterus, and in suppressing ovulation it reduces the stimulation of the uterine lining. In fact, the lining of the uterus does not fully develop during these Pill-induced cycles and, in some women, looks very thin, with little growth of the basal endometrium. Consequently, instead of referring to it as menstruation, doctors call the bleeding that occurs each month "withdrawal bleeding" because much less blood and tissue are shed than during a normally occurring period.

The Pill is probably as risk free as any medication available. (See Chapter 7.) If you suffer from severe menstrual cramps and also need contraception, your doctor will probably prescribe the Pill. Even women who are not sexually active prefer to use it as treatment for menstrual pain.

If neither of these therapies works on its own, most women will find relief in a combination of the Pill with one of the antiprostaglandins. If you try the combination and the pain persists, consult your doctor to see if some other condition is causing the pain. Sometimes, stronger short-term medication, such as Tylenol with codeine, can be helpful. In those relatively few cases in which the pain persists, surgical procedures, such as cutting the nerves to the uterus (presacral neurectomy), might be advised.

There are other techniques, such as relaxation exercises and biofeedback, that help some women handle menstrual pain, but you have to learn them from a skilled professional. It is best to visit a pain clinic that deals with such problems.

Proper diet and nutrition have special implications during menstruation. (See Chapter 6.) Become aware of diet patterns that seem to be associated with menstrual pain and modify them.

SECONDARY DYSMENORRHEA

Painful periods that start later in life are almost always caused by some developing abnormality of the reproductive tract, which is often not a serious condition. This includes fibroids, endometriosis, and uterine polyps. If your painful periods are of recent origin, be sure to consult a physician to find out what the problem may be and to see what remedies are available. Similarly, pain that occurs prior to the menstrual cycle is usually a sign of some pelvic-based problem that can be alleviated, often endometriosis or fibroids. (See Chapter 12.)

Mittelschmerz

As we have noted, *mittelschmerz* refers to pain that occurs during ovulation, in the middle of the menstrual cycle. When you ovulate and the follicle ruptures, releasing an egg, a tiny amount of bleeding takes place. Occasionally, probably by chance, there is enough bleeding for some blood and fluid to spill onto the peritoneal lining of the pelvis, causing pain. If felt at all, the discomfort is only mild; some women, however, experience more severe pain, sometimes every month. Once women develop beyond puberty, many find that mild *mittelschmerz* is a handy way to pinpoint the time of ovulation, either to prevent or encourage conception, but severe pain might require medication, such as Demerol or codeine.

It is sometimes difficult to differentiate *mittelschmerz* pain from that caused by an ovarian cyst or, if the pain is on the right side, from appendicitis. Doctors infer the diagnosis when the episode of pain occurs just at mid-cycle. It usually disappears by itself or can be relieved with medication, except in the very rare instance when a woman experiences massive bleeding that does not stop, in which case surgery is in order.

Some women experience pain with menstruation later in life. During the regeneration process of the uterine lining, the glands that are formed tend to go deeper and deeper into the smooth muscle wall of the uterus. These glands then bleed into the uterine wall so that, by the time a woman is in her 40s, she might have painful cramps because of this type of bleeding, called adenomyosis. The methods that alleviate pain in younger women are not as helpful. If the pain is severe, the only treatment is a hysterectomy. (See Chapter 14.)

THE ABSENCE OF MENSTRUATION

The absence of menstruation (amenorrhea) occurs in two forms: primary amenorrhea, in which a girl never begins to menstruate, and secondary amenorrhea, in which menstruation ceases after it has started.

PRIMARY AMENORRHEA

Although most young women are somewhat apprehensive about the arrival of menstruation, they are usually more concerned if they are the last among their peers to menstruate. Such concern is almost always unfounded, but if by the age of 14 a girl shows no evidence of beginning breast development (to indicate that the ovaries are making estrogen), or if she has not had a period by the time she is 16, a specialist should be consulted to determine if there is a medical problem. It is often reassuring to a young girl to be checked even earlier than this.

Although delayed puberty can signal chromosomal abnormalities or birth defects in the uterus or ovaries, primary amenorrhea is a very rare condition. Obvious abnormalities in development, such as the lack of normal external genitals or a closed hymen that will not permit menstrual flow to escape outside the vagina, will usually have been discovered by the pediatrician soon after birth. But a doctor may not detect other developmental problems—for example, the absence of ovaries or a uterus—until a girl fails to menstruate. Problems with the glands in the brain, responsible for releasing the required hormones, can also delay menstruation. A tumor of the pituitary gland, for example, might be responsible.

The most frequent cause of primary amenorrhea is failure to ovulate. Unable to produce sufficient estrogen and progesterone to permit the uterine wall to build up, the ovaries do not function to promote the conditions that produce menstruation, and none takes place. Clinicians usually diagnose and treat this abnormality by prescribing a synthetic progestin (Provera, for example) to be taken for 10 to 14 days each month. It usually produces bleeding within two to seven days after the last prescribed dose has been taken every month. It is very important to be certain that no pregnancy has occurred, because Provera causes serious harm to a fetus. Therefore, the doctor should do a pregnancy test before prescribing Provera.

If you are sexually active and don't want to become pregnant, you will need to use birth control from the time you begin taking such medication, because it can produce ovulation at any time. If you take a synthetic progestin and you still don't have a period, or if you bleed at another time, you should notify your doctor.

An improperly functioning hypothalamus is another possible

cause of primary amenorrhea. If your hypothalamus fails to produce GnRH, your pituitary will not make FSH and LH and your ovaries won't generate estrogen and progesterone. Stress is one explanation for this reversal of the normal endocrine function. Another might be weight loss from a chronic illness, severe dieting, or intensive athletic training. This is why female athletes and dancers sometimes experience amenorrhea, as well as young women who suffer from anorexia nervosa, an illness that distorts a woman's perception of her body image and leads to self-inflicted, serious—and sometimes fatal—weight loss. The kind of weight loss that can produce hypothalamic malfunctioning is not simply a matter of pounds taken off; it also involves body composition. If your body fat drops below 20 percent of your total body weight, amenorrhea is likely. One possible consequence of prolonged amenorrhea is the loss of bone density and an increased risk of osteoporosis.

Treatment

Doctors do not generally use GnRH to induce the release of FSH and LH because, unless you want to become pregnant, it is not necessary for you to ovulate. If you decide to have a child, you can take drugs that stimulate ovulation. Instead, amenorrhea is treated with the same estrogen-replacement therapy (ERT) prescribed for postmenopausal women. (See Chapter 15.) Birth control pills, which also provide pregnancy protection, are likewise prescribed.

SECONDARY AMENORRHEA

Secondary amenorrhea, in which menstruation ceases after periods have begun, is not a condition to be ignored, and you should consult a doctor about it as soon as possible. One of its consequences is that the ovary produces a steady stream of estrogen without the benefits of the maturing effect of the progesterone, which the ovary normally produces only after ovulation. If estrogen levels become moderate to high, this can stimulate the uterine lining and increase your vulnerability to precancerous conditions, such as the uncontrolled growth of the lining of the uterus (adenomatous hyperplasia) or to uterine cancer itself. (See Chapter 13.)

Pregnancy

The most common cause of secondary amenorrhea is pregnancy, occurring either normally in the uterus or abnormally in one of the fallopian tubes as a tubal (ectopic) pregnancy. When the placenta begins to develop, it produces the hormone hCG, which stops ovulation and thus prevents further periods. Even if you feel almost certain that you aren't pregnant, your doctor will probably order a pregnancy test, because experience with secondary amenorrhea has shown that, more often than not, conception has taken place.

Stress

Another frequent cause of secondary amenorrhea is stress, which affects the proper functioning of the hypothalamus and its ability to produce hormones. If stress is established as the cause, your periods should return as your life situation improves. The extreme weight loss that can cause primary amenorrhea can also make your periods cease once they have begun. Losing large amounts of weight as a result of strenuous exercise or dieting, as well as the kind of weight loss and misperception of one's body image associated with anorexia nervosa, may be related to the loss of the usual estrogen storage in fat cells.

The Pill

It is not unusual to skip periods while taking the OCP. If you think you may have missed taking any pills, or if you have any other symptoms of pregnancy, it is important to get a pregnancy test.

Ovarian Cysts

Simple ovarian cysts, the kind that occur when the follicle does not rupture during ovulation but instead keeps growing, can often cause amenorrhea. In this situation, the growing follicle produces large amounts of female hormones and interferes with the cycling mechanism. This usually goes away within two to three months, and normal periods will resume. Simple ovarian cysts do not indicate any underlying abnormality and do not interfere with fertility

unless an overzealous surgeon removes an ovary unnecessarily—
a phenomenon from which you can protect yourself by seeking a
second opinion and otherwise researching the necessity for such
a procedure if it is recommended. A woman who has repeated
cysts, or one who has only a single remaining ovary, may do well
to stay on the oral contraceptive pill and thus suppress ovulation
until she wants to become pregnant.

Polycystic Ovaries

Polycystic ovaries (PCO) are ovaries filled with little cysts, which
usually result from abnormalities in the hypothalamus, adrenals,
or ovaries. This condition sometimes produces periods that occur
irregularly, from every two to every nine months. While examination does not show which gland is causing the problem, a battery
of hormone tests helps to pinpoint the diagnosis—a procedure that
is, unfortunately, very expensive. Often doctors prescribe OCPs
as temporary correctives for the hormonal imbalances in this condition.

Previous Infection

A uterine lining scarred by previous infection—from an IUD or
a postpartum infection—can also interrupt menstruation.

Ovarian Failure

Ovarian failure, which is another major cause of secondary
amenorrhea, may take place in women at any time after periods
have started, from the teens to the 50s. After the age of 40, the
condition is considered normal menopause. A gynecologist can
make this diagnosis by measuring the blood level of the follicle-
stimulating hormone, which becomes greatly elevated when the
pituitary tries to compel the failing ovaries to ovulate. Whether the
ovaries fail early or late, it is usually prudent for women to consult
a doctor and take estrogen, but it is particularly important to do
so if the ovaries fail early in life, because the consequent loss of
estrogen increases the risk of developing cardiovascular disease
and osteoporosis. (See Chapter 15.)

Benign Tumors (Adenomas)

Benign tumors of the pituitary gland, called adenomas, produce excess amounts of the hormone prolactin, which can interfere with menstrual periods and also occasionally cause the breasts to produce a little milk. A blood test for prolactin can determine whether this condition is present. Although large tumors sometimes require surgery, doctors can treat smaller ones with the drug bromocriptine.

Thyroid

Thyroid abnormalities can also cause secondary amenorrhea, but this happens rarely. Very high or very low thyroid hormone levels can alter the menstrual pattern by making the pituitary gland produce extra thyroid-stimulating hormone, which can increase the level of prolactin and suppress menstruation.

PREMENSTRUAL SYNDROME (PMS)

Premenstrual syndrome is a condition, still poorly defined, that is related to the menstrual cycle. Many women notice body changes and mood alterations prior to their menstrual periods. While most of us note relatively mild cyclical fluctuations during our fertile years, others report severe symptoms. In the days before their periods begin, some women become virtually incapacitated. Psychiatrists call PMS pre–luteal phase dysphoria, a term that denotes agitation and anguish.

Investigators are still looking for ways to categorize the symptoms that women experience in order to acquire a better understanding of the phenomenon. Unfortunately, as with any symptomatology that varies greatly from individual to individual, this has been very difficult to do. Those women who report symptoms of PMS do not necessarily experience them in the same way with each cycle, and the symptoms often change as women age, which presents further barriers to understanding.

The physical signs of PMS include abdominal bloating, breast tenderness, constipation, and severe headaches; some women develop migraines. The psychological symptoms can range from mild to severe depression and irritability.

At the moment, we have very little factual information about what causes PMS. One theory supposes that it occurs because of a deficiency of progesterone. Another assumes that low levels of vitamin B_6 and magnesium are responsible. A third says that an excess of prostaglandin hormones precipitates the condition because prostaglandins stimulate the uterine muscle to contract and because antiprostaglandin medications have been effective in relieving painful menstruation. Still another conjecture is that an inadequate level of endorphins, natural painkillers produced by the brain, is the culprit; the reasoning behind this assumption is that changing endorphin levels alter brain sensitivity to pain and other neural signals that affect mood. Endorphins may influence how we excrete fluids, explaining the fluid buildup that is also a PMS symptom, but only continuing research can determine if any of these hypotheses plays a role in premenstrual syndrome.

Although there are many fads in the treatment of PMS, women who suffer severe depression or other emotional difficulties before their periods should consult a mental health professional for relief. For some women, an increased awareness that their depression and irritability are associated with their menstrual cycle and, therefore, short-term discomfort, can help them maintain their equilibrium and minimize stress in interpersonal relations. Other problems should be treated symptomatically. If pain is the chief complaint, your doctor can prescribe pain relief medication; if you experience swelling (edema), you should cut down on salt and sugar in your diet and ask your doctor about the advisability of prescribing a diuretic to get rid of excess fluid; if you have the jitters, you should cut down on caffeine by limiting your intake of chocolate, coffee, tea, and caffeine-containing soft drinks. You should also start a regular exercise program; this may help ease your symptoms by improving your overall physical condition.

Because PMS is connected to the menstrual cycle, we have to learn much more about the many regulatory pathways involved in the brain function and the regulation of the cycle before we can arrive at effective and dependable cures. This is scant assurance indeed, but while many PMS clinics have sprung up around the country in the absence of certain and effective treatment, it is not clear whether they offer any better therapy than that offered in a placebo treatment regime or in a woman's own special attention to proper diet, exercise, and awareness of mood fluctuations during her entire cycle.

4

The Breast

Susan Love, M.D., and Kathleen Mayzel, M.D.

THE ANATOMY OF THE BREAST

Romanticized and even fetishized as it has been throughout history, the female breast, an important element in women's sexuality, is basically a milk-producing organ. At the cellular level, lobules that make milk connect to ducts that transport the milk out to the nipple. One-third of the breast is composed of fat, which surrounds the lobules and ducts; the remaining two-thirds is composed of breast tissue. The amount of fat in the breast is what accounts for the wide range of differences in women's breast size. The actual size of our breasts is determined by our genes.

What varies as we gain or lose weight is not the breast tissue, but the fat content of the breast. Consequently, the only way to make your breasts larger or smaller is to alter your weight. Contrary to claims made by many advertisers, there is no exercise that can make the breasts either smaller or larger. Exercise changes the breast only as it contributes to weight loss; it is the weight loss, not the exercise, that causes the change. The assertion that large breasts are more likely to develop cancer is another myth.

Our breasts develop during puberty after the hypothalamus has signaled the pituitary gland to begin secreting hormones. This process usually takes place between the ages of eight and 13, and one to two years before a girl starts to menstruate. First the nipple begins to grow, followed by the appearance of a mound of breast tissue, which develops below the nipple. (See Chapter 3.) It is normal for one breast to be larger than the other. Although this may be disturbing to some women, it is worth remembering that while the difference may be quite apparent to you when you look in the mirror while naked, it is entirely unnoticeable when you are dressed.

The next event that alters the breast is pregnancy. As the breasts gradually become tender and enlarged, the nipples increase in size and the areolas darken in color. Nursing stretches the breasts as they fill with milk; breast size decreases once a woman stops nursing. The contention that breast-feeding has an impact on whether or not a woman is likely to develop cancer is another myth in this most myth-prone of areas.

As for the "support" that bra advertisers proclaim, wearing a bra is neither harmful nor helpful; whether or not you wear one at any time in your life should be your personal decision, based on what makes you comfortable. Bras have no effect on breast muscles because, except for those in the nipples, none exist in the breast: All the muscles in the area are behind the breast, in the chest wall. Running or exercising without wearing a bra cannot cause sagging breasts; if breasts sag, they do so in proportion to the fat they contain, which increases with age. The only physical corrective for sagging breasts is plastic surgery.

Cosmetic surgery on the breast is a very personal decision. Women must be aware that surgery to increase the size of their breasts, called augmentation mammoplasty, involves the insertion of a silicone or saline implant behind the breast tissue or the pectoralis major muscle, which interferes with subsequent mammography and thus the possible detection of breast cancer. This is a serious drawback, and if you are contemplating this surgery, you should think through your decision carefully, particularly if there is a history of breast cancer in your family. On the other hand, surgery to reduce the size of the breasts does not interfere with the ability of a mammogram to detect breast cancer. Nevertheless, surgery of any kind poses risks that must be carefully considered before any decision is made.

The breasts sit on the pectoralis major muscle of the chest wall (see Fig 4.1). We have noted that breast tissue extends far beyond the area of the breasts themselves: from the collarbone (clavicle) down to the muscle covering the middle of the abdomen, known as the rectus abdominis muscle, over to the breastbone (sternum) in the middle of the chest, and up to the armpit, or the axilla. The axillary lymph nodes are under the armpit, and some of the lymphatic fluid that normally drains the breast tissue passes into them.

BREAST CARE

Although some studies have suggested there may be a relation between breast cancer and a high-fat diet, a recent study of nurses conducted by the public health department at Harvard Medical School did not show this correlation. However, the Harvard study did show that a moderate alcohol intake—three drinks a week— was associated with a slightly increased risk of breast cancer. It's a fact, however, that a high-fat diet can lead to overweight and obesity. Therefore, you should limit your consumption of meat and dairy products by balancing them with eating high-fiber foods (see Chapter 6) and attend to the following procedures to maintain health.

SELF-EXAMINATION

Because breast cancer continues to occur in one out of every nine women in the United States, it is genuinely important for you to examine your breasts once a month. Many women who have good intentions about doing this don't because they don't know exactly what to look for or because they are uneasy about what they might find. But once you learn the procedure and make it routine, you'll find that it's an easy way of demystifying the subject. Remember that many apparent irregularities are perfectly normal; the trick is to learn the characteristics of your own breasts, so that you can easily detect any changes that might be important.

The best time to do the examination is about a week after your menstrual period, because the breasts are the least lumpy at that time. For women who have entered menopause and have stopped getting their periods, the first day of the month is an easy date to

Anterolateral Dissection

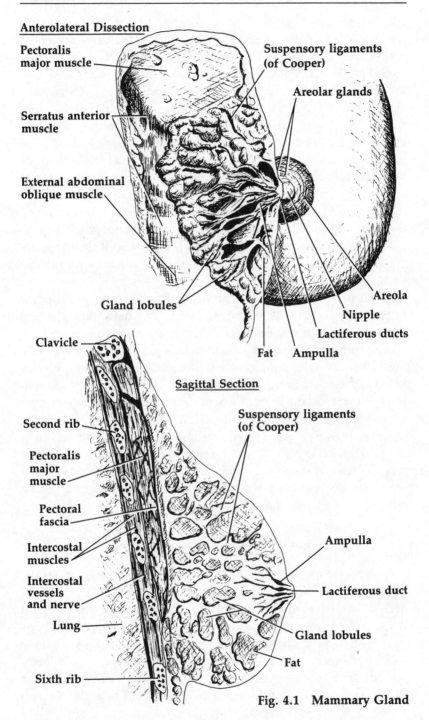

Pectoralis
major muscle

Suspensory ligaments
(of Cooper)

Areolar glands

Serratus anterior
muscle

External abdominal
oblique muscle

Gland lobules

Areola

Nipple

Lactiferous ducts

Fat   Ampulla

Clavicle

Sagittal Section

Second rib

Suspensory ligaments
(of Cooper)

Pectoralis
major
muscle

Pectoral
fascia

Ampulla

Intercostal
muscles

Intercostal
vessels
and nerve

Lactiferous duct

Lung

Gland lobules

Fat

Sixth rib

Fig. 4.1   Mammary Gland

set. Raise one arm above your head and, with the flat portion of the fingertips of the other hand, gently feel (palpate) the entire breast. You can do this by starting at the nipple and making increasingly larger circles until you've covered the entire breast; or you can start at the top of the breast and proceed horizontally across it, moving down until you have felt the entire breast. You should also feel the area above the breasts, up to the collarbone and along the breastbone to the abdominal wall muscle. However, you should leave the examination of your armpits to the doctor's annual breast examination. It is extremely difficult for a woman to evaluate this area; it contains muscle that women can mistake for lumps, and the lymph nodes in your armpits are often enlarged because they contain benign nodes. You should not check for nipple discharge by squeezing your nipples, because it is only spontaneous discharge from the nipples that indicates a possible problem.

If you perform regular self-exams, you will become accustomed to the normal "feel" of your breasts and can detect any changes that may occur. If you find a new lump or lumpy area, it's best to allow another menstrual period to complete its course before seeking further examination, as many of these lumps or lumpy areas will disappear. Although any lump or change tends to arouse concern, it is important to remember that the vast majority of lumps are benign (noncancerous) and also that all breast cancers are extremely slow-growing, so that one month makes no difference in the success of any treatment required. This means that women who do have a just-discovered cancerous lump have time to research the alternatives and get a second medical opinion regarding what treatment they should pursue.

PHYSICIAN'S EXAMINATION

A physician or other health-care provider should always feel the breasts as part of a routine physical examination. Many women find it easiest to combine this examination with their gynecological workup. For women age 40 and older, yearly breast examinations by a medical professional are recommended. If you have a family history of breast cancer, these annual examinations should begin at an earlier age. The examination should not be a cursory one; the physician or other health-care provider should take the time to examine both breasts in a manner similar to that of the breast self-examination. This may be done when you are sitting or lying down, or both. The doctor will also examine the armpits.

MAMMOGRAMS

Mammograms are X rays of the breasts. In routine mammography exams, the X-ray technician takes two views of each breast, one horizontally and one vertically. The mammogram machine gently compresses the breast in order to obtain an accurate picture with a minimum of radiation exposure, so the procedure may be slightly uncomfortable. Sometimes, additional views are necessary to clarify a finding.

The American Cancer Society recommends that women have one baseline mammogram between the ages of 35 and 40; a mammogram every one to two years between the ages of 40 and 50; and yearly mammograms over age 50. We do not recommend routine mammograms for women under the age of 35 because normal breast tissue is dense, with more tissue than fat, making mammograms more difficult to interpret since X rays don't penetrate tissue as easily as they do fat. However, if you are under 40 and you have a lump that is considered suspicious, or have had such a lump, or if your mother or sister developed breast cancer early in life, your doctor may wish to start yearly mammograms at an earlier age. Be aware that although large breasts don't make diagnosis more difficult, detecting breast cancer in young women whose breasts are dense—as opposed to large—is sometimes difficult.

How concerned should you be about the possibility of receiving harmful radiation from a mammogram? The method of film screen mammography used today involves a very low dose of radiation, approximately equivalent to the amount of exposure to atmospheric radiation that you receive when you fly cross-country. Nevertheless, the risk of developing breast cancer from exposure to radiation is higher in women under 35 than it is in older women. Researchers learned this by studying Japanese women who were in Hiroshima and Nagasaki when the first atomic bombs were dropped during World War II. Of the women who developed breast cancer apparently as a result of being exposed to the massive amounts of radiation, almost all were young. Although researchers still are uncertain as to why this is so, it probably reflects the fact that breast cells in younger women are dividing faster in response to their higher levels of estrogen.

Because there is not a high incidence of false positive results, ideally screening mammography will identify a breast cancer before you or your physician can feel it by examination. Mammography, however, is imperfect, and a "normal" mammogram does not necessarily mean that everything is fine. Not only are the density and the extent of breast tissue difficult to capture adequately on film, but because normal breast tissue can appear dense on X-ray film, abnormal conditions can sometimes be hidden by it. Be sure that the mammography you have is administered by an office or a center where the equipment used is up-to-date, and, more important, that your mammograms are performed and read by professionals with proper experience in the field. It is wise to have your mammograms done at the same office or center every year so that comparisons can be made; if you switch locations, you should obtain your old films and bring them with you to the new center.

Because no test or experience is foolproof, it is wise to combine regular mammography with an annual breast examination by a physician or other health-care provider, even as you continue the monthly self-examinations that account for by far the highest percentage of all breast cancers detected.

FIBROCYSTIC DISEASE

Fibrocystic disease is a catch-all term that has been used over the years to describe a variety of breast conditions. Lumpy breasts, painful breasts, and cysts of the breast were all grouped together and referred to under this label. Radiologists who work with breast X rays have used the term to describe what is, in fact, simply the normal, dense breast tissue seen on mammograms; in reporting on breast biopsies, pathologists have used it to characterize a variety of normal changes on the cellular level. Specialists discourage using this term today, preferring instead that doctors actually describe the breast problem, if any, they are seeing. The conditions that have been grouped together in the past and referred to as fibrocystic disease do not place a woman at increased risk for developing breast cancer.

BREAST LUMPS AND THEIR DIAGNOSIS

PHYSIOLOGIC NODULARITY

The majority of breast lumps are benign, not cancerous. In fact, the most common type of breast lump is not really a lump at all, but a condition called physiologic nodularity, which means simply normal lumpiness. As your body undergoes cyclical hormone changes every month, your breasts respond by developing lumpy areas. These lumpy areas usually increase in size and tenderness immediately before the menstrual period, then decrease in size and sensitivity after the menstrual period has begun, which is why self-examination is most accurate about a week after your period.

Lumpy breasts are normal and don't need any treatment. A true or dominant lump differs from an ordinary breast lump in that it does not change significantly during the menstrual cycle. It is these dominant, unchanging lumps that need further evaluation. Keep in mind that a dominant lump can be a cyst, a benign tumor such as a fibroadenoma, or a malignant tumor—that is, breast cancer. How to distinguish one from another can be clarified by understanding what characterizes each of them.

CYST

A cyst is a fluid-filled sac, most common in women in their 30s; it is a lump that sometimes can appear very suddenly—that is, "overnight." Sometimes the nodular areas in the breasts are erroneously referred to as cysts. The doctor can often aspirate a cyst right in the office by placing a needle with an attached syringe into the lump and drawing out (aspirating) the fluid. The process is no more painful than having blood drawn. Physicians should aspirate all dominant lumps. There is a major difference in draining cysts in the breasts and those in the abdomen; breast cysts are almost never malignant, and there is no proof that aspirating the rare malignant breast cyst will spread tumor cells anywhere else in the body. If the lump is a cyst, it will then disappear; the cyst fluid does not need to be studied under a microscope because the results of such fluid studies are highly inaccurate. Often the cells in cyst fluid have been floating around for a long time and are, in fact, dead cells. As a result, they can appear falsely abnormal under the microscope.

Examination by ultrasound (sonogram), in which the doctor elicits on-screen images of the body through the echoes from sound waves, can also diagnose a cyst. The procedure is sometimes useful to view densities reported on a mammogram that the doctor cannot feel. If ultrasound examination determines that the lump is a cyst, the doctor need not remove it, because cysts are benign.

SOLID LUMP

If a lump is not a cyst, it is a solid mass, which can be either benign or malignant. A common benign tumor in young women is a fibroadenoma, which is a smooth mass that moves around easily, feeling to the touch much like a marble. Surgeons usually recommend removing it to make certain that it is indeed a fibroadenoma, as opposed to a malignant lump masquerading as one. Malignant lumps are described later in this chapter.

BIOPSY

Assuming that the doctor has determined the lump is not a cyst, a biopsy—removing some or all of the lump and examining samples under a microscope—can determine if a solid mass is benign or malignant. The most common type is an excisional biopsy, which removes the entire lump. This procedure is performed in a hospital operating room under local or general anesthesia. An excisional biopsy done under local anesthesia carries little risk. General anesthesia, however, adds a degree of danger to any operative procedure.

Another type of biopsy is a fine-needle aspirate, which is different from the simple aspiration of a cyst. Although the technique is the same in both procedures, a simple cyst aspiration removes fluid; a fine-needle aspirate removes cells. In addition, the doctor may have to insert the needle several times when doing a fine-needle aspirate, while one insertion is all that is required for a successful simple aspiration.

The physician can do a fine-needle aspirate in the office by placing the needle with an attached syringe into the lump and removing some cells, which are then examined under the microscope. The advantage of the fine-needle aspirate is that, if it is positive, indicating the presence of cancer, a woman can discuss her options for treatment with her doctor immediately and thus save herself from an excisional biopsy. Keep in mind that a negative result to a fine-needle aspirate is not considered definitive; an excisional biopsy will still be necessary. Usually it takes from 24 to 48 hours to process a biopsy. With a fine-needle biopsy, however, the findings can come back very quickly, sometimes the same day.

If your doctor recommends a biopsy, be sure to ask the following questions:

1. What kind of biopsy do you recommend? Will a fine-needle aspirate be useful?
2. If you recommend an excisional biopsy, will you use local or general anesthesia? Why? Do I have a choice about the anesthesia?
3. When will the result of the biopsy be available, and how soon can I have it? May I call you or will you call me?
4. Will a "frozen biopsy" (frozen section) be done so that a reading will be available in less than two hours? What percent of frozen sections done at your hospital correlate correctly with the final pathology report?
5. When will I be able to talk with you about the result of the biopsy and my treatment options?

MAMMOGRAPHIC FINDINGS

Sometimes a mammogram will show abnormal areas that are too small to feel, such as calcifications, which are microscopic deposits of calcium in the breast. (Calcification is unrelated to how much calcium or milk product a woman consumes.) The vast majority of breast calcifications—about 85 percent—are benign and occur as the result of the normal aging process. Sometimes, however, they can be an early sign of breast cancer, and the presence of certain patterns requires further investigation—for example, a cluster (e.g., a group of five or more); a linear pattern; or a cluster that increases in size on sequential mammograms. Surgeons should biopsy any suspicious calcifications using the wire localization technique. This procedure starts in the hospital's X-ray department, where a radiologist places a small needle into the area in question. A thin wire is then threaded through the needle and into the suspicious area. Once this has been done, the woman is taken to the operating room where, using the wire as a guide, the surgeon removes the questionable area, using either local or general anesthesia.

OTHER BREAST CONDITIONS

BREAST PAIN

Breast pain, which doctors call mastalgia, is a very common condition. Most breast pain is cyclical, caused by monthly hormonal changes. The breasts are more sensitive immediately before the menstrual period, and the tenderness usually abates after bleeding begins. Unfortunately, few remedies exist to eliminate this kind of breast pain. If your pain is relatively severe and over-the-counter painkillers give you some relief, by all means use them. It should be somewhat reassuring to note that painful breasts are not usually associated with underlying breast cancer.

Recent controlled studies have exonerated the methylxanthines found in caffeine and chocolate as a cause of breast pain. Similarly, among the many claims made for vitamin E was that it alleviated breast pain by working on a cellular level to change certain hormonal pathways. Recent clinical studies have disproved this as well.

NIPPLE DISCHARGES

Most women have some discharge when they squeeze their nipples. This is normal. The type of discharge that needs further evaluation is a discharge from one breast that occurs spontaneously, noticeable as a spot on the bra or nightgown.

If you have a spontaneous nipple discharge, your doctor should evaluate it by examining your breast and ordering a mammogram. The doctor may also test the discharge for the presence of blood and/or send it for cytology, a microscopic study that establishes the presence or absence of specific cell types. In addition, the doctor may refer you to a specially trained radiologist for a ductogram. This procedure involves injecting radiopaque dye into a small catheter or tube that has been placed into the duct that is discharging and then doing a mammogram, which outlines the ductal system and identifies any abnormality that may be present. The physician uses the ductogram to select the best plan for obtaining a biopsy of the area.

The most common cause of nipple discharge is an intraductal papilloma, a small benign tumor that extends into the opening (lumen) of the duct. Rarely, in fewer than 4 percent of cases, is a nipple discharge an early sign of breast cancer.

BREAST CANCER

No disease frightens women more than breast cancer, primarily because the therapy has been so radical and disfiguring and the mortality rate so high. But the actual risk of developing breast cancer in your lifetime, commonly quoted today as one in nine, is actually not so great, because this method of computing assumes that every woman is at equal risk and that every woman will live to be 110. To cast all this in more realistic terms, the chance of getting breast cancer for the average 40-year-old woman is one in 1,000 per year, or .001 percent, and for the average 50-year-old woman, the figure doubles to .002 percent. While far too many women still die of breast cancer, the cure rates for early cancers are very high, over 75 percent. Be sure you have read the earlier section on breast lumps before continuing with this section.

Certain factors do increase a woman's risk of developing breast cancer. They include a family history of breast cancer in a mother or sister, a first pregnancy that occurs after age 35, having experienced the onset of the first menstrual period before the age of 10, or experiencing menopause after the age of 55. These risk factors don't mean that a woman will develop breast cancer; they are simply an indication of the need for regular mammography and breast examination.

In the past, radical mastectomy, the most deforming kind of breast surgery, was widely employed in the treatment of breast cancer; as recently as the early 1970s, 48 percent of all breast cancer patients suffered this radical surgery, compared with 5.7 percent in 1981–82. Feminists saw the overuse of unnecessarily deforming surgery as an important health issue, and their research and protests, along with other studies that showed lumpectomy and other forms of mastectomy had equally good survival rates, were an important influence on doctors in substantially changing their approach to cancer treatment.

Breast cancer appears either in the lobules that make milk or in the ducts that transport the milk to the nipple. Ninety percent of breast cancer is ductal in origin, while approximately 10 percent starts in the lobules.

LOBULAR CARCINOMA IN SITU

Lobular carcinoma in situ is not breast cancer but an increase in the number of cells lining the milk-producing lobules of the breast. Because it produces no abnormalities in the breast, doctors usually discover it as an incidental finding during a biopsy for another reason. While not a cancer, the condition is an indicator or marker of an increased risk that a woman will subsequently develop breast cancer; the likelihood is that about 25 percent of women with lobular carcinoma in situ will develop invasive breast cancer in either breast over the next 25 to 30 years.

Given these figures, treatment consists of either following the breasts carefully to detect any sign of cancer or removing both breasts to prevent cancer from developing. If a woman chooses to have both breasts removed, then the surgeon must perform bilateral total mastectomies, which involve removing all the breast tissue, including the nipples. If the woman elects close observation, she must have annual mammograms and a breast examination by a physician once or twice a year.

Because the chance of developing cancer as a result of this condition is still relatively low, and because breast cancer is slow-growing, we recommend the close-following option, which is what the vast majority of women who must make this difficult decision choose. Occasionally, a woman cannot live with the kind of uncertainty that this choice produces, and for her bilateral total mastectomy may be the only option possible.

DUCTAL CARCINOMA IN SITU, OR INTRADUCTAL CARCINOMA

The cells lining the duct walls of the breast are normally positioned in a single layer. When the cells divide or form more than one layer, the resulting condition is referred to as ductal hyperplasia. The next step on the hyperplasia continuum is atypical ductal hyperplasia; here, the cells multiply and look somewhat abnormal. Atypical ductal hyperplasia, diagnosed through a biopsy, *slightly* increases a woman's risk of developing breast cancer over her lifetime. When the cells become even more atypical but still remain inside the duct wall, the condition is described as intraductal carcinoma, or ductal carcinoma in situ.

Ductal carcinoma in situ is a type of noninvasive breast cancer or precancer in which the atypical cells remain within the ductal system. They can spread extensively throughout the ductal system of the breast, but they do not extend outside it or go elsewhere in the body. Annual mammograms sometimes detect this type of carcinoma.

When the abnormal cells extend outside the duct wall or invade the tissue surrounding the duct wall, the condition is referred to as infiltrating ductal carcinoma, or invasive ductal carcinoma. Only 25 to 30 percent of intraductal carcinoma goes on to become invasive ductal carcinoma.

The standard treatment for ductal carcinoma in situ has always been a total mastectomy—removing all the breast tissue—which results in a cure rate close to 99 percent. However, total mastectomy does seem to constitute drastic, and sometimes unnecessarily drastic, treatment for precancer. Recently, surgeons have begun using a far less aggressive approach to ductal carcinoma in situ. They now attempt to remove all of the involved tissue with a wide excision—a partial mastectomy. This procedure also involves removing additional breast tissue from around the original biopsy site to be as certain as possible that all of the ductal carcinoma in situ cells have been excised. If the partial mastectomy reveals no additional ductal carcinoma in situ cells, or indicates only a small number of ductal carcinoma in situ cells that do not extend to the edge of the tissue that was removed, then future treatment can be confined to either close observation or radiation therapy.

Close observation includes regular mammograms, at least once a year, and breast examination by a physician twice a year. If doctors add radiation therapy to the wide excision approach, this usually requires six and a half weeks of daily treatment. At this point we have insufficient data to determine which of these treatments offers better results. Currently, a national study is under way, sponsored by the National Surgical Adjuvant Breast and Bowel Project (NSABBP), which is investigating whether patients with ductal carcinoma in situ who receive wide excision alone do as well as those who receive radiation therapy in addition to wide excision. The patients in the study are selected at random to preserve objectivity. When the results of this study become available in the near future, they should contribute substantially to our knowledge.

If a partial mastectomy reveals extensive ductal carcinoma in situ, or if the margins are revealed as "dirty"—that is, with tumor cells extending to the edge of the removed tissue—then the best treatment is a total mastectomy.

INVASIVE CANCER

Infiltrating or invasive ductal carcinoma involves tumor cells that have spread beyond the ductal system within the breast. Infiltrating or invasive lobular carcinoma originates in the lobules but has spread beyond them into the adjacent breast tissue. The treatment for infiltrating ductal and infiltrating lobular carcinoma is the same.

Invasive cancer has the potential to spread elsewhere in the body, a process that is called metastasis. Although this does not always happen, the next step after breast cancer has been diagnosed is usually a staging workup to ensure that the cancer has not spread beyond the breast. Not all physicians believe that staging is necessary for early breast cancer—that is, for small tumors that are less than two centimeters in diameter—because the incidence of such cancers spreading elsewhere in the body is very low.

STAGING

When breast cancer spreads, it commonly goes to the bone, lungs, or liver. Therefore, the staging workup usually consists of a bone scan, a chest X ray, blood tests to determine liver function, and a special blood test—called a CEA level—that looks for a carcinoembryonic antigen marker, an enzyme that is occasionally elevated in women with breast cancer.

A bone scan, which is done in a hospital's nuclear medicine department, consists of injecting a small amount of radioactive dye into one of the veins of the hand or arm. The dye spreads throughout the skeletal system in approximately two hours, allowing the radiologist to take pictures of the entire skeleton. Sometimes the radiologist also takes X rays of particular bones in order to correlate the bone scan with the X rays. The chest X ray required by staging is simply a routine two-view X ray of the lung. Remember that staging might not be indicated for tumors that are less than two centimeters in diameter. If these tests are all negative, it does not mean that no cancer cells have spread; the cells may simply be too small for the radiologist to detect with the staging tests.

OTHER TESTS

Another indicator of distant spread is the condition of the axillary lymph nodes under the arms. If tumor cells are present in the underarm (axillary) lymph nodes, it indicates that microscopic tumor cells may have spread elsewhere in the body but were too small for the staging tests to identify. Even the absence of cancer cells in the lymph nodes is not a 100 percent accurate indication. Thirty percent of women with negative nodes have microscopic disease elsewhere, and 35 percent of women with positive nodes do not.

Another useful tool in determining the possibility of distant microscopic metastases is observing the characteristics of the primary tumor itself. Using microscopic study, doctors can identify some characteristics that may indicate the cancer has indeed spread: (1) tumor cells invading the lymphatic vessel at the primary site; (2) poorly differentiated tumor cells in the primary tumor; (3) a tumor larger than five centimeters (two inches) in diameter; and (4) estrogen-receptor-negative tumor cells, which are cells without estrogen-receptor binding sites on them.

TREATMENT

LUMPECTOMY AND RADIATION THERAPY

One way of treating breast cancer involves a lumpectomy, also called a partial mastectomy, which is followed by radiation therapy to the breast. The surgeon removes the tumor as well as some additional breast tissue from around the original biopsy site in order to obtain a margin of normal breast tissue from around the site of the tumor. At the same time, but through a separate incision at the lower end of the armpit, the surgeon will do an axillary dissection, removing five to 15 lymph nodes of the 30 to 40 that are present in the axilla. Radiation therapy to the breast follows, usually for approximately six and a half weeks, five days a week. Each treatment lasts for about 15 minutes. For the first five weeks, the radiation therapist irradiates the entire breast. During the last week and a half, the tumor area becomes the focus of additional treatment; for this, a different machine is used and a higher dose of radiation is given. The main side effect from radiation therapy is fatigue. The skin over the breast may also become slightly sunburned. It is rare for patients to experience serious long-term effects, but permanent swelling of the arm sometimes occurs.

MASTECTOMY

If the tumor is to be removed, and if it is too large to be excised with a clean area of tissue around it—known medically as negative margins—then the surgeon will perform a modified radical mastectomy.

"Simple mastectomy" and "total mastectomy" are two terms for the same procedure: removal of the entire breast. A modified radical mastectomy removes the entire breast plus some or all of the axillary lymph nodes. A radical mastectomy takes all breast tissue, the muscle that covers the chest and connects to the upper arm (pectoralis major muscle), and all axillary lymph nodes. It is the most deforming type of breast surgery and, as noted earlier, doctors use it very rarely today. If a surgeon recommends a radical mastectomy, it is particularly important for you to keep a written record of the reasons given and to be sure to secure additional opinions before consenting to this surgery.

If your doctor recommends a mastectomy, ask these questions:

1. What are my other options for treatment?
2. What's your opinion about the relative effectiveness of these treatments?
3. Why are you recommending a mastectomy? What about lumpectomy and radiation?
4. Will I need chemotherapy?

If you aren't satisfied with the options your doctor offers, be sure to seek additional opinions. *Remember, you have the time to do this.* If your doctor says you should have the mastectomy, for example, and you want to be certain that a lumpectomy or other treatment may be viable, seek additional opinions from physicians who are not colleagues of your doctor and will therefore not necessarily share his or her philosophy. Although most women feel it is easier to talk to a woman physician about breast cancer, there is no evidence that female doctors are more sympathetic to women cancer patients than male doctors.

CHEMOTHERAPY

If microscopic cancer seems to be present elsewhere in the body, women are usually given chemotherapy or hormonal therapy in addition to any surgery that may be undertaken to remove the originally diagnosed cancer.

Chemotherapy is intended to destroy those cancer cells that are inaccessible by surgery. Because the chemicals used are very powerful, side effects, sometimes severe, are common.

The most frequent types of chemotherapy for premenopausal women is a combination of three drugs with the initials CMF. This stands for Cytoxan, methotrexate, and 5 fluorouracil. Methotrexate and 5 fluorouracil are administered intravenously, while Cytoxan can be given either orally or intravenously. The treatment extends over a six-month period in three-week cycles. The side effects from this type of chemotherapy may involve some nausea and vomiting, fatigue, and some temporary loss of hair.

Another regime of chemotherapy, known as CAF, involves Cytoxan, given by mouth or intravenously, and Adriamycin and 5 fluorouracil, administered intravenously. This is stronger treatment and has more significant side effects. Hair loss, usually temporary, always occurs with this kind of chemotherapy; nausea and vomiting sometimes do. In addition, Adriamycin can sometimes cause damage to the heart muscle.

Doctors cannot determine if chemotherapy is effective in individual patients until the cancer either returns or the patient remains free of a recurrence. The most recent overview of the effectiveness of chemotherapy, however, shows that premenopausal women with positive nodes survive longer if they receive chemotherapy than do women who don't receive it.

The role chemotherapy (or hormone therapy) should play in women whose lymph nodes are negative is a matter of controversy. The vast majority (75 to 80 percent) of women with negative lymph nodes are cured by mastectomy or lumpectomy and radiation and would not benefit from chemotherapy or hormone therapy. However, as we have noted, the inspection of lymph nodes is not a perfect indicator of whether a cancer has spread. The potential benefit of chemotherapy to women with negative nodes is small, if it exists at all, especially when weighed against the possible long-term risks of chemotherapy, one of which is an increased chance of developing leukemia. If your lymph nodes are negative, you and your doctor should give serious consideration to these facts before deciding whether you are a candidate for chemotherapy.

HORMONE THERAPY

Hormone therapy for breast cancer usually employs an estrogen-blocker (tamoxifen) administered by pill. This drug binds or attaches to estrogen-receptor sites on the breast cancer cell and stops the cell from dividing. The pathologist can test the tumor at the time of the original biopsy to determine the estrogen-receptor status of a tumor cell. Women who have stopped menstruating, whose tumor cells are positive for estrogen-receptor cells, and who have positive lymph nodes are usually prescribed tamoxifen; studies have shown a survival benefit in postmenopausal women who have estrogen-receptor cells and take this drug. The duration of therapy with tamoxifen is still controversial and now ranges anywhere from two years to the rest of a woman's life. The possible side effects of tamoxifen for postmenopausal women include occasional but sometimes severe hot flashes, depression, and uterine bleeding. Recent European studies have indicated that there may be a slightly increased risk of uterine cancer and that there may be a possible benefit in protecting women from osteoporosis. However, these findings are based on very early data that need to be corroborated by additional studies.

Always keep in mind that the prognosis for breast cancer is very good. Cancer specialists can cure 75 to 80 percent of women with early-stage disease. And they can now do it with less deforming treatments and a better cosmetic result than at any time in the past. The continuing research that is at last under way on breast cancer will make future treatments even more successful.

BREAST RECONSTRUCTION

A plastic surgeon can reconstruct the breast at the time of mastectomy, or this surgery can be performed at a later date. The advantages of immediate reconstruction are that you need only one surgery and one administration of anesthesia, and you do not have to go through a period of time dealing with your absent breast and the prospect of another operation. The disadvantages include a longer hospital stay—five to seven days, as opposed to three to five days, and lengthier surgery; for example, if a woman elects a reconstruction using a muscle flap (described below), the combined mastectomy and reconstruction can extend the surgery and the time under anesthesia to as long as eight hours. Not all women can tolerate such extended surgery. In addition, because the procedure requires a general surgeon and a plastic surgeon, it can be difficult to coordinate the schedules of both. Furthermore, some plastic surgeons will not do an immediate reconstruction. Thus the timing decision must be a personal one, based on your own inclinations after considering the advantages and disadvantages, your health and ability to tolerate extended surgery, and the advice of both your general and plastic surgeons.

The two types of reconstructive surgery now available consist of silicone or saline implants or the attachment of rotation flaps made of muscle.

In silicone implants done under general anesthesia, a plastic sac filled with liquid silicone is placed under the pectoralis major muscle that covers the chest wall, allowing the muscle and overlying skin to expand over the implant and form a breast mound. Sometimes the muscle and skin cannot accommodate the implant, in which case the plastic surgeon places a tissue-expander beneath the pectoralis major muscle. The expander is a plastic sac holding a small amount of saline (saltwater). A valve placed under the skin surface allows the surgeon to inject additional saline over a period of two to three months, an office procedure, slowly expanding the overlying skin and muscle. In a subsequent operation, the surgeon places the silicone implant under the muscle and removes the expander.

More than 2 million women have received breast implants, 80 percent for cosmetic reasons and the rest for breast reconstruction after mastectomy or injury. Because silicone breast implants have been used since the 1960s, and the law governing such devices was not enacted until 1976, the Food and Drug Administration (FDA) has not regulated them. This changed in April 1991, when the FDA required manufacturers of silicone breast implants to submit data within three months proving that their products are both safe and effective. The agency took this action because of emerging health concerns about the side effects of breast implants, which, in addition to false mammography results, include infection, pain, hardening of the surrounding breast tissue, silicone leakage, and implant failure.

Specifically, reports that the polyurethane foam used to coat one type of silicone breast implant might break down into 2-toluene diamine (TDA), which has been shown to cause cancer in laboratory animals, caused Surgitek, the manufacturer of the polyurethane-coated devices *Meme* and *Replicon*, to take them off the market until the FDA's review was complete. A very small amount of TDA was found in the milk of one nursing mother who had a polyurethane-coated breast implant, but the doctor who discovered it did not believe it posed a health threat to her infant.

On July 31, 1991, an FDA advisory panel recommended that the approximately 200,000 American women with polyurethane-coated implants not have them removed because the dangers inherent in the surgery are greater than the possible risk of cancer, which appears to be minimal. The FDA has required Surgitek to conduct additional studies to assess the danger from TDA.

As for silicone implants in general, FDA Commissioner David A. Kessler, M.D., advised women who are considering using them to get all available information on their risks from the package insert that comes with each implant, from their doctors, or by writing to the FDA at 5600 Fishers Lane, Rockville, MD 20857. Meanwhile, the agency has set up a special team of scientists to review the information that has been submitted by six manufacturers of 10 implants by the end of January 1992. The agency also plans to require the manufacturers of saline-filled breast implants to submit safety and effectiveness data soon. In addition, the FDA has removed one unapproved breast implant, Misti Gold, manufactured by Bioplasty, Inc., of St. Paul, Minnesota, from the market, warning surgeons who may still have this implant on hand not to use it.

The second type of breast reconstruction, also done under general anesthesia, entails the insertion of rotation flaps that are made from the woman's own muscles. Plastic surgeons create these flaps by using either the rectus abdominis muscle that covers the front of the abdominal wall or the latissimus dorsi muscle that goes back behind the shoulder. In a single procedure, the surgeon removes the muscle and overlying skin, with their blood supply intact, and tunnels under the skin into the area of the mastectomy, forming a breast mound. In a second procedure at a later time, the surgeon can create a nipple-areola complex either by using skin from the inner thigh or with a new method that employs tattooing.

Women elect breast reconstruction for different reasons. A reconstructed breast allows a woman to feel "balanced" without having to place a prosthesis or artificial breast in her bra. Reconstruction is particularly important for women who prefer not to wear bras. It should be noted, however, that a reconstructed breast doesn't look or feel like a normal breast, especially in terms of sensation. Also, complications can arise from reconstruction. The silicone implant is, after all, a "foreign" object, and the woman's body may "reject" it. Such a rejection, which happens in 5 to 10 percent of cases, is usually signaled by an infection. In another 5 to 10 percent of cases, encapsulation—hardening of the implant—occurs.

The disadvantage of the rotation flap procedure is that because it moves muscle from another area of the body to the site of the mastectomy, it not only leaves a scar in the place from which the muscle was removed but also produces a loss of the normal function of that particular muscle. The rectus abdominis muscle normally helps support the abdominal wall, for example, and its removal may increase the risk of hernia formation; removing the latissimus dorsi muscle may affect shoulder motion. Be sure to weigh the pros and cons of reconstruction carefully, and beware of succumbing to the enthusiasm of either friends or medical professionals in evaluating whether either of these alternatives is right for you.

ESTROGEN-REPLACEMENT THERAPY AND THE BREAST

Estrogen-replacement therapy (ERT) is a controversial issue for older women. Physicians sometimes prescribe ERT for the relief of such postmenopausal symptoms as hot flashes—flushes and, sometimes, sweating—and vaginal dryness; for the prevention of osteoporosis, a crippling bone disease affecting 25 percent of women over 60; and for a potential reduction in the risk of heart disease, which rises dramatically for women after menopause. (See Chapter 15.)

Breast tissue is normally responsive to estrogen stimulation; therefore, the addition of postmenopausal estrogen fools the breast into thinking it is still premenopausal by providing it with estrogen. As a result, the breasts may become tender, lumpy, and develop cysts. A recent Swedish study shows that women on long-term ERT are at slightly increased risk of developing breast cancer, and the Harvard nurses' study has confirmed that conclusion by finding an increased risk for estrogen users. This is a risk that some researchers still consider small when compared to estrogen's protective benefits in the areas of cardiovascular disease and osteoporosis. Given all these findings, however, women should pay particular attention to evaluating the benefits and liabilities of ERT and consider it in the perspective of their own medical history, as well as their family history. If your female relatives have or have had breast cancer, ERT may not be for you. However, a woman suffering from severe hot flashes and vaginal dryness, for which estrogen is the only available therapy, may decide to accept it, in spite of having relatives with breast cancer, because she needs relief from debilitating symptoms. On the other hand, if there is a lot of heart disease and osteoporosis in your family, you may want to consider ERT. Like so much else in medicine, this too must be a personal decision.

5

Female Sexuality

Mary Jane Gray, M.D.

We know very little about early human beings and even less about the sexual interactions between primitive men and women. Other primates shed scant light in this area because patterns vary, from the monogamous gibbons living in nuclear families to the extended kinship systems, with their promiscuous males, of the chimpanzees and gorillas.

If the history of human sexual interaction is itself vague, then the sexual behavior of our species has always ranged widely, depending on a great variety of cultural influences. The ancient Jews embraced the concept of monogamy, especially for women. They clearly understood both the reproductive and the pleasurable aspects of sex and believed that intercourse between man and wife was good and a joy to God. Beginning with Paul's message to the early Christians that it is better to marry than to burn, sex became a potential source of guilt. Augustine focused on sex as sin and taught that intercourse was moral only if the intent was procreation, a view that has remained a theme in the Roman Catholic Church until today. Luther, a married man himself, stressed the concept of sex within marriage, and Protestants have, to varying degrees, officially held to this line. Variations of attitude toward sexual pleasure and purpose, ritual and taboo, both within and outside of marriage, vary broadly among different cultures, religions, and geographic areas. In a world of such diversity there is no one accepted standard of sexual behavior.

SEXUAL DEVELOPMENT

The moment of fertilization determines our biological sex—that is, whether the fetus is male or female. Since all eggs in the human female contain X chromosomes, a person's sexual destiny is determined by whether a sperm bearing an X chromosome fertilizes the egg to create the double X female (XX), or whether one carrying a Y chromosome gets to the egg first, producing the male XY combination. Researchers have recently found that, although slightly more sperm carry the X chromosome, the Y chromosome seems to have a stronger fertilization ability, managing to penetrate more than half of all eggs.

The sex of a developing fetus can now be discovered by taking a piece of placenta at eight weeks of pregnancy and subjecting it to chromosomal studies. Although there have been many attempts to control the sex of a fetus—by putting semen in a centrifuge in order to separate X and Y sperm, by changing the acidity of the vagina, and by timing intercourse to occur just before or just after ovulation—these methods have met with only slight success and leave a large element of chance in determining whether the fetus will be male or female.

For the first eight weeks after fertilization, development of the gonads (testes or ovaries) and reproductive tract is the same for both the male and the female fetus. Then the Y chromosome directs the growth of the gonad into a testis that produces testosterone, which, in turn, controls the formation of the male reproductive tract, with its ducts and external genitalia. If no testosterone is produced, the development is female, regardless of whether or not ovaries and estrogens are present. If a pregnant woman carrying a female infant receives male hormones, the infant may be masculinized. The male infant, on the other hand, is always exposed to high levels of estrogen from the mother but is rarely influenced by it. Throughout life, ovaries and testes retain the capacity to produce both male and female hormones and do so to varying degrees.

Since male and female fetuses start out the same, it is easy to understand that abnormal hormonal patterns may mislead sexual development so that an infant can be born with ambiguous genitalia. If this occurs and the sex of the baby is not immediately obvious, it is a matter for concern, tests, and consultation. In addition to determining the chromosomal sex of the infant and whether it has ovaries or testes, specialists must find the cause of the problem to assess future potential for fertility and sexual functioning at puberty. Surgery can do wonders to alter the genitals to fit the indicated chromosomal sex and make rearing the child as normal as possible, but parents and doctors must arrive at a firm plan before they tell friends and family the sex of the newborn. The less confusion there is among those who will be close to the child, the less uncertainty will exist in the developing youngster's mind about his or her sexual identity.

Such a situation underlines that there are many aspects to sex, among them sex according to chromosomes, sex according to gonads (testes or ovaries), sex as identified by external appearance, and the sex the individual is convinced he or she is. Gender identity is the internal private sense we have of ourselves; gender role is the way we act to convey our sex to the world; and gender behavior consists of specific sexual acts. We all learn gender roles from our experiences as very young children, and after the age of two they can be altered only with great difficulty. When all of the factors of gender agree, life is easier for the individual in his or her world.

Sexual orientation refers to whether a person is sexually attracted to the opposite sex and is heterosexual, or is attracted to the same sex and is homosexual, or gay, the term that has come into wide use to disassociate homosexuality from the pejorative associations visited on it by cultural ignorance. Some individuals find both sexes attractive and are bisexual. Still others are attracted to one sex at a certain time in their lives and another at a different stage. Regardless of how we identify our sexual orientation, it's wise to remember that most of us can feel sexual attraction to people of both sexes. Sexual orientation may or may not involve sexual activity. Sex researcher Alfred Kinsey found a continuum of sexual behavior, from exclusively heterosexual to exclusively homosexual, with approximately 40 percent of males and 20 percent of females stating that they have had some homosexual activity. At least half of homosexually oriented individuals are or have been married.

INFANCY

At birth, female infants have slightly swollen vaginal lips and a thick discharge from the opening of the vagina; both sexes have breast swelling under the nipples. These features reflect the high maternal hormone levels to which the infant has recently been exposed and disappear over the first few days of life. They underscore the fact that both internal and external reproductive organs are capable of such hormonal response from birth to death. Physical stimulation of the penis, such as that which occurs during circumcision, for example, can produce an erection in the male infant, and recent ultrasound studies have documented erections occurring while the fetus is still in the uterus. We know, therefore, that the sexual organs are not quiescent even at birth, and soon the infant discovers while exploring other parts of the body that touching the genitals may produce pleasurable sensations. The way parents react (or overreact) to such normal explorations may profoundly affect the child's attitudes toward his or her body and, later, toward sex. Since exploring genitalia is a normal and healthy part of infancy, parents should not pay any more attention to it than to other normal infant behavior; they certainly should not indicate it is wrong.

Immediately after birth, infants experience the gratification of relating to another human being by snuggling close to their mothers' warm bodies and either suckling at the breast or being held closely while receiving nourishment from a bottle. Suckling is an important source of pleasure to both a nursing mother and an infant. A little later, the infant becomes aware of the quality of interaction between his or her parents and other caregivers, and of the atmosphere of love, or the lack of it, in the home. This, too, forms the background for the later development of the kind of loving relationships that foster good sexual functioning.

CHILDHOOD

While childhood is usually a period of relative sexual calm, it is nonetheless a time of curiosity and exploration. When children ask questions about the differences between boys and girls and where babies come from, parents should answer calmly and factually with information appropriate to the child's age. Correct information, warmly offered, will avoid confusion in the youngster's mind and will promote a healthy attitude toward sex.

One of the ways children express their sexual curiosity is by exploring their own bodies and those of their young friends, often in the guise of such games as "playing doctor." Most of this exploration is harmless, but parents usually want to establish some socially acceptable limits. Parents should teach their children at an early age the difference between what they may do in private and what is acceptable in public. Parents need to know, however, that masturbating, the self-stimulation of the genitals, is normal and causes no harm, no matter how uncomfortable it may make them feel. Children should be taught the proper names for their genitals so that parents are not complicit in perpetuating any sexual taboos that may have existed in their own original families.

Sexual stimulation of children by adolescents or adults, however, including parents, is quite another matter. Recent studies show that between 15 and 40 percent of children under the age of 14 have suffered some sort of sexual abuse. It is not clear whether the actual incidence of abuse is increasing or whether physicians, teachers, and social workers have simply become more aware of the prevalence of this severe problem. Most young children who are sexually abused are subjected to genital touching or further sexual activity by relatives, acquaintances, or trusted others. Sometimes it is stepfathers and stepbrothers who initiate these acts, although biological fathers and brothers can do so as well. Girls are sexually abused more often than boys. If parents, teachers, or others suspect that a child is being sexually abused, they should immediately seek professional advice about how to protect the child and to sort out the issues. It is also important to have a competent, caring doctor examine the youngster, not only to treat possible visible symptoms but also because sexually transmitted diseases (STDs) are very frequent in children subjected to sexual abuse. Long-term problems for youngsters who have suffered sexual abuse include depression, eating disorders, chronic pelvic pain, low self-esteem, and difficulty responding sexually in later years. Children who are victims of incest—sexual abuse by members of their immediate families—suffer these effects profoundly in later life and may need continuing counseling to help alleviate them. It is particularly important for parents and health-care providers to understand that the sexual abuse of children cuts across all class and income levels.

ADOLESCENCE

Puberty, the time of initial sexual development, heralds the onset of adolescence. Among the many potential traumas of this period is that of finding one's body, formerly comfortable and controllable, suddenly changing in size, shape, feeling, and configuration. The growth spurt occurs with startling speed, often leaving a tall, gangling body without sufficient muscle mass to regulate it. With all these changes, it is no surprise that adolescents are constantly wondering if they are "normal" and turning to their peers, who are going through roughly the same experience, for confirmation that they indeed are typical. Since there are wide differences in timetables for these changes and a great deal of anatomical variation, the answers they receive are not always accurate or sufficiently reassuring.

Female sexual development generally proceeds in an orderly manner, first charted by British pediatrician J. M. Tanner. (See Chapters 3 and 4.) All young women need a matter-of-fact explanation of menstruation well in advance of its occurrence. (See Chapter 3.) Even once this has taken place, the event is usually a surprise that most women remember for the rest of their lives. The prospect and the actuality of dealing with a flow that may occur at often unpredictable moments for the next 40 years is frequently a source of embarrassment to adolescents, but its onset should be a matter of pride in having reached a developmental marker: the beginning of fertility. (The adolescent male, with a penis that is not under his control, has different but analogous problems.)

The most important developmental task for the teenage girl is to establish her own identity as separate from her family. This process rarely proceeds smoothly, as the struggle to separate often leads to erratic rebellion. In turning to their peers for support, teenagers also become vulnerable to pressures to experiment with alcohol, other drugs, and sex. Gradually, they begin to establish their own values, based on their convictions and experience and on their early teaching, but this is a continuing and sometimes stormy process, and often they must make decisions in areas that they have not yet thought through.

Part of establishing identity lies in authenticating a person's sexual character and sexual values. Despite the normalcy of the process, the hormonal surges of puberty bring on sexual feelings and fantasies and, often, guilt. Our society sends young people extremely mixed messages about sex. Even parental instructions often seem confusing, such as "Look pretty, be popular, but don't get sexually involved." Such messages are almost totally obscured by those from television and the movies, where sexual intercourse is either constantly depicted or implied without ever raising the issues of contraception or of STDs, pregnancy, or other consequences. While love and clear direction from home can help to protect young people from sexual involvement that occurs too early in their lives, parents must stay aware about whatever sexual activity prevails among their children's peer groups, at school and elsewhere, and make certain that young people are informed accordingly in terms of protection against pregnancy and STDs. Disapproval of, or ignorance about, a daughter's or son's sexual activity, no matter how premature parents may judge it to be, is no assurance that an adolescent will not be sexually active. On the contrary, these attitudes, implicitly conveyed, sometimes push the adolescent into sexual activity.

Establishing a sexual identity is a task for all individuals. It involves role models, fantasies, and many other factors that researchers have still to understand clearly. By the early teens, however, and probably long before, most individuals "know" that they are either attracted by their own or the opposite sex, and this is such a "core" knowledge that it does not change easily, if at all. This does not mean, however, that the sexual experimentation between same-sex adolescents necessarily signifies homosexuality. Experimentation is normal and should not be regarded with disapproval or concern.

For most young people, the sexual activity that accompanies developing a sexual identity first takes the form of masturbation. Masturbating is almost universal. Highly pleasurable, it allows the individual to become acquainted with her physical responses to sexual stimulation in a controlled and private environment. Young women masturbate in a variety of ways: through sexual fantasies;

by stimulating their nipples and stroking their breasts with their fingertips and the palms of their hands; by caressing the clitoris and all the other sensitive spots on the vulva with their hands, or rubbing this responsive area against a pillow; by touching favorite spots on their bodies while in the bathtub, or a hot tub, under flowing or pulsing water; or by using a vibrator. Most women, contrary to popular belief, do not insert anything into the vagina when masturbating.

Sadly, for some 20 percent or more of young people, sexual activity has already involved being molested as a child. As we have noted, the effects of this abuse vary in kind and intensity, depending on its extent, the circumstances under which it occurred, who the abuser was, and the help that was available to allow the child to understand and deal with what happened. Sexual abuse can be said to have taken place whenever a child is used for the sexual pleasure of an older person—including a friend, stranger, or family member—and ranges from inappropriate touching, kissing, hugging, or stroking to actual intercourse or oral sex.

Teenagers often seek security and a sense of their own worth and attractiveness through forming intense relationships with others. Ideally, these progress slowly, from being able to talk to each other to touching, kissing, petting, and, finally, perhaps, to closer sexual contact. But when the pressure for sexual experience outdistances the ability to discuss what is happening, trouble lies ahead.

Other stresses often combine with peer pressure to push adolescents in the direction of intercourse. Those particularly likely to have early intercourse are adolescents from single-parent homes; those whose parents are constantly fighting; kids who are not doing well in school; teens who feel depressed about the future; and those who are using drugs. Sometimes first experiences with alcohol and drugs, usually unplanned, dull the thought processes and judgment enough for the young person to acquiesce in behavior that would be unacceptable under other circumstances.

In accord with the trend in our society toward earlier and earlier sexual involvement, 60 percent of women have had intercourse by the age of 18. Intercourse before the age of 16 to 18 is almost always premature. The relationships in which it occurs are rarely strong enough to withstand the emotional complexities intercourse entails, and teenagers have not yet developed the skills needed to anticipate the consequences of their actions. Premature sex is self-centered, concerned with getting instead of giving, and often is a means to obtaining selfish ends, such as acceptance, power, and popularity. There is often pressure on the partner, usually the young girl, to "put out" or be abandoned, and if she is one of the last of her peer group to have intercourse, this pressure is experienced as even more severe. A youngster engaged in such sex, which very often is contrary to the code by which the adolescent was reared and takes place before he or she has had time to establish a new one, is usually surrounded by guilt, and the young person feels the need to conceal the activity from parents, a fact that makes for stressed family ties.

Those who are responsible for sex education in our public schools have seen the folly of the purely factual, or "plumbing," approach to sex instruction. The same general principles that govern behavior in other areas can be applied to sex.

Premature sex is also unconcerned about pregnancy, relying on magical "it can't happen to me" fantasies. Statistics underscore just how truly "fantastic" this approach really is. There are 1.2 million teen pregnancies in the United States every year, and 16 percent of all teens become pregnant. Of these, 50 percent obtain abortions; 25 percent give birth to the baby but do not marry; and 25 percent marry, but of these marriages, about 80 percent eventually end in divorce. The younger the couple when they begin intercourse, the figures show, the less likely they are to use contraception. On average, a young teen couple will have intercourse for a year before they seek out reliable birth control, a finding that demonstrates that the availability of contraception is not the deciding factor in young people's beginning to have sex. The more committed a boy and girl are to each other and the more experienced, the more likely it is that they will use some form of pregnancy protection. Although similar levels of sexual activity prevail among the youth of Western European nations, the pregnancy rates are far lower there (see Fig. 5.1; see also Chapter 7).

Much speculation has taken place about the failure of the young to use contraceptives. Certainly teenage girls engage in the mechanism of denial of risk—a combination of considering themselves "too young" to have a baby and a genuine inability to realize that the outcome of the evening's activity may well be intercourse. Old cultural myths about the delights of young women's being swept

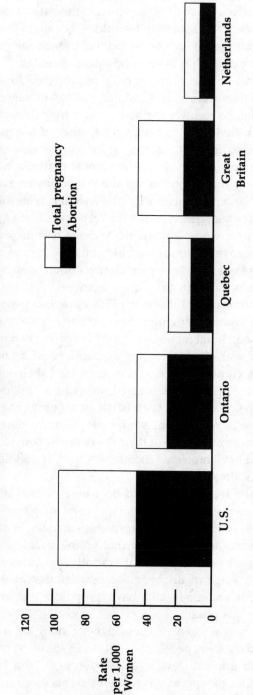

Figure 5.1   Teenage (ages 15–19) Total Pregnancy
and Abortion Rate in Three Countries and Two Canadian Provinces

Source: Elise P. Jones, et al., "Unintended Pregnancy, Contraceptive Practice and Family Planning Services in Developed
Countries," *Family Planning Perspectives*, vol. 20, no. 2 (March/April 1988), © The Alan Guttmacher Institute.

off their feet by amorous young men contribute to this passive—and often tragic—stance that it would be wrong to prepare for the event. To young women who are in thrall to such dangerous myths, sex is immoral if it has been anticipated, although "I was carried away" seems to make unplanned, unprotected lovemaking romantic and thus acceptable. In addition, many teenagers are simply ignorant of contraceptive methods, and if they do know anything about them, they tend to have a false sense of the risks involved in unprotected intercourse and an inaccurate idea about contraceptives, which they think are dangerous, particularly the Pill and the IUD. Very young couples are often embarrassed even to broach the subject of birth control with one another, with the result that each assumes the other is taking the responsibility to guard against unwanted pregnancy. Finally, adolescents fear they will find the same disapproving attitudes at birth control clinics as at home and therefore are reluctant to request contraception, which would most certainly be prescribed, from these agencies.

Sexually transmitted diseases (STDs) are also a major problem among the young. Although most sexually active young people engage in sequential monogamy, they may have two or three partners over a year, thus increasing exposure to possible infection as the years accumulate. Teens have increased their knowledge of AIDS, but they have not increased their use of condoms. Because there is usually a 10-year span between acquiring the AIDS virus and dying as a result of it, young people are well into their 20s before the deaths of some of their peers finally convince them that they should have protected themselves, and by that time immense damage has already been done.

Ideally, the teen years should be a time of gradual sexual maturing and increasing familiarity with burgeoning emotions, strong sexual drives, and the physical responses to them. Some specialists in adolescence have suggested that young people might pursue relationships based on physical warmth and caressing, even to climax, as a stage in discovery—a practice that incurs far fewer risks than intercourse—and have proposed the name "outercourse" for this phase.

Giving young women the support they require to enter the sexual sphere at their own pace rather than as victims of peer pressure alone, or of implicit threats of abandonment by a beloved, is a crucial task for parents at this time. If parents confuse this support with expressing condemnation, anxiety, or anger, the results will be painful for all involved.

Boys and girls need to develop skills so that they can have friendships and romances based on caring and trust, not exploitation. This can lay the foundation for developing the caring, committed, adult relationships of the future.

ADULT SEXUALITY

The boundary between adolescence and adulthood is a developmental one that is not related to age. The female sexual drive tends to lag behind that of the male during the teen years, very likely because of the burden of prohibitions placed on girls growing up in our society; in reality, the sex drive of females is probably just as strong as that of males. To reach maturity valuing one's sexuality without using it in hurtful ways is a great gift; so is using it at the right time and in healthy ways. Increasing years, however, bring greater expectations and the strong desire to function well and pleasurably in the sexual area.

Almost 50 years ago, in interviews with white, middle-class Americans, Alfred Kinsey found that men and women functioned more similarly in the sexual sphere than had been previously believed. He also found that women were increasingly likely to reach orgasm with advancing age and experience, and that while 90 percent of women will reach orgasm at least once during coitus in a lifetime, fewer than 50 percent were consistently orgasmic. Kinsey was the first to publicize the fact that women are frequently capable of multiple orgasms, a truth documented by William H. Masters and Virginia E. Johnson and implemented by Mary Jane Sherfey in her theory that women's intense and still-unbridled sex drive in prehistoric times posed a threat to men.

Masters and Johnson were the first researchers who studied human sexual responses in a detailed scientific manner, using large numbers of subjects and publishing the results in scientific journals. While their writing has been criticized in some quarters for imparting a mechanical quality to sexuality in terms of describing the sexual capabilities of its subjects, it is enormously useful in outlining for us the facts of human sexuality.

Masters and Johnson divided the sexual response into four

phases: The *excitement* phase produces the engorgement of all the organs in the vulva and profuse vaginal lubrication in the female and erection of the penis in the male. In addition, a woman's clitoris, breasts, and nipples enlarge. As blood vessels near the skin dilate, there may be a pink flush on the body and face. In the *plateau* phase, both sexes experience an increasing pulse rate and heightened blood pressure, rapid respiration, and escalating muscular tension. The clitoris may disappear under the clitoral hood, and the upper vagina increases in length and width, while even more blood may flow to the area and produce a deep red or wine color in the inner and outer lips. During *orgasm*, the third phase, the male ejaculates sperm and both partners experience rapid contractions of the pelvic muscles, accompanied by intense feelings of pleasure. In the fourth phase, called *resolution*, the pelvic organs gradually return to the prestimulated state. Males usually cannot repeat the cycle without a resting interval, which increases in length as they age. Some women, on the other hand, if stimulated promptly, can proceed again to orgasm without passing through the phase of resolution (see Table 5.1).

Masters and Johnson emphasized the similarities of the male and female response, reminding us that the genitalia of the two sexes start from the same tissues in the embryo. They also took issue with Freud's doctrine of vaginal versus clitoral orgasm. Freud proclaimed what he called the vaginal orgasm to be more mature and thus of a higher quality than the clitoral orgasm. Masters and Johnson found that an orgasm was an orgasm, regardless of whether a woman produced it by stimulating her clitoris herself, by having a male or female partner stimulate it directly, or by having it stimulated indirectly by the penis in the vagina. Certainly the sexual act is hardly a purely mechanical matter, and a great variety of circumstances affects the quality of sexual experience, but the body's basic physiologic responses appear to be based on the same reflex, whether stimulation is by masturbation, by a partner, or as a result of intercourse.

Every person asks: Am I normal sexually? Most of us at one time or another have expended a great deal of anxiety about such issues as the conventional frequency of intercourse, the conventional length of intercourse, the appropriateness of various sexual positions, and the practice of the various types of intercourse. There is no "right" way to have sex. Frequency of intercourse, for ex-

Table 5.1 Phases of Sexual Response

	Female	Male
1. Excitement Phase		
Breasts	Nipple erection	Similar (less marked)
Skin	Rash, flush	Delayed reaction
Muscles	Increased tone	Increased tone
Heart rate	Increases	Increases
Blood pressure	Increases	Increases
Genitalia	Clitoris engorged	Erection of penis
	Vagina lubricates and distends	Tensing and thickening of scrotal skin
	Engorgement of labia	Elevation of testicles
2. Plateau Phase		
Breasts	Increase in size	Inconsistent
Skin	Well-developed flush	Rash, flush
Muscles	Voluntary and involuntary tension	Same
Respiration	Beginning increase	Same
Heart rate	100–175	100–175
Blood pressure	Increases	Increases
Genitalia	Elevation of clitoris	Increase erection
	Change in shape of vagina	Increase in size of testes, further elevation
	Elevation of uterus	
3. Orgasmic Phase		
Skin	Well-developed flush	Same
Muscles	Involuntary contraction and spasm, loss of control	Same
Respiration	Up to 40/minute	Same
Heart rate	100–180	Same
Blood pressure	Increased elevation	Same
Genitalia	Vaginal and uterine contractions every .8 seconds	Expulsive contraction of penile urethra every .8 seconds

	Female	Male
4. Resolution Phase		
Breasts	Return to normal	Loss of nipple erection
Skin	Rapid loss of flush	Same
Muscles	Slow loss of tone	Same
Respiration Heart rate Blood pressure }	Return to normal	Same
Perspiration	Widespread	Inconsistent
Genitalia	Loss of engorgement Gaping of cervix	Loss of engorgement first rapid, then slowly

Source: Adapted from William H. Masters and Virginia E. Johnson, *Human Sexual Response* (Boston: Little, Brown, 1966).

---

ample, becomes an issue only when a person who wants sex twice a day pairs off with someone who is happiest with sex twice a month. Even then, such situations are best handled in terms of how well individuals are able to work out their differences than they are in identifying the differences as "sexual" problems. Sexual positions are as varied as the imagination and flexibility of the pair permit. Similarly, oral stimulation to climax or rectal intercourse may occur between same-sex or different-sex partners. While anal intercourse is normal and pleasurable to many people of both sexes, it seems to be associated with (usually minor) tearing of the rectal tissue, which permits easier transmission of the AIDS virus than other forms of intercourse. When contemplating this type of love-making, couples should be aware of the increased risk of contracting AIDS.

Self-stimulation, or masturbation, is usually both pleasant and harmless. About 80 percent of women and even more men engage in this activity either frequently or occasionally. Although no such reason is necessary to enjoy it, masturbating certainly helps to relieve tension in a relationship when one spouse is ill or when the frequency of the partners' desires for intercourse varies widely. Although in our society there is still a large residue of guilt associated with masturbation, enlightenment about its pleasures, benefits, and common practice is gradually making its way into most levels of our culture.

More important questions in the realm of sexual activity are: Does what I am doing bring pleasure to my partner and to me? Does it harm me or my partner? Does it strengthen bonds between us?

Women have been under great pressure in recent years to conform to outside standards of sexual performance. Researcher Shere Hite confirmed in the 1970s what Kinsey and others as far back as Edith Hamilton in the 1920s had found: Only 30 percent of women regularly have orgasm with intercourse. Another 20 percent reach orgasm if their partners add clitoral stimulation, but these women often stated that their partners refused to help them climax. All female orgasms rely on clitoral stimulation. This fact, coupled with the Masters and Johnson finding that vaginal stimulation is transferred only indirectly to the clitoris and the fact that 95 percent of women can reach orgasm with self-stimulation, suggests that a woman's climax depends to some extent on her partner's ability to arouse and please her. Men must understand that a woman needs foreplay, clitoral stimulation, and sufficient time to become aroused before penetration and that what produces his orgasm is not necessarily the same as what produces hers.

On the other hand, insisting that a woman reach a climax if she is satisfied without one is also unreasonable; although many women who do not reach orgasm during intercourse feel deprived and some are left tense and irritable, others find the pleasures of being held and caressed and of stimulating their partners entirely satisfying. As women have struggled to overcome old sex-role stereotyping and have become more open and assertive about letting their sexual partners know what their particular sexual needs are, it seems likely that the research findings about the female orgasm will change substantially.

One way you can enhance your sexual pleasure is by strengthening and sensitizing the vaginal muscles by routinely practicing Kegel exercises. These extremely useful exercises can be performed literally anywhere and at any time, and are equally useful in improving bladder control and restoring tone to your vaginal muscles after childbirth. You can identify these muscles by spreading your legs apart and starting, then stopping, the flow of urine.

Start by contracting and drawing up the muscles of the pelvic floor; hold for three seconds, then relax. Do this five times. Repeat during the day until you work up to 10 groups of five contractions each. You can do this exercise when you are lying down or sitting up.

Next, try to raise the entire pelvic area by imagining that you are moving your uterus and bladder up toward your stomach. When you have pulled them as high as you can, gradually relax the muscles so they move down slowly, relaxing when they return to their normal position. Then tense up slightly so that the pelvic floor is slightly tense. (This step-by-step, up-and-down motion is similar to the one used to strengthen the abdominal muscles, where, lying on your back, you gradually raise and then lower your shoulders, feeling the tug on the abdominals.) When you have mastered this, raise the whole pelvic area, as though you were sucking fluid into your vagina, then relax; repeat these contractions five times. Work up to doing this exercise four to six times a day.

The contemporary woman must decide what it is that she needs and wants from sex and be able to communicate it to her potential partner as they exchange sexual histories. In this AIDS-threatening era, such a discussion is imperative and, for the modern woman, even fashionable. Many new couples contemplating sexual involvement seek screenings for STDs from their respective doctors. Because this kind of evaluation is, unfortunately, no guarantee of continuing good health, every sensible woman knows that a sexual partner cannot be chosen lightly and that using a condom should be a standard part of all sexual encounters. Condoms do not guarantee protection from sexually transmissible diseases, but they play an important part in "safer sex." Clearly more vital is establishing a monogamous relationship with a partner who is also monogamous.

SEXUAL PROBLEMS

RELATIONSHIP PROBLEMS

Many problems that manifest themselves as sexual are really problems of the relationship itself. If a woman has serious reservations about her partner, cannot communicate with him, feels continually angry or hurt, or believes that he doesn't care about the effect his actions have on her and on their life as a couple, there is little hope that the sex will be any better than any other aspect of the relationship. If, however, such a couple has enough of a commitment to their partnership so that both are willing to seek counseling, then they can hope to improve their overall interaction and, as a result, their sex life.

ABSENT LIBIDO

Lack of sexual desire, or libido, is the most common sexual problem. As delineated by Helen Kaplan, it has many causes. When the condition has always been present and the person has never experienced any interest in sex, it is often part of a broader inability to accept pleasure, and as such it may be difficult to treat. A lack of sexual desire in a person who has previously enjoyed sex is most frequently one of the symptoms of depression, and becomes less and less severe as the depression lifts; this can often be accomplished with the help of antidepressant medications.

Fatigue, acute and chronic illness, and many of the medications used to treat chronic illness can also affect a person's interest in sex, sometimes to a great extent. Examples of such medications include thiazides and beta-adrenergic blocking agents used for the treatment of high blood pressure, and antidepressant drugs. Women who have had their ovaries removed sometimes complain that they have less interest in sex than previously, even though they are receiving estrogen. Adding very low doses of testosterone may help alleviate this situation, as there is evidence that sexual desire in the female—as well as in the male—is somewhat dependent on testosterone.

INABILITY TO REACH ORGASM

Although many women come to orgasm quickly, some 5 to 10 percent have never had an orgasm and another large group rarely have one with intercourse. Paul Gebhardt found some correlation between a woman's ability to have an orgasm and many other factors, such as the happiness of her parents' marriage, her ability to trust, her own currently happy marriage, more than 20 minutes of foreplay, and at least 15 minutes of penile penetration—a broad spectrum indeed.

If you are unable to have an orgasm, your gynecologist or a sex therapist may be of help. Masters and Johnson found that simply relearning techniques involving pleasurable touching and en-

hanced communication skills in informing partners about what
feels good are more effective in treating this problem than psychotherapy. Some women have found the stimulation of a vibrator
effective. In any case, counseling that provides straightforward
answers to questions about sex is often very useful, even to women
who believe their own knowledge about orgasm is sophisticated
and up-to-date.

PAINFUL SEX

Painful sex (dyspareunia) is a problem almost all women encounter at some time. A lack of adequate lubrication during the
excitement phase of intercourse causes painful friction between the
penis and the vagina, which brings on vaginal pain. If your partner
is not stimulating you adequately or you feel a lack of desire, you
need to let your partner know what arouses you or you may have
to discuss what is holding you back, if you know what it is. Or,
you may need a different partner. This situation, if ignored, easily
becomes a syndrome, for pain itself—or the anticipation of pain—
inhibits the natural lubrication that arousal initiates, and the cycle
becomes self-perpetuating. Sometimes you can interrupt this cycle
by using one of the vaginal lubricants available at a drugstore
without prescription, such as Lubrin, Astroglide, or Replens. Be
sure to choose one that uses a water base, not petroleum jelly,
because your natural secretions are water-based.

One of the normal changes that comes with aging in the female
is a decrease in vaginal lubrication, which reflects the declining
level of estrogen that takes place with menopause. If it causes
painful intercourse, this is a strong indication of the need for some
extra estrogen, but be sure to consider the potential risks of estrogen before deciding to use it (see Chapter 15). One relatively new
lubricating product is a moisturizing gel tampon that is inserted
three times a week to provide a continuous moist layer in the
vagina. Sold over-the-counter, it is also far more expensive than
ordinary vaginal lubricating gels.

Another major cause of painful intercourse is vaginitis, a term
that refers to a wide range of vaginal infections, the most common
of which is a yeast infection. If you experience pain with intercourse
under circumstances that are otherwise the same—that is, you still
want sex and your feelings toward your partner haven't changed—

then ask your health-care provider to check for a yeast infection, which usually can be easily treated. Other infections, such as trichomonas or bacterial vaginosis, can also cause an irritated vagina and consequent pain during intercourse. Another cause of vaginitis is allergies—to soaps, lotions, douches, and medications. (See Chapter 11 for more on infections and sexually transmitted diseases.)

VAGINISMUS

Women whose first pelvic examination or first attempts at intercourse were traumatic may develop involuntary, painful spasms of the muscles at the vaginal opening with any further attempts at penetration. This condition is called vaginismus, and it can be overcome with the help of a health-care provider who has had experience in treating the problem. Therapy involves initially desensitizing the woman to touch in the area, using simple tasks carried out at home.

AGING

As we reach the age of menopause and beyond, we may find that we need extra vaginal lubrication to help produce sufficient moisture for intercourse. This does not mean that women cannot continue to enjoy sex as long as they like; some women report even greater sexual pleasure after menopause, partially because the possibility of an unwanted pregnancy has now been removed (see Chapter 15). Women should be aware, however, that the aging process affects the male quite differently. He tends to be interested in having sex less frequently and to require more stimulation to achieve and maintain an erection. In addition, he may not ejaculate every time he has intercourse. Should this happen, there is no need to persist in attempting to help him ejaculate, because there are no adverse medical consequences in simply letting the erection subside. When a couple remains in good health, however, there is no reason why they should not continue to enjoy sex into their 70s and 80s. Although chronic illness may interfere with sexual functioning, sexual dysfunction among older women and men is more often caused by the medications they take for their illnesses—those for high blood pressure, for example—than by the illness itself. Frequently, doctors can either change such medications or lower their dose if patients bring the problem to their attention. Discussing sex with your health-care provider should be something you do freely at every age. If the doctor seems uncomfortable discussing it with you, the problem is the doctor's, and if your persistence doesn't help, try to find another practitioner, one who's more at ease about these matters.

SEXUAL PROBLEMS AND GAY WOMEN

Gay women may have the same relationship problems as their heterosexual sisters, but they have no unplanned pregnancies and few STDs. Unlike gay men, gay women are generally monogamous or serially monogamous, with established long-term relationships and fewer sexual partners, so they are not at high risk for AIDS. They are at somewhat greater risk than heterosexual women for depression and alcoholism, however, because of the disproportionate pressures they suffer from society's harsh attitudes toward their sexuality.

PROBLEMS WITH PREGNANCY

There is no reason to avoid intercourse during a normal pregnancy. (See Chapter 9.) Intercourse does not cause miscarriage or premature labor, but if you have unexplained bleeding or pain, you should postpone intercourse until you can discuss the problem with your physician. As the pregnancy progresses and the pregnant uterus begins to get in the way of conventional lovemaking, the couple will need to experiment with different positions in order to find one that is comfortable. Some women notice a definite decrease in sexual desire during pregnancy. Even so, it is good to hold and be held and to love and comfort each other. Some women, particularly those who did not plan the pregnancy and are leery of childbearing, find they are even more interested in sex because they no longer have to worry about becoming pregnant. Whichever your own inclination, pregnancy is a time to strengthen marital bonds, because couples need them once the baby arrives.

Caution: Once the bag of water has broken or labor has begun, it is best not to have intercourse. Also, throughout pregnancy, it is dangerous for your partner to blow into your vagina; air can make its way into your circulatory system and cause death.

Ask your health-care provider when it's advisable for you to resume intercourse after delivery. This will depend on the number of stitches you had if you had vaginal tears or were given an episiotomy, on the lack of complications, as well as on the method of contraception you use.

COMPULSIVE SEX

Recently, psychiatrists and sex therapists have become concerned about the occasional problem of greatly heightened sexual interest, or compulsive sex, although there is a difference of opinion as to whether the condition exists as a separate entity, exclusive of such conditions as manic-depression, for example. Some therapists have treated patients with a compulsive interest in and need for sex with a discussion and support group approach similar to the one used by Alcoholics Anonymous and other such organizations.

RAPE

Rape is a crime of violence as much as it is a severe sexual offense, and the incidence of reported attacks appears to be increasing. Recent surveys suggest that at least 30 percent of girls have been assaulted by the age of 18 and that almost 50 percent of women either have been raped or have been the object of a rape attempt sometime in their lives. (This may not indicate an enormous increase; Edith Hamilton reported in 1929 that 37 percent of women had been sexually abused by the age of 16.) For all ages, it is likely that the victim knows the rapist. Considering the high incidence of what has come to be termed *date rape*—a term that tends to trivialize the seriousness of the offense—it is a matter of dismay, but not surprise, that 51 percent of college males say that, if they knew they could get away with it, they would force intercourse on their dates.

If a woman is able to offer resistance to rape, she may reduce the chance of sexual contact, but this increases the likelihood that she will be harmed physically.

The legal definition of rape has two elements. Sexual contact must have taken place, although not necessarily with penetration or ejaculation, and the contact must have been made against the woman's will. Rape may still be the most underreported of all crimes, because many of the women who are its victims feel dirty and shamed by it and want to go away and hide rather than face emergency rooms and police interrogation. It has taken many years for our health-care system to respond with the kind of support that women so traumatized require, but today most personnel in hospital emergency rooms are trained to be supportive of the rape victim. Most call on the services of a local rape crisis center as well as a medical team. While many police departments have become more enlightened in this area, some are not as advanced as others.

If you have been assaulted or raped, there are a number of reasons why you should go immediately to an emergency room. The first is legal. If you intend to bring charges against the assailant, then evidence of trauma, the presence of sperm and fluid used to ascertain the blood type of the rapist, and the possible presence of foreign pubic hairs must be obtained within the first 24 hours—the sooner the better. Don't go home and shower and douche before seeing the doctor; most states have a system for filing a "blind" report of rape, which means that the facts of the case go on record and law enforcement personnel collect evidence and mobilize support people, but the victim has time to consider whether or not she wishes to report the name of her assailant, if she knows it, and to file charges against him.

Rapists may also be infected with one or more STDs, and a doctor can prescribe antibiotics to protect you against your contracting some of them as a routine matter. If penetration has taken place, you can become pregnant if you are not taking the oral contraceptive pill; therefore, doctors usually recommend that you take a brief course of oral contraceptives to serve as a morning-after pill to try to prevent pregnancy. The physician will also examine you for possible injuries. Although these are usually superficial and rarely produce lasting physical damage, it is important to have them evaluated and treated. In most cities, trained personnel from the local rape crisis center are on call day and night to come and stay with you as your advocate.

What are the long-term results of rape? Recent medical findings reveal that many women who have been raped experience a long-term increase in pelvic pain, sexual dysfunction, and a variety of gynecologic problems. Pregnancy and STDs do occur, but not very frequently, especially if you take preventive measures immediately after the assault. Much more common are the emotional consequences. You may suffer from nightmares and experience an understandable aversion to sex, but these symptoms gradually fade. Your relationship with your spouse or partner may also become very tenuous. Many men need counseling to educate them about the fact that the energy and rage they direct against their partner's rapist is useful only when it is transformed into loving support for her at this time; otherwise, it is as if he has "stolen" the experience from her and is acting out his own selfish response instead of using his energy on her behalf. Feelings of helplessness often engender such a response from a rape victim's loved ones, and this is a syndrome to be recognized and redirected.

Often women blame themselves for having been raped, reasoning that if only they had behaved differently, the rape would not have occurred. *Do not succumb to this kind of thinking.* You may need counseling to help with the healing process; if so, look for a referral to a counselor who is trained in this field.

Anyone who stays in the presence of contemptuous talk about women without objecting to it, if possible, is implicitly condoning the atmosphere that nourishes the high incidence of rape in our society. Men—and women—who would never themselves act violently toward women convey complicity toward such violence if they allow others to express it verbally without asserting themselves and pointing out, as calmly as they can, how wrong attitudes that denigrate and diminish women truly are.

6

The Special Nutritional Needs of Women

Artemis P. Simopoulos, M.D.

A variety of genetic, behavioral, and environmental factors affect the health of the individual and the general population. Although nutrition is only one environmental factor, it is enormously important in determining our level of well-being. One reason for the current interest in nutrition is that, unlike our genetic heritage and other environmental factors, it is something we can control.

There is no longer much question that proper nutrition and exercise not only nourish our bodies but also help us achieve our best possible physical and psychological state. Aerobic exercise allows women to become lean while they eat more, find it easier to relax, sleep better, meet physical emergencies with greater comfort and safety, have finer posture and a more attractive figure, develop less osteoporosis, and, some say, enjoy superior sex lives.

But trying to reach these goals confronts us with a major obstacle: the lack of knowledge about nutrition for women. Of the many clinical trials and intervention studies relating diet to coronary heart disease and hypertension during the last 20 years, almost all involved middle-aged men, and this despite the fact that hypertension is more common in women than in men. Even more troublesome is the fact that authorities have inappropriately applied data from these studies to women of all ages. Women get heart disease much later than men, and researchers should be investigating this fact rather than assuming that it is simply a result of a decrease in estrogen following menopause. Further testing is needed to precisely define the need for estrogens in the prevention of heart disease and their role in cancer.

THE NUTRITIONALLY ADEQUATE DIET

The U.S. Department of Health and Human Services in conjunction with the Department of Agriculture issued updated dietary guidelines in 1990 that provide basic principles for a nutritionally adequate diet. They are:

- Eat a variety of foods.
- Maintain healthy weight.
- Choose a diet low in fat, saturated fat, and cholesterol.
- Eat plenty of vegetables, fruits, and grain products.
- Use sugars only in moderation.
- Use salt and sodium only in moderation.
- If you drink alcoholic beverages, do so in moderation.

Adult women consume an average of 1,900 to 2,200 calories daily. Relatively inactive women need fewer calories and active women more to maintain a desirable body weight; differences in energy requirements are based on both the pattern of a person's activity and the body composition that results from that pattern of activity.

A nutritionally sound diet must have variety, balance, and moderation. Balance means not only eating foods from each of the four food groups (described below), but also balancing how much you eat against how active you are. Although this diet is appropriate for all healthy Americans, it does not apply to persons with special dietary needs because of diseases and conditions that interfere with normal nutrition. No dietary guideline can guarantee well-being, since one's health depends on many factors, including heredity, life-style, personality traits, mental fitness and attitude, and environment. Food *alone* cannot make us well, but good eating habits can help us stay healthy.

The first guideline, "Eat a variety of foods," is important because no one food contains all the necessary nutrients in the proper amounts to maintain health—except, of course, human milk during the first three months of life. The Recommended Dietary Allowances (RDA), devised by the National Research Council of the National Academy of Sciences (NAS), outlines the nutrient requirements of women and men. You can meet these requirements by eating a variety of foods from the four food groups:

- meats, poultry, fish, eggs, and legumes (beans and peas)
- vegetables and fruits
- breads, pastas, and cereals
- milk, cheese, and yogurt

For example, many fruits and vegetables are good sources of vitamins A and C; breads and cereals provide the B vitamins and iron; dairy products contain much of the required calcium; and meat, fish, poultry, and legumes supply protein.

The second government guideline, "Maintain healthy weight," does not distinguish the weight range between men and women and, therefore, is not a useful guide for women. The term *desirable body weight*, which was used in the 1985 version of the dietary guidelines, is more scientific, despite the fact that doctors lack adequate data that relate weight to illness and rely instead on available statistics that associate body weight and mortality. Most American women have a fairly adequate diet but consume more calories than they expend. As a result, the average woman is 20 percent above the range of desirable body weight (see Table 6.1).

Understanding the distribution of calories in the food you eat is a first step to controlling your weight. Of the fats, protein, and carbohydrates that provide energy from food, fat has nine calories per gram and is a dense source of calories compared to carbohydrate and protein, both of which contain four calories per gram. Alcohol, with seven calories per gram, is highly caloric, and limiting its use is an important contribution to good nutrition.

One important way to achieve a desirable weight, as well as other vital benefits, is to limit the amount of fat in your diet. No more than 30 percent of your total calories should come from fat. The process you follow in achieving this is rather like budgeting: You have so many calories to spend each day, and you have to learn how to calculate your "fat allowance." For example, if you

Table 6.1 Desirable Body Weight Ranges*

Height Without Shoes	Weight Without Clothes	
	Men (pounds)	Women (pounds)
4'10"		92–121
4'11"		95–124
5'0"		98–127
5'1"	105–134	101–130
5'2"	108–137	104–134
5'3"	111–141	107–138
5'4"	114–145	110–142
5'5"	117–149	114–146
5'6"	121–154	118–150
5'7"	125–159	122–154
5'8"	129–163	126–159
5'9"	133–167	130–164
5'10"	137–172	134–169
5'11"	141–177	
6'0"	145–182	
6'1"	149–187	
6'2"	153–192	
6'3"	157–197	

*For women 18–25 years of age, subtract one pound for each year under 25. Adapted from the 1959 Metropolitan Desirable Weight Table. Table reproduced from 1985 Dietary Guidelines (US DHHS and USDA, Washington, D.C., Home and Garden Bulletin No. 232).

consume 2,000 calories daily, 30 percent of the total will let you spend 600 fat calories a day. Thus, you may decide that a three-ounce piece of London broil, which contains 12 grams of fat, a total of 108 fat calories, is too expensive and you'd rather switch to haddock, with its one gram of fat (see Table 6.2). You can figure out the percentage of fat calories for any food if you know the number of calories and grams of fat the food contains. The formula is simple: Multiply the number of grams of fat by 9, multiply that figure by 100, and then divide by the total number of calories in the food. The calculation for our piece of London broil looks like this: $12 \times 9 = 108 \times 100 = 10,800$ divided by 208 (total calories) = 52 percent, the percentage of caloric content of this meat that is fat.

But controlling fat intake doesn't mean you must become a math-

Table 6.2 An Easy Way to Figure Your Fat Intake: Count Grams

The list will help you follow the recommendation to eat no more than 30 percent of calories as fat. Thirty percent for someone who consumes 1,500 calories a day averages out to a maximum of 50 grams. For every 100 calories above that, the daily fat allowance rises by about 3 grams.

Meat, Fish, Poultry, and Eggs	Grams of fat	Total calories
Beef (3 oz. trimmed of removable fat)		
corned beef	16	213
eye of round, roasted (select)	5	151
London broil, braised (choice)	12	208
porterhouse steak, broiled (choice)	9	185
rib, broiled (prime)	16	238
rib eye (Delmonico) steak, broiled (choice)	10	191
T-bone steak, broiled (choice)	9	182
top loin steak, broiled (select)	6	162
wedge-bone sirloin steak, broiled (choice)	8	180
Luncheon meats (1 slice)		
Louis Rich 96% Fat Free Turkey Pastrami	0	25
Louis Rich Oven-Roasted Turkey Breast	0	30
Oscar Mayer Bologna	4	50
Oscar Mayer Hard Salami	3	35
Oscar Mayer 95% Fat Free Smoked Cooked Ham	1	25
Weaver Chicken Frank with Cheese	12	140
Seafood (3 oz. cooked unless otherwise indicated)		
anchovies, canned in oil, drained, 5	2	42
Atlantic cod	1	89
haddock	1	95
lobster	1	83
salmon, pink, canned with bone and liquid	5	118
smoked salmon (lox)	4	99
swordfish	4	132
tuna, canned in oil and drained	7	158
tuna, canned in water and drained	0	111
shrimp	1	84
shrimp, breaded and fried	10	206
Poultry (3 oz. roasted unless otherwise indicated)		
chicken breast, meat with skin	7	165
chicken breast, meat only	3	142
chicken drumstick, meat with skin, batter dipped and fried, 1 average	11	193

chicken drumstick, meat only, 1 average	2	76
chicken wing, meat only, 1 average	2	43
turkey, light meat with skin	7	168
turkey, light meat only	3	133
turkey, dark meat with skin	10	188
turkey, dark meat only	6	160

Eggs

1 large	5	75
Fleischmann's Egg Beaters, ¼ cup	0	25
Morningstar Scramblers, ¼ cup	3	60

Milk and Dairy Products

Milk (1 cup)

whole	8	150
2% fat	5	120
1% fat	3	100
skim	0	90
buttermilk	2	99

Cream (1 tbsp.)

half and half	2	20
heavy whipping cream	6	52
sour cream	3	26

Cheese

American, 1 oz.	9	106
cheddar, 1 oz.	9	114
cottage cheese, creamed, 1 cup	9	217
cottage cheese, 1% fat, 1 cup	2	164
cream cheese, 1 oz.	10	99
mozzarella, 1 oz.	6	80
mozzarella, part-skim, 1 oz.	5	72
parmesan, grated, 1 tbsp.	2	23
ricotta, ½ cup	16	216
ricotta, part-skim, ½ cup	10	171
Swiss, 1 oz.	8	107
Weight Watchers American Pasteurized Process Cheese Product, 1 slice	2	45

Yogurt

Colombo, plain, 8 oz.	7	150
Colombo, plain nonfat lite, 8 oz.	0	110
Dannon Fresh Flavors (coffee, lemon, vanilla), 8 oz.	3	200
Dannon Original (all flavors), 8 oz.	3	240
Yoplait Original (all flavors), 6 oz.	3	190

Food from Grains	Grams of fat	Total calories
Breads		
bagel, 1	1	163
English muffin, 1	1	135
whole-wheat bread, 1 slice	1	61
Cereals		
General Mills' Cheerios, 1¼ cups	2	110
Kellogg's Corn Flakes, 1 cup	0	100
Kellogg's Raisin Bran, ¾ cup	1	120
Nabisco Cream of Wheat, quick, 1 cup cooked	0	100
Nabisco Shredded Wheat, 1 biscuit	0	80
Old-Fashioned Quaker Oatmeal, ⅔ cup cooked	2	100
Quaker 100% Natural, ¼ cup	5	130
Quaker Puffed Rice, 1 cup	0	50
Crackers		
Sunshine Cheez-It Snack Crackers, 12	4	70
Nabisco Honey Maid Honey Grahams, 1 sheet	1	60
Nabisco Ritz, 4	4	70
oyster crackers, 10	1	33
Other		
pasta, 1 cup cooked	1	159
white rice, 1 cup cooked	0	223
pancakes, 4" plain	2	62
waffles, 7" plain	8	206
French toast, 1 slice	7	153
Dunkin' Donuts Oat Bran Muffin, plain	11	350
Sara Lee Golden Corn Muffin	13	250
Fruits and Vegetables		
apple, 1 medium	1	81
banana, 1 medium	1	105
fruit cocktail, canned in heavy syrup, ½ cup	0	93
orange, 1 medium	0	65
raisins, ⅓ cup	0	150
avocado, ½ medium	15	153
broccoli, ½ cup cooked	0	23
carrot, raw, 1 medium	0	31
corn, canned, ½ cup	1	66
green beans, ½ cup cooked	0	22
peas, ½ cup cooked	0	67

Beans, Nuts, and Seeds	Grams of fat	Total calories
kidney beans, ½ cup boiled	0	113
lentils, ½ cup boiled	0	116
cashews, dry roasted, ¼ cup	16	197
coconut meat, dried, sweetened, flaked, ¼ cup	6	88
peanuts, dry roasted, ¼ cup	18	207
peanut butter, 1 tbsp.	8	95
pistachios, dry roasted, ¼ cup	17	194
sesame seeds, dry-roasted, ¼ cup	21	221
tahini (sesame butter), 1 tbsp.	7	86
walnuts, black, dried, chopped, ¼ cup	18	190

Spreads and Oils

butter, 1 tsp.	4	36
whipped butter, 1 tsp.	3	27
margarine, stick & tub, 1 tsp.	4	34
diet margarine, tub, 1 tsp.	2	17
vegetable oil (corn, cottonseed, olive, peanut, canola, safflower, sesame, soybean, sunflower), 1 tbsp.	14	120 (average)
vegetable oil spray, 2.5-second spray	1	6

Salad Dressings

blue cheese, 1 tbsp.	8	77
French, 1 tbsp.	6	67
Italian, 1 tbsp.	7	69
Russian, 1 tbsp.	8	76
thousand island, 1 tbsp.	6	59

Soups

Campbell's Chicken Noodle, 1 cup	2	70
Campbell's Cream of Mushroom, 1 cup	7	100
Lipton Noodle, 1 cup	2	70
Progresso Green Split Pea, 1 cup	3	152
Progresso Beef Minestrone, 1 cup	3	135
Ramen Pride Oriental Noodles & Pork Flavor, 10 oz.	8	198

Sweets	Grams of fat	Total calories
Cadbury's Milk Chocolate with Fruit & Nuts, 1 oz.	8	150
Hershey Chocolate Kisses, 5 pieces	8	125
Snicker's Bar, 2.16 oz.	14	290
Three Musketeers Bar, 2.13 oz.	9	260
angel food cake, 1/12 cake	0	126
brownie with nuts (3 × 1 × 7/8")	6	97
cheesecake, 1/8 cake	13	278
Hostess Ding Dong, 1	9	170
Hostess Twinkie, 1	5	160
pound cake, 1/2" slice	6	150
Almost Home Chocolate Chip Cookie, 2	5	130
Fig Newton, 1	1	50
Nabisco Gingersnaps, 4	3	120
apple pie, 1/8	12	282
banana cream pie, 1/8	12	233
pumpkin pie, 1/8	13	241
chocolate pudding, 1 cup	12	385
Dunkin' Donuts Plain Cake Ring	22	319
Nature Valley Granola Bar	5	120
Sara Lee Cheese Danish	8	130

Frozen Desserts

Ice cream

	Grams of fat	Total calories
Breyers, vanilla fudge twirl, 1/2 cup	8	160
Häagen Dazs, chocolate chocolate chip, 1/2 cup	18	290
Sealtest, vanilla, chocolate, or strawberry, 1/2 cup	6	140

Other

	Grams of fat	Total calories
Dole Fruit 'N Yogurt Bar	0	70
Dole Fruit sorbet, strawberry, 1/2 cup	0	100
Eskimo Pie, 3-oz. bar	12	180
Jell-O Chocolate Pudding Pop	2	80
Light n' Lively Ice Milk, heavenly hash, 1/2 cup	3	120
orange sherbet, 1/2 cup	3	92
Popsicle Ice Pop	0	50
Tofutti, wildberry supreme, 1/2 cup	12	210
Yoplait Frozen Yogurt, 3 fl. oz.	2	90

Meat, Fish, Poultry, and Eggs	Grams of fat	Total calories
Toppings		
chocolate syrup, 2 tbsp.	1	92
fudge topping, 2 tbsp.	5	124
whipped cream, pressurized, 2 tbsp.	1	16
Dry Snack Foods		
Lay's Bar-B-Q Flavored Potato Chips, 1 oz.	9	150
Orville Redenbacher's Natural Microwave Popping Corn, 4 cups popped	7	110
popcorn, air-popped, 1 cup popped	0	23
Pringle's Light Potato Chips, 1 oz.	8	150
pretzels, 1 oz.	1	111
Ruffles Potato Chips, 1 oz.	10	150

Sources: *Tufts University Diet and Nutrition Letter*, October 1989. USDA Handbooks 8, Bowes and Church's *Food Values of Portions Commonly Used*, 15th edition, manufacturers' product information. Values for fat and calorie content have been rounded to the nearest whole number. "Less than a gram of fat" on labels was rounded to zero.

ematician, carrying your calculator under one arm and tables of fat content under the other. You'll quickly come to recognize the foods with high fat content and to avoid or ration them accordingly. They include fatty meats; chicken skin; any food that is breaded and fried; whole milk; many cheeses; all cooking oils; all cookies, candies, pies, ice cream, and cakes (except angel food); nuts; avocado; potato chips; and most other crunchy snack foods. However, not all fats are alike, and some foods with high fat content are helpful.

HOW DIFFERENT FATS WORK

Fats actually contribute about 40 percent of the calories consumed by most Americans. Our digestive juices break down fats into fatty acids which, along with ingested cholesterol, are absorbed by the body. Fats remain inside our fat cells mainly as energy stores or as components of cell membranes. There is currently great interest in fats, as researchers work to learn more about how certain of them contribute to heart disease and other illnesses that plague Western society.

There are three kinds of fats, each with a different structure. Saturated fat, such as that found in lard and butter, raises serum cholesterol and thus promotes the plaque deposits on arterial walls that cause heart attacks. In fact, animal products such as beef, veal, pork, lamb, poultry, fish and shellfish, tallow and lard, whole milk and whole milk products, and eggs deliver more than half of the total fat to U.S. diets, three-quarters of the saturated, or hydrogenated, fat, and all of the cholesterol. One government health survey showed that the American devotion to hamburgers has made ground beef the single biggest contributor of fat to the American diet.

The second class of fats is polyunsaturated fatty acids. Although researchers originally thought polyunsaturated fat was a single entity, we now know that there are two separate families. One of these, omega-6, is found in the seeds of plants, such as corn and sunflowers. Through technological advances in the ability to extract oil from corn and other plant seeds, omega-6 has become a readily available and plentiful part of the American diet in the form of corn and other vegetable oils and margarine. The other polyunsaturated fatty acid, known as omega-3, is found in deep-sea, cold-water fish, such as sardines, bluefish, mackerel, salmon, and herring; canola, linseed, flaxseed, and walnut oils; walnuts, soybeans, and butternuts; fruits, such as avocados, raw raspberries, and strawberries; and green leafy vegetables, such as spinach, buttercrunch, red-leaf lettuce, and purslane, a wild green leafy vegetable that some farmers are now beginning to grow in the United States. The third class are monounsaturates, such as olive oil and peanut oil.

Since the late 1950s, when researchers discovered that corn oil lowers serum cholesterol, there has been a race to get consumers to replace butter and lard with corn and other vegetable oils, because scientists believed polyunsaturated fatty acids lowered cholesterol more effectively than monounsaturated fatty acids. This led to an increased amount of omega-6 fatty acids in the American diet. At that time, there was not much information, although some studies did indicate that sardine and cod liver oils, which contain omega-3, also lower cholesterol and triglycerides (another type of fat) and prevent blood clotting.

We estimate that the present Western diet is "deficient" in omega-3 fatty acids, with the ratio of omega-6 to omega-3 somewhere between 10 and 14 to one, instead of one to one, which we believe was the case with earlier societies that fed on wild animals and plants. While we do not know the ideal ratio of omega-6 to omega-3 fatty acids, there is no question that Americans consume six to 10 times the amount of omega-6 needed for optimal health.

In addition, properly controlled studies over the past few years have indicated that a diet rich in monounsaturated fat is as effective as a diet abundant in polyunsaturated fatty acids in lowering low-density lipoprotein (LDL) cholesterol, the "bad" cholesterol that promotes plaque deposits. Olive oil has the added advantage of not decreasing high-density lipoprotein (HDL), which, because it removes cholesterol from artery walls, is known as the "good" cholesterol.

Women usually have higher levels of HDL cholesterol than men and are less prone to cardiovascular disease at the same level of total cholesterol. Studies have shown that a low HDL is a better predictor of heart attacks in women than is total cholesterol. It stands to reason then that women should choose a diet and life-style that will increase HDL. Olive oil does not usually lower HDL; in fact, it raises HDL in most people. Fish oils or eating fish also increases HDL in some, but not all, people. Corn oil, on the other hand, lowers HDL. Weight loss through diet or exercise increases HDL, as does exercise even without weight loss.

Saturated (or hydrogenated) fats, monounsaturated fatty acids, and cholesterol are called nonessential fatty acids because the human body makes them. Polyunsaturated fatty acids, on the other hand, are essential fatty acids because the body cannot manufacture them but must obtain them directly from the diet.

HEALTH EFFECTS OF OMEGA-6
AND OMEGA-3 FATTY ACIDS

Omega-6 and omega-3 fatty acids work differently in the body. Omega-6 fatty acids produce substances that constrict blood vessels, clump platelets (the disk-shaped structures in the blood), and form blood clots, which precipitate heart attacks. They also stimulate white cells that are involved in inflammation, contributing to the development of arthritis.

Omega-3 fatty acids, on the other hand, produce substances that dilate or relax blood vessels, prevent clumping of platelets and clot formation, and thus delay injury to the blood vessel walls. For these reasons, populations that eat fish have less heart disease. Eating fish, or taking fish oils, appears to prevent heart attacks and lower blood pressure in patients with mild forms of hypertension. And because their properties work against inflammation, fish oil containing omega-3 fatty acids has been used to treat patients with rheumatoid arthritis, psoriasis, and ulcerative colitis with encouraging results.

Omega-3 fatty acids appear to strengthen drug effects when used in conjunction with them, and this combination may lead to a decrease in the dosage required, which, in turn, may lessen the toxic side effects of such drugs. In addition, animal studies have shown that two of the omega-3s, those found in linseed oil and fish oil, slow down the growth of tumors, whereas omega-6 does not; in fact, corn oil promotes tumor growth in many animal models.

OTHER IMPORTANT NUTRIENTS

CARBOHYDRATES

Carbohydrates, in the form of sugars and starches, are the major source of energy and account for 46.4 percent of the energy in the diet of adult women in the United States. The estimated average intake of carbohydrates by adults is 287 grams for males and 117 grams for females. Grain products provide about 41 percent of carbohydrates, while fruits and vegetables account for 23 percent. These foods also supply minerals, vitamins, and fiber. To compensate for the reduction of fat in your diet, you should increase the amount of fruit, vegetables, legumes, and whole-grain cereals you eat. All of these complex carbohydrates not only give you important nutrients, they also boost the amount of fiber in your diet, which softens the stool, increases its bulk, and promotes healthy elimination. The additional mass of softer stool may also dilute carcinogens, and the rapid passage through the large intestine (colon) reduces the amount of time that potential carcinogens in the stool can interact with the mucosal surface of the colon and initiate disease.

PROTEIN

Women need about 45 grams of protein a day. The body makes protein from amino acids and can produce almost half of them; the others, referred to as essential amino acids, must come from the daily diet. Our bodies do not store protein for long.

Animal protein, which contains all the essential amino acids, includes fish, poultry, meat, milk, eggs, and cheese. One ounce of meat, fish, or poultry contains six to eight grams of protein, while a quart of milk contains 32 grams (see Table 6.3). Although vegetable protein—found in beans, seeds, nuts, and grains—is incomplete in terms of the protein the body requires, certain combinations make it complete: mixing whole grains, cereals, and flours, for example, with either legumes (beans, lentils, chick-peas), nuts, or seeds. Eating beans and rice together supplies 43 percent more protein than consuming them separately; combining yeast

Table 6.3 Protein and Caloric Value of Common Foods

Foods	Amount	Grams Protein	Calories
Beef			
sirloin, broiled			
lean & fat	3.0 oz.	23	240
lean	2.5 oz.	22	150
ground			
lean	3.0 oz.	21	230
regular	3.0 oz.	20	245
Veal			
cutlet	3.0 oz.	23	185
Lamb			
roast			
lean & fat	3.0 oz.	22	205
lean	2.6 oz.	20	140
Liver, fried	3.0 oz.	23	185
Pork			
loin chop, broiled			
lean & fat	3.1 oz.	24	275
lean	2.5 oz.	23	165
Poultry			
fried, flour coated			
½ breast	3.5 oz.	31	220
drumstick	1.7 oz.	13	120
roast			
½ breast	3.0 oz.	27	140
drumstick	1.6 oz.	12	75
Fish			
crabmeat, canned	1 cup	23	135
flounder, sole—baked, with lemon juice			
with butter, margarine	3.0 oz.	16	120
without fat	3.0 oz.	17	80
haddock, breaded, fried	3.0 oz.	17	175
halibut, broiled, with butter & lemon juice	3.0 oz.	20	140
salmon, pink			
canned	3.0 oz.	17	120
baked	3.0 oz.	21	140
tuna, canned in oil	3.0 oz.	24	165
Cheese			
Camembert wedge	1.3 oz.	8	115
Cheddar	1.0 oz.	7	115
Cottage, creamed			
4% fat, large curd	1 cup	28	235
2% fat, large curd	1 cup	31	205
uncreamed	1 cup	25	125
Swiss	1.0 oz.	8	105
Eggs			
raw, whole, no shell	1	6	80
Yogurt, with milk solids			
low-fat with fruit	8.0 oz.	10	230
plain	8.0 oz.	12	145
nonfat	8.0 oz.	13	125

Foods	Amount	Grams Protein	Calories
Legumes			
Beans, cooked			
Great Northern	1 cup	14	210
navy	1 cup	15	225
red Kidney	1 cup	15	230
soy	1 cup	20	235
lima	1 cup	16	260
lentils	1 cup	16	215
Nuts			
almonds	1.0 oz.	6	165
cashews	1.0 oz.	4	165
peanuts	1.0 oz.	8	165
peanut butter	1 tbsp.	5	95
pecans	1.0 oz.	2	190
sunflower seeds	1.0 oz.	6	160
Greens, cooked			
asparagus			
frozen	1 cup	5	50
fresh	1 cup	5	45
broccoli			
frozen	1 cup	6	50
fresh	1 cup	5	45
Brussels sprouts			
frozen	1 cup	6	65
fresh	1 cup	4	60
kale			
frozen	1 cup	4	40
fresh	1 cup	2	40
peas, frozen	1 cup	8	125
spinach, cooked			
frozen	1 cup	6	55
fresh	1 cup	5	40
spirulina (seaweed), dried	1.0 oz.	16	80
Grains			
Breads			
French	1 slice	3	100
wheat	1 slice	2	65
rye	1 slice	2	65
pumpernickel	1 slice	3	80
Cereals			
oatmeal	1 cup	6	145
bran flakes, 40%	¾ cup	4	90
Grape-Nuts	¼ cup	3	100
Special K	1⅓ cup	6	110
Rice, cooked			
brown	1 cup	5	230
white, enriched	1 cup	4	225
Spaghetti			
firm	1 cup	7	190
tender	1 cup	5	155

Source: "Nutritive Value of Foods," *Home & Garden Bulletin* 72 (1981).

and rice increases available protein by 57 percent over eating them individually; and mixing rice and sesame seeds boosts protein by 21 percent (see Table 6.4).

CALCIUM

From adolescence to age 24 or 25, women need 1,200 milligrams of calcium daily, because peak bone mass is probably not attained before age 25. After 25, 800 milligrams a day is an appropriate amount, except during pregnancy and lactation, when the daily requirement increases to 1,200 milligrams. Postmenopausal women at risk for osteoporosis need 1,200 to 1,500 milligrams daily. (See the section on osteoporosis later in this chapter.)

IRON

The iron requirement for both sexes is 15 milligrams daily, which healthy people can get from their diet by eating 30 to 90 grams of meat, poultry, or fish, all of which contain highly absorbable heme iron. Foods containing 25 to 75 milligrams of vitamin C improve the absorption of nonheme iron from vegetable sources. Women who eat little or no animal protein and whose diets are low in vitamin C may require higher amounts of iron or vitamin C as supplements.

SODIUM

We estimate that minimum sodium requirements range from 120 milligrams in the first six months of life to 500 milligrams a day in adulthood. You need an extra 69 milligrams daily during pregnancy and 135 milligrams a day during lactation. Ten percent of our salt intake exists naturally in food, and we add another 15 percent when cooking, while 75 percent comes from processed foods. Normal adults can handle much larger amounts, 10 times the minimum requirement, without any difficulty. However, if you have a family history of high blood pressure, you should ration your salt intake, because salt tends to increase blood pressure in individuals sensitive to it.

Table 6.4 Complementary Vegetable Proteins

By balancing the strengths of one plant protein food with the weaknesses of another, these food combinations bolster their overall protein value.

Cereal Grains and Legumes

- rice with black bean sauce
- split pea soup and cornbread
- lentil barley soup
- baked beans and brown bread
- cracked wheat and bean salad
- tofu (soybean curd) with rice
- beans and tortillas

Legumes and Seeds/Nuts

- garbanzo bean and tahini (sesame-seed paste) dip
- roasted soybeans, sunflower seeds, and peanut snack mix
- peanut butter and sunflower-seed sandwich or cookies

Rice and Seeds

- sesame-seed-and-rice pilaf (or pudding made with these ingredients)

From Alice White, *The Total Nutrition Guide for Mother and Baby: From Pregnancy Through the First Three Years* (New York: Ballantine, 1983).

THE MENSTRUAL CYCLE AND FOOD INTAKE

During adolescence, girls gain an average of 45 pounds, 20 of which are fat, compared to a 57-pound weight gain for boys, only six of them fat. This additional fat is natural and necessary, preparing a female for pregnancy. Throughout her reproductive life, a woman's body experiences the effects of hormonal changes in an average 28-day menstrual cycle.

The menstrual cycle consists of four phases:

- menstrual, when bleeding occurs
- follicular, when the ovaries produce follicles

- periovulatory, when the ovaries release egg(s)
- luteal, the last part of the cycle before menstruation, when the egg either implants or sheds from the wall of the uterus

Estrogen levels are high and progesterone is low around the time of ovulation. During the luteal phase, this situation reverses, with progesterone high and estrogen low. This is significant because these hormones affect our appetites for food in the different phases of the menstrual cycle.

Animal studies have shown that food intake is *low* around the time of ovulation, when estrogen levels are *high* relative to progesterone. Food intake is *high* and body weight increases during the luteal phase before menstruation, a time when estrogen levels are *low*.

In women, the results of various studies agree with the animal research but vary in how much women actually increase the number of calories they eat. A recent study carefully quantified the relationship of food intake to the menstrual cycle in seven women between the ages of 24 and 43. The women used portable tape recorders to measure the food they ate accurately over one entire cycle. They consumed 283 more calories a day during the luteal phase than during the periovulatory phase, and 214 more calories daily during the luteal phase than during the follicular phase. There was no difference in food intake in either the menstrual, follicular, or periovulatory phase. Thus caloric consumption was highest during the luteal phase, followed by the follicular phase.

Earlier studies found greater differences in the number of calories consumed, averaging, in fact, 500 calories per day more during 10 premenstrual days compared with 10 postmenstrual days. However, the measurement of food intake in these studies was not as accurate as it was in the more recent research. In fact, despite the use of lengthy questionnaires, the dietary histories kept by most people are notoriously inaccurate. When researchers compared an objective measure of dietary intake with estimations of dietary intake from dietary records kept by subjects living at home rather than in institutions, they found that two-thirds of the individuals significantly underestimated their caloric intake. This finding, which has long been suspected, makes the results of many nutritional studies questionable.

Other investigators studying the basal metabolic rate (BMR), the rate at which the body burns calories when at rest, found that the BMR *increased* just before menstruation and decreased to its lowest point during ovulation. The differences in the BMR between these two phases was 359 calories daily. These changes in BMR are consistent with the differences found in food. What researchers don't know, however, is whether women eat more because their basal metabolic rate increases, or if the BMR speeds up in response to the additional food. Still other studies have shown that there is a rise in daily energy expenditure of sedentary women during the luteal phase.

From studies such as these, we can see that a series of relationships occurs between the hormonal status of women and how much food they consume, as well as between the number of calories they eat and the amount of energy they expend. These findings are important because, during the luteal phase, women on diets either will not lose weight, will lose less, or will gain weight. If you are dieting, don't become discouraged and abandon your weight-loss efforts because of this built-in hormonal need for more food right before you menstruate.

In addition to changes in food intake, some earlier studies showed a greater craving for sweets during various phases of the menstrual cycle. Although more recent studies failed to find significant differences in sugar consumption, there was a tendency toward increases in sugar intake during the luteal phase.

NUTRITION DURING PREGNANCY AND LACTATION

In the past, most of the interest in the nutritional status of pregnant women focused on how it affected the growth of the fetus and the outcome of the pregnancy—that is, whether a woman gave birth to a healthy, full-term baby of normal weight. Only recently has research turned to the devastating effect of excess weight gain during pregnancy on obesity in the mother.

A woman's nutritional status prior to and during her pregnancy is but one of many important factors that influence fetal growth and birth weight. Others include genetic factors, infections, placental abnormalities, toxins, work environment, maternal obesity, diabetes, toxemia, hypertension, alcohol intake, and smoking.

Anything that interferes with the delivery of nutrients to the fetus, or with the ability of the fetus to adapt to physiological changes that occur during pregnancy—congenital defects and chromosomal abnormalities, for example—can cause fetal malnutrition.

Doctors cannot define the ideal diet for the pregnant woman because ethical considerations preclude the necessary experiments. Obviously, researchers cannot deliberately feed one group of pregnant women an inadequate diet in order to compare their infants with those of well-fed mothers. However, investigators can come up with an estimation of nutritional requirements, using data obtained from studies of changes in body composition and metabolism; clinical observations measuring alterations in total body weight, body water, body density, oxygen consumption, and the amount of protein, fat, carbohydrates, vitamins, and minerals consumed during pregnancy; and the assessment of newborn size.

In the United States, nutrient standards have long been based on the RDA. Authorities know that individuals of similar age, sex, and activity level may have different nutrient needs because of their diverse genetic and environmental factors. They don't know the needs of each individual, of course, and to make sure that the nutrients recommended fulfill the dietary requirements of all, the RDAs have been set at the upper end of the range of requirements of the group as a whole. This heightened level has led to recommendations for increases in food intake far above those needed for normal pregnancy in an already overnourished population. Remember that the average American woman is already 20 percent above her desirable body weight. When excessive weight gain during pregnancy is added to this, it becomes clear that women are at particularly greater risk of overweight and obesity.

ENERGY

Your energy needs increase during pregnancy because your body is getting ready for the growth of the fetus and the placenta as well as for lactation. Usually women gain 27.5 pounds during a full-term pregnancy; the average weight of a newborn infant in the United States is 7.26 pounds. In 1971, experts estimated that women consume an extra 80,000 calories over the nine months of pregnancy, or approximately 300 extra calories a day. The World Health Organization (WHO) has used this figure in setting dietary standards for pregnant women. Since then, other studies have shown that additional caloric needs can range from 45,000 to 110,000 during the entire course of a pregnancy.

Because of the difficulty most women have in losing the excessive weight they gained during pregnancy, we recommend that if you are a typical, well-nourished American woman, you need no more than 45,000 extra calories during the entire nine months. This number of calories is adequate to support a full-term pregnancy. You require no extra food during the first trimester; during the second and third trimesters you should eat an additional 300 calories a day.

While these are good general guidelines, doctors, midwives, and nutritionists must carefully consider the degree of obesity or leanness of the expectant mother prior to pregnancy in giving dietary advice to *individual* women. A woman's nutritional status during pregnancy is more likely to be compromised if she is less than 16 years old, is economically deprived, is underweight, if she gains less than two pounds a month during the second and third trimesters, if she is pregnant for the third time in two years, and if she smokes, drinks, or uses drugs. When lean mothers—those who weigh less than 110 pounds and gain less than 10 pounds during pregnancy—are compared to women of average weight and average weight gain, the results show that they give birth to an excessive number of low-birth-weight (LBW) infants—under five and a half pounds. LBW infants have a much higher incidence of illness and death than do normal-weight infants, who weigh between seven and eight and a half pounds. Adolescents who are 15 years old or younger when they conceive are at particular risk, since many of them have not finished growing themselves and need extra nutrients over and beyond those required to nourish the fetus. Youngsters in this age group, who give birth to about 30,000 babies annually in the United States, experience more than twice the prematurity rate of mothers who are 20 to 24 years old and have a high proportion of LBW newborns. Among girls who are 14 or 15 years old, adequate prenatal care and improved nutrition are of special importance if their rates of premature births are to be reduced.

PROTEIN

Because protein builds all body tissue, including brain cells—
which start developing rapidly during the second half of pregnancy
and continue growing until the baby is 18 months old—it has
particular importance during pregnancy. The NAS advocates 76
grams of protein daily for a pregnant woman. During lactation, a
woman needs 60 grams of protein a day for the first six months
and 57 grams daily for the second six months.

FOLATE (FOLIC ACID AND FOLACIN)

Several lines of evidence suggest a relationship between the
amount of folic acid, a B vitamin, women consume early in pregnancy and the presence of neural tube defects (NTDs) in their
babies. Infants born with NTDs suffer serious malformations of the
brain and spinal cord. About half of these newborns die; surviving
children experience paralysis, and many are mentally retarded. In
the United States, NTDs occur about once in every 1,000 births. In
the United Kingdom, which has a high incidence of NTDs, neural
tube defects are more common among people of very low income,
whose diet tends to be poor. Several reports also link NTDs in
newborns with mothers who used the folate antagonist aminop-
terin for cancer during pregnancy. Retrospective studies of women
at the end of pregnancy have shown that those whose infants had
neural tube defects consumed lower levels of folate, ascorbic acid,
and riboflavin than those with unaffected children.

You need 800 micrograms a day of folate during pregnancy and
500 micrograms daily when breast-feeding. In a study of 22,776
women who had either alpha fetoprotein screening or amniocentesis—two common prenatal tests—those women who took a multivitamin supplement containing folic acid while planning a
pregnancy and during the first six weeks after conception had 50
to 70 percent fewer babies with neural tube defects. The prevalence
of NTDs was 3.6 for each 1,000 babies born to women who did *not*
take a multivitamin prior to or during the first trimester, compared
with only 0.9 per 1,000 infants of women who took folate during
the first six weeks of their pregnancies. Among the women with
a previous NTD child, the difference was much more striking: 13
babies per 1,000 births among mothers who did not receive folate

supplementation, compared to 3.5 per 1,000 for those who did.

Many foods contain folate, including liver and kidney, dark green leafy vegetables, asparagus, yeast, nuts, legumes, and whole grains (see Table 6.5). Since this vitamin can be destroyed in cooking water, you should steam, broil, or stir-fry when preparing folate-containing foods. In addition, two drugs used to control epilepsy—phenobarbital and Dilantin—destroy folic acid. Whether or not you have used these drugs, you should take a multivitamin supplement containing folate during pregnancy.

CALCIUM

Pregnancy also requires that you increase your consumption of calcium, to 1,200 milligrams a day. Four eight-ounce glasses of milk daily provide this total calcium requirement; this amount of milk also provides 32 grams of protein, several B vitamins, and, if fortified, vitamins A and D. If you are concerned about weight gain, you can reduce the 150 calories in a glass of whole milk by using a low-fat variety, such as 2 percent at 120 calories per eight ounces; 1 percent at 100 calories; and skim milk at 86 calories. This is why milk is a nutritional bargain; it contains a great deal of nourishment for relatively few calories (see Table 6.6).

The National Institute of Child Health and Human Development is conducting a study to determine if calcium supplementation during pregnancy prevents premature birth and preeclampsia, a serious disease of pregnancy.

IRON

Your need for iron doubles during pregnancy. This increased requirement cannot be met by the iron content of the conventional American diet or by the existing iron stores of many women. Therefore, doctors and midwives recommend 30 to 60 milligrams of supplemental iron during the last two trimesters of pregnancy. Iron needs during lactation are not substantially different from those of nonpregnant women, but you should continue taking an iron supplement for two to three months after giving birth, to replenish stores depleted by the pregnancy.

Because the body absorbs iron more efficiently from food than from supplements, you may want to get part of your iron needs

Table 6.5 Good Sources of Folate

Food	Selected Serving Size	Percentage of U.S. RDA[1]
Breads, Cereals, and Other Grain Products		
English muffin, whole-wheat	1	+
Pita bread, whole-wheat	1 small	+
Ready-to-eat cereals, fortified	1 oz.	+ +
Wheat germ, plain	2 tbsp.	+
Fruits		
Grapefruit and orange juice, frozen, reconstituted	¾ cup	+
Orange juice		
fresh	¾ cup	+
frozen, reconstituted	¾ cup	+
Vegetables		
Artichoke, globe (french), cooked	1 medium	+
Asparagus, cooked	½ cup	+
Beets, cooked	½ cup	+
Broccoli, cooked	½ cup	+
Brussels sprouts, cooked	½ cup	+
Cauliflower, cooked	½ cup	+
Chinese cabbage, cooked	½ cup	+
Corn, cream style, cooked	½ cup	+
Endive, chicory, escarole, or romaine; raw	1 cup	+
Mustard greens, cooked	½ cup	+
Okra, cooked	½ cup	+
Parsnips, cooked	½ cup	+
Peas, green, cooked	½ cup	+
Spinach		
cooked	½ cup	+ +
raw	1 cup	+
Turnip greens, cooked	½ cup	+
Meat, Poultry, Fish, and Alternatives		
Meat and Poultry		
Liver, braised		
beef or calf	3 oz.	+ + +
pork	3 oz.	+ +
chicken or turkey	½ cup diced	+ + +
Fish and Seafood		
Crabmeat, steamed	3 oz.	+

Food	Selected Serving Size	Percentage of U.S. RDA[1]
Dry Beans, Peas, and Lentils		
Beans, cooked		
Bayo, black, brown, calico, chick-peas (garbanzo beans), lima, mexican, pinto, or white	½ cup	+
Black-eyed peas (cowpeas)	½ cup	+ + +
Red kidney	½ cup	+ +
Lentils, cooked	½ cup	+ + +
Peas, split, green or yellow, cooked	½ cup	+

[1]A selected serving size contains—

+ 10–24 percent of the U.S. RDA for adults and children over 4 years of age

+ + 25–39 percent of the U.S. RDA for adults and children over 4 years of age

+ + + 40 percent or more of the U.S. RDA for adults and children over 4 years of age

Source: USDA

from your diet by consuming ready-to-eat and cooked cereals that have been fortified with iron, liver, clams, oysters, and soybeans (see Table 6.7).

CRAVINGS

Some women experience cravings for certain foods, such as pickles, a choice that may reflect the pregnant body's need for extra salt. A heightened desire for ice, clay, or cornstarch can indicate a deficiency in iron or other nutrients. It is important to consult your caregiver if you experience these symptoms so your diet can be adjusted to eliminate any deficiencies.

WEIGHT GAIN IN PREGNANCY AND FUTURE OBESITY

Most women say that their first substantial weight gain as adults occurred during their first pregnancy, with further increases taking

Table 6.6 Good Sources of Calcium

Food	Selected Serving Size	Percentage of U.S. RDA[1]
Breads, Cereals, and Other Grain Products		
English muffin, plain with raisins	1	+
Muffin, bran	1 med.	+
Oatmeal, instant, fortified, prepared	⅔ cup	+
Pancakes, plain, fruit, buckwheat, or whole-wheat	2 4-in. pancakes	+
Waffles		
Bran, cornmeal, or fruit	2 4-in. squares	+
Plain	2 4-in. squares	+ +
Vegetables		
Broccoli, cooked	½ cup	+
Spinach, cooked	½ cup	+
Turnip greens, cooked	½ cup	+
Meat, Poultry, Fish, and Alternatives		
Fish and Seafood		
Mackerel, canned, drained	3 oz.	+
Ocean perch, baked or broiled	3 oz.	+
Salmon, canned, drained	3 oz.	+
Dry Beans, Peas, and Lentils		
Tofu (bean curd)[2]	½ cup cubed	+ +
Milk, Cheese, and Yogurt		
Cheese, natural		
Blue, brick, camembert, feta, gouda, monterey, mozzarella, muenster, provolone, or roquefort	1 oz.	+
Gruyere or swiss	1 oz.	+ +
Parmesan (hard) or romano	1 oz.	+ +
Cheese, process, cheddar or swiss	¾ oz.	+
Cheese, ricotta	½ cup	+ +
Ice cream or ice milk, soft-serve	½ cup	+
Milk		
Buttermilk	1 cup	+ +
Chocolate	1 cup	+ +
Dry, nonfat, reconstituted	1 cup	+ +
Evaporated, whole or skim, diluted	1 cup	+ +
Lowfat or skim	1 cup	+ +
Whole	1 cup	+ +

Food	Selected Serving Size	Percentage of U.S. RDA[1]
Yogurt		
Flavored or fruit, made with whole or lowfat milk	8 oz.	+ +
Frozen	8 oz.	+ +
Plain		
Made with whole milk	8 oz.	+ +
Made with lowfat or nonfat milk	8 oz.	+ + +

[1]A selected serving size contains—

+   10–24 percent of the U.S. RDA for adults and children over 4 years of age

+ +   25–39 percent of the U.S. RDA for adults and children over 4 years of age

+ + +   40 percent or more of the U.S. RDA for adults and children over 4 years of age

[2]If made with calcium sulfate.

Source: USDA

place with each subsequent pregnancy. Therefore, failure to return to prepregnancy weight after childbirth is of great concern to women. Since the average American woman is already overweight, the NAS committee's recommended weight gain of 25 to 30 pounds during pregnancy may be too high for the majority of women (see Fig. 6.1).

Similarly, although women do require extra energy when they are breast-feeding, they may be consuming more calories than they actually need. The usual recommendation during lactation is an extra 500 calories a day. Since a woman burns about 600 calories daily producing enough breast milk for her infant, even with the recommended extra intake, she will slowly lose weight as she breast-feeds. However, there is actually no need for any extra calories during the first three months of lactation, because the body has prepared for nursing by storing calories as fat in the hips and upper arms. Studies and observations of well-nourished lactating women in the United States indicate that they can successfully nurse their infants on 2,000 to 2,220 calories a day. Other researchers have reported effective lactation with various degrees of weight

Table 6.7 Good Sources of Iron

Food	Selected Serving Size	Percentage of U.S. RDA[1]
Breads, Cereals, and Other Grain Products[2]		
Bagel, plain, pumpernickel, or whole-wheat	1 med.	+
Farina, regular or quick, cooked	⅔ cup	+ +
Muffin, bran	1 med.	+
Noodles, cooked	1 cup	+
Oatmeal, instant, fortified, prepared	⅔ cup	+ +
Pita bread, plain or whole-wheat	1 small	+
Pretzel, soft	1	+
Ready-to-eat cereals, fortified	1 oz.	+ +
Rice, white, regular or converted, cooked	⅔ cup	+
Fruits		
Apricots, dried, cooked, unsweetened	½ cup	+
Vegetables		
Beans, lima, cooked	½ cup	+
Spinach, cooked	½ cup	+
Meat, Poultry, Fish, and Alternatives		
Meat and Poultry		
Beef		
Brisket, braised, lean only	3 oz.	+
Ground; extra lean, lean, or regular; baked or broiled	1 patty	+
Pot roast, braised, lean only	3 oz.	+
Roast, rib, roasted, lean only	3 oz.	+
Shortribs, braised, lean only	3 oz.	+
Steak, baked, broiled, or braised; lean only	3 oz.	+
Stew meat, simmered, lean only	3 oz.	+
Liver, braised		
Beef	3 oz.	+ +
Calf	3 oz.	+
Pork	3 oz.	+ + +
Chicken or turkey	½ cup diced	+ +
Liverwurst	1 oz.	+
Tongue, braised	3 oz.	+
Turkey, dark meat, roasted, without skin	3 oz.	+

Food	Selected Serving Size	Percentage of U.S. RDA[1]
Fish and Seafood		
Clams; steamed, boiled, or canned; drained	3 oz.	+ + +
Mackerel, canned, drained	3 oz.	+
Mussels, steamed, boiled, or poached	3 oz.	+
Oysters		
Baked, broiled, or steamed	3 oz.	+ +
Canned, undrained	3 oz.	+ +
Shrimp; broiled, steamed, boiled, or canned; drained	3 oz.	+
Trout, baked or broiled	3 oz.	+
Dry Beans, Peas, and Lentils		
Beans; black-eyed peas (cowpeas), chick-peas (garbanzo beans), red kidney, or white; cooked	½ cup	+
Lentils, cooked	½ cup	+
Soybeans	½ cup	+ +
Nuts and Seeds		
Pine nuts (pignolias)	2 tbsp.	+
Pumpkin or squash seeds, hulled, roasted	2 tbsp.	+

[1]A selected serving size contains—

+   10–24 percent of the U.S. RDA for adults and children over 4 years of age

+ +   25–39 percent of the U.S. RDA for adults and children over 4 years of age

+ + +   40 percent or more of the U.S. RDA for adults and children over 4 years of age

[2]Breads, pasta, and cereals are enriched unless otherwise noted.

Source: USDA

---

loss in well-nourished lactating women on diets ranging from 1,900 to 2,900 calories daily, depending on their physical activity. Milk production was not diminished in adequately nourished women on intakes of *less than* 2,000 calories daily, with an average production of 25 ounces daily during the first six months and 20 ounces during the second half-year. These findings emphasize that current

Percentage of population

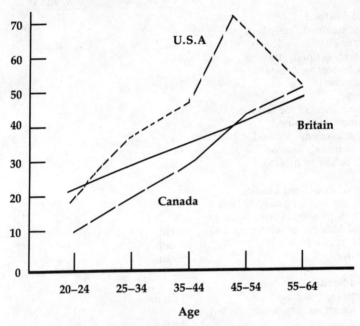

Source: W. J. Millar and T. Stephens, "Prevalence of Excessive Body Weight (BMI > 25), Females, Ages 20–64, Britain (1980), Canada (1981), United States (1976–80)," *American Journal of Public Health* 77 (1984): 38.

recommendations for caloric intake during lactation are too high.

One recent study investigated changes in body weight and in fat deposits under the skin occurring after delivery in lactating versus nonlactating women. It examined these changes in relation to how many calories the women consumed, how much energy they expended, their ages, number of pregnancies, and their pre-pregnancy weight. The study found that the most important difference between the two groups was in fat distribution. The women who breast-fed lost fat in their hip and shoulder regions, indicating that lactating women mobilize their fat differently and get into shape earlier than women who don't nurse their infants. However, the research also concluded that the women who were breast-feeding were eating too much, so that the number of calories lost in breast milk was not enough to permit weight loss. Other studies have also shown that breast-feeding does not always promote weight loss in well-nourished women.

All of these findings suggest that the National Research Council's RDA of 2,500 calories a day for the lactating woman is excessive. In conclusion, ideally a woman should control the amount of weight gained before pregnancy, gain no more than 22–24.5 pounds during pregnancy, breast-feed but not increase caloric intake during the first three months after birth, and increase caloric intake by only an additional 500 calories daily thereafter.

INFANT ALLERGIES DURING NURSING

Infants at high risk for having allergic reactions are those with a family history of allergy and/or those with elevated levels of immunoglobulin E (IgE) in the cord blood (IgE is one of five classes of antibodies). Some studies have shown that infants with two allergic parents have a 60 to 80 percent chance of developing allergies, and that infants with elevated IgE in the cord blood have an 8 percent chance of developing an allergy. Other research confirms that dietary restrictions in nursing mothers can prevent some allergic dermatitis and gastrointestinal (GI) symptoms, but that dietary restrictions do not avert respiratory allergies, although they may postpone the development of breathing problems. In a study of 221 infants at high risk for allergy, 97 were breast-fed and the mothers of 49 of them were on a restricted diet, eliminating highly allergenic foods such as milk, eggs, fish, and peanuts. The infants of mothers on restricted diets were only half as likely to develop allergic dermatitis by 18 months of age as were the infants of those mothers on nonrestricted diets.

As a result of such findings, we recommend that lactating mothers of infants at high risk for developing allergic reactions try to eliminate major allergens from their diets. There is no evidence, however, that restriction of a mother's diet during pregnancy will help prevent allergies from developing in the future.

OBESITY

Why all the concern about excessive weight gain during adolescence and pregnancy? The answer is simple—and very disturbing. Obesity is the most serious disorder in Western societies; we are literally eating ourselves to death. In developed countries, the problem of overconsumption starts early, with children as young as seven exhibiting a trend toward increasing height and weight as a result. Not only is the U.S. population becoming heavier, but our average caloric intake has also increased. The U.S. Department of Agriculture's (USDA) most recent survey of food consumption was conducted in 1985. It investigated 1,503 women ranging in age from 19 to 50 and 548 of their children between the ages of one and five, using personal interviews to obtain a one-day recall of everything the participants ate. This information was compared with data collected in a comparable manner for individuals of the same ages in the Nationwide Food Consumption Survey in 1977–78. The results indicated that, while there was a decrease in the mean amount of meat, poultry, and fish eaten by both women and their children in 1985 compared to 1977, there was an increase in the total number of calories consumed over the same eight years. This finding shows that, although people followed the general recommendation to decrease the amount of meat they ate, they also reduced the amount of fish and poultry in their diets. In addition, they ate more of other foods, increasing their caloric intake.

HOW MUCH WEIGHT IS TOO MUCH?

Obesity means having too much body fat in relation to the bone, muscle, and other elements that contribute to your total body weight. For healthy functioning, men's body weight should be 15 percent fat and women's 19 percent. Men whose body fat exceeds 20 percent of their weight and women with a body fat over 30 percent of their total pounds are considered obese.

A number of reference standards exist for measuring obesity. The best is one that relates weight and the location of body fat to illness (morbidity). Since no such national data have been collected in the United States, the next best standard is body weight in relation to mortality.

The term *desirable body weight* is the weight range associated with the *lowest mortality* as determined in a table developed by the Metropolitan Life Insurance Company in 1959 (Table 6.1). The table presents a range of weights for men and women for a particular height. Individuals whose weight is above the range for their height are considered obese.

Another standard for estimating the presence of obesity is the body mass index (BMI), determined by the ratio of weight (W) in kilograms to height (H) in meters squared ($W/H^2 = kg/m^2$). BMI is a more accurate index of obesity than the Metropolitan Weight Table, because obesity has a relatively high correlation with how much of one's body mass is composed of fat and a relatively low correlation with height. In the absence of the skinfold measurements used in clinics, which are an even more accurate gauge, BMI is the most satisfactory index of obesity based on weight and height available.

BMI is not an easy calculation for Americans because we still think in terms of pounds, feet, and inches rather than kilograms, meters, and centimeters. In order to calculate your BMI, you must first transpose your weight in pounds to kilograms by multiplying by .45. Thus, a 123-pound woman weighs 55.35 kilograms (123 × .45 = 55.35). You then transpose your height to centimeters by multiplying it by 2.5. If the same 123-pound woman is 64 inches (5 feet 4 inches) tall, she would measure 160 centimeters (64 × 2.5 = 160) or 1.6 meters, since there are 100 centimeters in a meter. You then square your height by multiplying 1.6 by itself, which equals 2.56. The calculation for obtaining the BMI of our 5-foot-4-

inch, 123-pound woman looks like this: 123 × .45 = 55.35 kilograms divided by 2.56 = a BMI of 21.62, well within the desirable
BMI for women, which ranges from 19 to 25, with a mean of 21.5.
Consulting Figure 6.2 to find your BMI will be easier than doing
this arithmetic.

FAT DISTRIBUTION

The number of extra pounds does not tell the whole story; *where*
fat settles in the body is equally important. In women, extra weight
typically settles in the upper thighs. While this is hardly advantageous, it is far less dangerous than the accumulation of fat in the
abdomen that obese men take on. There is conclusive statistical
evidence that associates abdominal obesity with a number of disorders in the way the body metabolizes insulin and fats, as well
as with noninsulin-dependent diabetes mellitus (NIDDM) and hypertension.

Doctors assess abdominal obesity by the ratio of waist-to-hip
circumference. The upper limit of normal occurs when the waist
measures 15 percent less than the hips. Having a waist measurement that *exceeds* that of the hips, besides being unattractive, is
detrimental to health.

VALIDATING DESIRABLE BODY WEIGHT

While the most extensive data relating body weight to mortality
come from the insurance companies, researchers also consider data
from the Framingham Heart Study—in which the population of
Framingham, Massachusetts, was followed for three decades to
find out what illnesses they contracted and what diseases caused
their deaths—as typical of the U.S. population as a whole in terms
of mortality. When epidemiologists looked at data from the study
to correlate the relationship of body weight to mortality, they used
Metropolitan Life relative weight (MRW), which expresses body
weight as a percentage of a person's desirable weight, as the standard. They found that minimum mortality occurred when the MRW
ranged from 100 to 109 percent—that is, when individuals were
not more than 9 percent above their desirable weight, or if they
had a BMI between 21.66 and 23.83.

Grade I obesity corresponds to a BMI of 25–29.9; grade II to a

Figure 6.2 Nomogram for Body Mass Index (Quetelet's Index) from 1959 and 1983 Metropolitan Life Insurance Tables

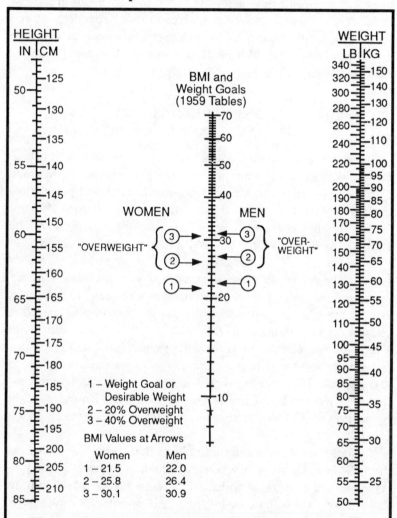

The ratio weight/height² (metric units) is read from the central scale after a straight edge is placed between height and body weight.

Instructions: Place a ruler across the table so that the left side is on your height and the right side is on your weight. Your BMI is the point the ruler touches on the middle line.

Source: B. T. Burton and W. R. Foster "Health Implications of Obesity: An NIH Consensus Development Conference." Reprinted from *Journal of the American Dietetic Association* 85 (1985):1117.

BMI of 30–40; and grade III to a BMI over 40, also known as morbid obesity. The health risks associated with obesity begin in the BMI range of 25–30, with differing degrees of risk depending on age, sex, and a family history of hypertension, diabetes, or disorders of fat metabolism. A BMI of 30 or more is considered risky regardless of whether these factors are present or not.

THE SERIOUSNESS AND
THE PREVALENCE OF OBESITY

Given the severe medical risks that come with obesity, it is troubling to note that Americans are more obese than other, comparable national populations. A study of noninstitutionalized populations in Canada, Great Britain, and the United States between 1976 and 1981 compared the prevalence of overweight and obesity. This study defined overweight as a BMI of 25.1 to 30, and obesity as a value exceeding 30. Among those studied, American men were found to be the most obese, especially at younger ages. The proportion of excessively heavy men reaches a plateau around age 50 in all three countries, possibly because the most obese men died off, leaving only those who were relatively less obese as survivors. The study found that the United States also has the highest proportion of excessively heavy women at all ages except between 20 and 24. The difference is greatest between American women and the other women between the ages of 45 and 54. Unlike men, the proportion of overweight or obese women did not level off by age 64.

Not only are Americans more obese than other nationals, but the U.S. population as a whole is becoming heavier. Three government health surveys conducted between 1960 and 1980 indicate that the average weight-for-height of the population continues to rise. The greatest increase occurred among those white and black females already most overweight. Women below the poverty line have a much higher prevalence of obesity between the ages of 25 and 55 than do women above the poverty line, demonstrating that race and income are independent predictors of overweight in women.

Moreover, these national surveys dramatically underestimate the extent of obesity in the American population. First, they employ statistical definitions to estimate overweight—such as the percent-above-average weight of a person—rather than using data relating body weight to the rate of illness and death of the survey population, as the Framingham Heart Study researchers did. Second, these statistics use the weight of people from the 20-to-29-year-old age group as desirable body weight, an arbitrary definition since it is clear that the U.S. population at ages 20 and 29 is already overweight. Any calculation based on this rationale, therefore, underestimates the prevalence of obesity, because the standard is higher and the difference between the standard and the overweight is consequently less. Thus the numbers the three studies report—32.6 million adult Americans who are overweight and another 11.5 million who are obese, or a total of 44.1 million—should be considered very low estimates rather than accurate findings.

Just how low is apparent if we calculate the prevalence of obesity on the basis of long-term prospective studies, using criteria that relate obesity to illness and death from cardiovascular disease, as the Framingham Heart Study does. This standard shows that 80 percent of the men over 40 and 70 percent of the women over 40 in the Framingham Heart Study are above the desirable weight range and are at increased risk for cardiovascular disease.

Another problem exists in the very definition of overweight and obesity: The BMI indicating the reading at which health problems start for both men and women is set too high. For example, a U.S. government survey obtained health and nutrition data between 1982 and 1984 on Mexican Americans, Cuban Americans, and Puerto Ricans, who together constitute approximately 76 percent of the Hispanic population in the United States. Men were considered "overweight" if their BMI was above 27.8, and "severely overweight" if it exceeded 31.1. For women, BMI cutoff points were 27.3 and 32.2, respectively. But in reality, we know that health problems occur long before people reach these BMIs. At a BMI of 27.3, for example, the risk for heart attack doubles.

The prevalence of overweight reported for Hispanic Americans in this survey was substantially higher than that of non-Hispanic Americans aged 20 to 74 years. Thirty-five to 40 percent of Hispanic women are overweight, compared to 25 percent of Caucasian American women. Only African American women, 44 percent of whom are overweight, scored higher. The same was true of severe overweight, with black women showing a substantially higher incidence (19 percent) of obesity than Hispanic American women.

Most of us gain weight as we become older, at least through middle age; therefore, the frequency of obesity among Hispanic American adults between the ages of 20 and 24, especially among women, is serious, because the risk of severe obesity and its implications will be even greater at middle age.

THE GENETICS OF OBESITY

Many studies of twins and adopted children tell us what we can easily see by casual observation: Obesity is hereditary. Obviously, the extent of obesity depends a great deal on the imbalance between how much we eat (energy intake) and how much we exercise (energy expenditure), but people who are genetically predisposed to obesity are most vulnerable to weight gain. Researchers have suggested the existence of several genetic and nongenetic forms of obesity, although they have not yet uncovered a specific gene. One recent study showed that obese children tend to have an increased number of fat cells and that childhood obesity more often than not leads to adult obesity. Obese children are more likely to have first-degree relatives who are fat than nonobese children. Studies of identical and fraternal twins indicate that 70 percent of the adult differences in body-mass index are genetic. And a recent Canadian study of identical twins has shown that genes control how the body uses excess calories. Some of us store these calories as muscle and remain lean, while others store them as fat and gain weight.

The variability in total energy expenditure and in the resting metabolic rate (RMR) also appear to be under genetic control. Studies have shown that a decrease in total energy expenditure (EE) or in RMR indicate an increased risk of weight gain in infants and adults.

Research has also shown that a lower metabolic rate in adults predicted an increase in body weight and body fat over a four-year period, and that the metabolic rate is strongly familial. Another study found that obese infants of obese mothers expend less energy as early as three months of age and that this lower energy expenditure at three months predicted an increase in body weight and body fat by the time these infants were two years old. This study indicates that clinicians can identify genetic risk from parental obesity early in life. As our knowledge of the role genes play in human obesity increases, doctors should be able to improve their ability to identify those individuals who are at risk and prescribe a diet and exercise program that will help prevent overweight before it starts or becomes entrenched.

In the meantime, there is ample evidence, based on the information derived from family history and measures of RMR and EE, to begin proper diet and physical activity in children to prevent weight gain, either by controlling calories for those with decreased RMR or by increasing activity for those with low energy expenditure.

THE ADVERSE EFFECTS OF OBESITY

Everyone who is plagued by obesity is at far higher risk for a number of debilitating diseases than their nonobese counterparts, and this irrefutable fact is the greatest incentive to weight control.

CORONARY HEART DISEASE

The most important—and one of the only—studies of the relationship between obesity and the risk of coronary heart disease in women involved 115,886 U.S. female nurses who were 30 to 55 years old in 1976 and free of coronary disease, stroke, and cancer. They were followed for eight years to learn the number and the nature of fatal and nonfatal heart attacks that would occur among them. During that period, 306 nonfatal heart attacks (myocardial infarctions) occurred; 83 deaths were attributed to coronary heart disease; and there were 216 cases of confirmed angina pectoris, the type of heart disease characterized by severe, sharp pain resulting from lack of oxygen to the heart muscle and often brought on by effort or excitement. The higher the weight as determined by the BMI standard, the greater the incidence in each of these categories of heart disease. More important, the study found that even mild to moderate overweight increased the chance of developing coronary heart disease in middle-aged women, with the frequency rising appreciably after a BMI of 23. This finding is consistent with the conclusions of the Framingham Heart Study and bears out what that study showed about male mortality: Men who were 20 percent above desirable weight (BMI = 26.0) suffered an elevated mortality rate from cardiovascular disease, indicating that even slight increases above desirable weight often have dire consequences.

HIGH BLOOD PRESSURE (HYPERTENSION)

Blood pressure readings reflect the force exerted by the blood against the body's arterial walls. The systolic pressure, the higher reading, measures this force when the heart is fully contracted; the diastolic, or lower number, measures it when the heart is relaxed. The formula mm/Hg reflects millimeters of mercury on the blood pressure cuff. Thus a reading of 120/80 means the measurer first heard the blood pulsing against the arterial walls at 120 (the systolic pressure) and last heard it at 80 (the diastolic pressure).

There is no question any longer that weight gain and increased blood pressure go hand in hand. In 1974, researchers showed that an increase in the Metropolitan Relative Weight of only 10 percent would predict a rise in systolic blood pressure of 7 mm/Hg. In 1983, investigators using the data from Framingham found that obese women in their 40s were *seven* times as likely to develop high blood pressure as were lean women of the same age.

In 1986, investigators compared the effectiveness of weight loss on blood pressure with the antihypertensive drug metoprolol (Lopressor, Apo-Metoprolol) and with a placebo in young overweight patients with high blood pressure. They found that an average weight loss of 18 pounds caused an average drop in blood pressure of 14/13 mm/Hg, compared with a decrease of 12/8 mm/Hg in the metoprolol group and 9/4 mm/Hg in the placebo group. If you are overweight and have hypertension, weight loss should lower your blood pressure.

DIABETES

Obesity is an established risk factor for noninsulin-dependent diabetes mellitus (NIDDM). Mexican Americans, with their higher prevalence of overweight, are two to four times more likely to develop NIDDM than Caucasian Americans, and they also do so several years earlier, presumably because they are overweight for longer periods of time, thus further increasing their susceptibility.

In 1972, a prospective study showed that moderate obesity, where patients' weight exceeded the norm by 45 percent or less, increased the risk of diabetes about tenfold. In those whose weights exceeded the standard by more than 45 percent, the risk jumped about 30 times. And a workshop on body weight, health, and longevity held in 1982 reported that a 10-pound weight loss improves the results of the glucose tolerance test and decreases the insulin requirements of the diabetic.

Although physicians know that weight loss decreases blood pressure, improves the glucose tolerance of the diabetic, and decreases insulin requirements, they do not know how weight gain or loss asserts its effects on human metabolism. Until research clarifies the various mechanisms involved, patients with NIDDM must make every effort to keep their weight within the desirable body weight range. This means eating less and exercising more, a regimen that is greatly preferable to treatment with drugs whose long-term effects are not known.

CANCER

We have fewer studies on the relationship between obesity and cancer in either men or women than we have for other diseases. Certainly no such long-term studies compare in scope to the Framingham Heart Study, with its 30-year follow-up. But recently the American Cancer Society carried out an analysis of data collected from 1959 to 1972 that confirmed the fact that those subjects who enjoyed greater longevity were close to, or 10 to 20 percent below, average weight.

This study described the mortality experiences according to variations in weight among 750,000 men and women drawn from the general population in large and small cities of 26 states; nonwhites, persons in the lowest socioeconomic segments, itinerants, and institutionalized individuals were somewhat underrepresented. The results showed that those who were 40 percent or more above average weight suffered high rates of death from cancer. Men primarily developed cancer of the colon and the rectum, while women experienced cancer of the gallbladder and biliary passages, breast, cervix, endometrium, uterus, and ovaries. In women between 50 and 70 years of age, those who were 40 percent above average weight had cancer mortality one and two-thirds times higher than did those of average weight, while for men the increased mortality rate was one-third to one-half higher.

Other research, including case control studies, has shown an association between overweight and breast cancer. One Dutch study found that the risk of breast cancer at age 65 was twice as high for heavier women as for lighter ones. The same was true of the incidence of breast cancer among Japanese women, although the total frequency was lower because even the heavier Japanese women weighed far less than those studied in Holland.

Researchers don't know how overweight functions to increase cancer risk, but a number of studies have pointed to estrogen as playing a role in the development of cancers of the uterus, cervix, breast, and ovaries, which account for half of all cancers in women. Fat (adipose) tissue is the major source of estrogen formation in postmenopausal women. Obese women also have increased levels of prolactin, androgens, and cortisol, although no association has yet been established between those and cancer.

NUTRITION AT MENOPAUSE AND BEYOND

At menopause, a woman's body undergoes significant changes, including the end of menstruation. (See Chapter 15.) We need less iron after menopause, and the RDA drops to 10–11 milligrams. If you already are getting the recommended 800 milligrams of calcium a day, there is no need to increase it unless you are at risk for osteoporosis. A recent study found that postmenopausal women who consumed 800 milligrams of calcium daily stopped the slow, steady erosion of bone in their hips, wrists, and spines. In addition women, particularly those who either don't live in sunny climates or are not exposed to sunlight on a daily basis, need more vitamin D than men.

Women also require more vitamin B_{12} after the age of 60 because of the greater prevalence of achlorhydria, the absence of hydrochloric acids from gastric secretions, which diminishes vitamin B_{12} absorption.

After menopause, the body's muscle mass begins to decrease and the basal metabolic rate lessens. To avoid weight gain, you should either eat less, particularly by reducing your fat intake; increase your physical activity by walking, swimming, playing tennis, running, or dancing; or do both. You should eat two to four servings of green, yellow, and orange fruits and vegetables daily, and consume no more than 1,900 to 2,000 calories a day.

This is a crucial time, since weight gain increases rapidly after menopause, as does the incidence of hypertension.

WOMEN'S SPECIAL SUSCEPTIBILITY TO ALCOHOL

Although alcohol is not a nutrient, it contains a high proportion of calories: seven per gram. When alcohol is consumed, three factors control the level it assumes in the blood and in other tissues in the body: the route of intake, its distribution, and the rate of elimination by the body. Long ago, investigators observed differences between how men and women "held their liquor," but they did not understand the mechanisms behind them. Today we do.

The liver is the principal site of alcohol metabolism; the primary enzymes involved are the alcohol dehydrogenases. Recent reports indicate that alcohol dehydrogenase in the lining of the stomach (gastric mucosa) may contribute substantially to alcohol metabolism and that this effect appears to be different in men and women. Many epidemiologic studies have shown that women are more susceptible than men to the adverse effects of alcohol. For example, women suffer liver damage earlier, after consuming smaller quantities of alcohol and for shorter periods of time, than their male counterparts. Because women have a larger lipid (fatty substance) content in their bodies and therefore less water than men, women may have higher blood alcohol levels because there is a smaller volume of water in which to distribute the alcohol. Because women also have a relatively lower rate of alcohol dehydrogenase activity in the stomach, their stomach secretions are less efficient at breaking down alcohol, and they have more alcohol available in their blood and body tissues than men do, even when drinking smaller amounts. This difference in the gastric metabolism of alcohol between men and women decreases among chronic alcoholics, both male and female.

Racial differences also play a role. There is some evidence that African American women are particularly susceptible to alcohol-induced liver damage, for example. The gastric alcohol dehydrogenase is low in both African American and Caucasian women.

Liver damage is not the only negative effect of alcohol in women. Even small quantities of alcohol can injure the fetus. The toxic effect of alcohol on fetal growth and development is particularly dangerous for nonalcoholic young women who do not know they are pregnant during the first trimester and consume relatively small quantities of alcohol. (See Chapter 9.)

Drinking alcohol after eating diminishes alcohol's ability to stay in the body and may be a protective mechanism, since it also reduces the amount of alcohol that passes into the liver and systemic circulation, as compared with alcohol consumed at other times. Researchers call this protective effect gastric first-pass metabolism, and it is decreased by fasting, which is why you should not drink on an empty stomach. Because the activity of gastric alcohol dehydrogenase returns to normal after a person stops drinking, the decrease in activity may be due to mucosal damage.

Since men and women process alcohol in the stomach differently, any standards set for safe levels of alcohol consumption must take these metabolic variations into consideration. Given equal amounts of alcohol, women show higher levels of alcohol in the general and capillary circulation than men and are, therefore, more vulnerable to experiencing problems with coordination, such as that demanded by driving. Fasting or prolonged alcohol abuse further exaggerates this difference. For all these reasons, it is important for women either to avoid alcohol or to carefully limit the amount they drink.

IRON DEFICIENCY ANEMIA

Nutrient deficiencies have practically been eliminated in the United States and other Western cultures with the exception of iron deficiency anemia, which is the most common dietary deficiency in the world.

The World Health Organization (WHO) defines iron deficiency anemia in terms of hemoglobin level. In people 14 years old and over, males are considered anemic if their hemoglobin level is below 13 grams per deciliter (g/dl) of blood and females are anemic if it is less than 12 g/dl. For pregnant women, values below 11 g/

dl for the first and third trimesters, and 10.5 g/dl for the second trimester, have been proposed.

The range of normal hemoglobin values is wide, extending from 13 to 16 g/dl in men and 12 to 16 g/dl in women. Using hemoglobin as an indicator of anemia, 2.5 to 4 percent of nonpregnant women ages 15 to 44 showed evidence of iron deficiency in the United States. The average iron intake of this population group was 10 to 11 milligrams daily in surveys conducted by a number of government agencies. Further analysis of this data, which took into account both the variation in iron intake by this population and iron losses by menstruating women, showed that 14 milligrams a day of iron is adequate to meet the needs of all women in this age group except the 5 percent who have "heavy" bleeding during their menstrual cycles. We recommend 15 milligrams of iron daily for this latter age group.

Women with iron deficiency anemia may tire easily. There is an association between hemoglobin concentration and both work capacity and decreased immune function. In children, iron deficiency anemia may cause decreased resistance to infection, apathy, a shortened attention span, and reduced ability to learn.

There is no evidence of much iron deficiency anemia among the elderly except for that associated with inflammatory bowel disease. Ten milligrams of iron daily is adequate for men and women in this age group.

SOURCES OF IRON

Many foods contain iron; the main dietary sources are meat, eggs, vegetables, and cereals, many of which are fortified with iron. The food consumption data from one government survey for women 18 to 24 years of age showed that for a daily iron intake of 10.7 milligrams, 30 percent of the iron came from meat, poultry, and fish and 25 percent from fortified cereals. The gastrointestinal tract absorbs iron efficiently from animal sources (heme iron), and absorption increases even more when we eat or drink foods rich in vitamin C (ascorbic acid).

Fruits, vegetables, and juices contain varying amounts of iron. Meat and ascorbic acid enhance the amount of iron absorbed from these foods (see Table 6.7).

NUTRITION AND ATHLETICS

Young women today understand that exercise and physical fitness are vital to health. The total calories we need to consume in fat, protein, and carbohydrate are closely related to the amount of physical activity we engage in; the more active we are, the more calories we need.

Keep in mind that as you begin or continue a physical conditioning program, your body's need for energy from these calories depends upon whether you want to maintain, lose, or gain weight. If you eat a typical Western diet, you receive enough protein, fat, carbohydrate, and calories from these dietary sources and don't need further supplementation to enhance physical performance.

Do you need vitamin and mineral supplements? Recent research suggests that vitamins E, C, and possibly A are used up during endurance exercises and supplementation may be necessary. What about the value of the so-called ergogenic aids that have been said to enhance athletic and work output, such as wheat germ, wheat germ oil, lecithin, honey, gelatin, phosphates, sunflower seeds, bee pollen, kelp, or brewer's yeast? It is now well established that a balanced diet provides all the nutrients necessary for good health and that such supplementary additions are unnecessary for most people. Such a diet contains the variety to provide the six vital types of nutrients: fats, carbohydrates, proteins, vitamins, minerals, and water. Since vitamins and minerals are present in a varied diet, and since they are not used to produce energy but instead burn it, supplementation has no role in enhancing physical performance.

The principal electrolyte deficits that must be corrected after profuse sweating are sodium and chloride. The concentration of electrolytes in sweat, and the total losses that occur with physical activity, vary widely from one individual to another, according to the degree of acclimatization, the amount of adrenaline the body produces, environmental temperature, and humidity. The quantity of sodium lost by an adult in sweat increases markedly under conditions of high physical work in high surrounding temperatures and may reach levels of *eight grams* per day as a result of profuse sweating. When you need more than *three liters* of water daily to replace sweat loss, you need extra sodium chloride in your diet.

We do not know the *precise* requirements for sodium and chloride. However, the suggested safe and adequate intake of sodium by adults is one to three grams, and of chloride from 1.7 to five grams. One teaspoon of salt contains two grams of sodium. During periods of regular exercise, the loss of these electrolytes is actually quite small and can be replaced with a normal dietary intake over the subsequent 24 hours. Even athletes who lose five to eight liters of sweat and require 13 to 15 grams of salt per day can obtain this salt from the foods consumed following the event. In fact, it is practically impossible not to get enough salt on the typical U.S. diet, since naturally occurring sodium amounts to about one gram daily and most Americans consume 10 to 15 grams of salt every day. You definitely do not need salt tablets, particularly since they frequently cause nausea, vomiting, and gastric distress.

However, it is essential to replace body fluids following strenuous exercise. Whenever you sweat profusely, you should drink liberal amounts of fluid before, during, and after exercise to prevent dehydration.

All healthy women, regardless of age, should exercise regularly and pay attention to their energy balance by weighing themselves twice a week. Brisk walking, the most convenient and least expensive sport, is valuable as an element in weight loss, improves cardiovascular and general fitness, decreases the risk of cancers of the reproductive system, maintains strong bones, and possibly slows down the loss of bone mass and the development of osteoporosis later in life.

EATING DISORDERS

The prevalence of eating disorders among women, particularly anorexia nervosa and bulimia, continues to increase. Current estimates indicate that anorexia nervosa and bulimia affect 10 to 15 percent of adolescent girls and young women. While both disorders, which sometimes coexist in the same person, bring anguish to those who suffer from them and to their families, their origins are still not well understood. Early recognition and treatment of both are important, but each poses a challenge to families and physicians.

Anorexia nervosa is a syndrome characterized by a disturbance in the perception of one's body image, an intense fear of becoming obese, and subsequent extreme weight loss. Bulimia is characterized by secretive binge-eating episodes followed by self-induced vomiting, the use of laxatives or diuretics, and fasting, also motivated by an intense preoccupation with body weight. Although bulimia is an entity distinct from anorexia nervosa, patients with anorexia sometimes have bulimic symptoms. Several reports have indicated that 44 to 55 percent of patients with anorexia will develop the symptoms of bulimia during the course of the disorder.

Both disorders have a psychiatric base and often escape early notice by parents and physicians because the patients appear healthy during the early stages.

ANOREXIA NERVOSA

Our knowledge of what *causes* eating disorders is still evolving. Most physicians consider anorexia nervosa an endocrine and psychologic disorder in which an obsessive fear of weight gain leads to faulty eating patterns, severe weight loss, and malnutrition. Anorectic patients have psychological, perceptual, and cognitive disturbances. Compared with the self-perceptions of normal thin persons, anorectic persons overestimate their body width—particularly the face, chest, waist, and hips—while their assessment of inanimate objects and of other people's bodies remains normal. They also distort their awareness of hunger, deny fatigue by being hyperactive, and fail to recognize their emotional stages, such as anger, anxiety, and depression. Some are unable to view situations in anything but extremes, and they interpret events and behavior in rigid and highly personalized ways.

Research suggests that certain sociocultural factors have strongly influenced the historical development of anorexia. One may be the change in the ideal physical image for women, from the plumpness of the previous century to the slimness of today. It may also be that the pressure on women to be successful, independent, and competitive while maintaining the traditional role of wife, homemaker, and mother creates a stressful family situation in which the disorder develops in those who are predisposed. The American Psychiatric Association has established the following diagnostic criteria for anorexia nervosa:

• intense fear of becoming obese, which does not diminish as weight loss progresses

- disturbance of body image, particularly claiming to "feel fat" even when emaciated
- weight loss of at least 25 percent of original body weight or, if under age 18, weight loss from original body weight plus projected weight gain based on growth charts to make 25 percent
- refusal to maintain body weight above a minimal normal weight for age and height
- no known physical illness that would account for the weight loss

Since severe weight loss can cause serious electrolyte imbalance, such as low levels of potassium and magnesium, it is vital that a young woman be brought for treatment before hospitalization becomes necessary. Any substantial weight loss not explained by a physical illness should alert family members to talk with their physician about referring the affected person for psychotherapy.

BULIMIA

Persons with bulimia engage in various compulsive acts and rituals to lose and control weight, including abstaining from food, vomiting, ingesting laxatives or diuretics, and exercising vigorously to the point of exhaustion. In addition to college-age women, people in certain occupational groups are vulnerable to this disorder, including jockeys, wrestlers, gymnasts, models, ballet dancers, actors, and actresses. As in anorexia, the majority of bulimics are women. One of the difficulties in recognizing the bulimic woman is that she appears physically healthy. Often she has developed anxiety and depression by the time her family recognizes the problem or she seeks medical treatment; in fact, about 5 percent of bulimics will have attempted suicide by then.

Most bulimic patients are preoccupied with eating. In one-third of the patients, binge-purge cycles interfere with work or social activities. The person susceptible to bulimia is usually a high achiever, exhibits marked dependence on her parents, is socially ambitious, and has difficulty establishing personal relationships. One study showed that 6 percent of bulimics first went through a period of rigid dieting and purging, followed by eating binges and purging.

The American Psychiatric Association has also established criteria for bulimia, which include the presence of recurrent binge eating and at least three of the following characteristics:

- the consumption of high-caloric, easily ingested food during a binge
- termination of eating episodes by abdominal pain, sleep, social interruption, or self-induced vomiting
- repeated attempts to lose weight through severely restrictive diets, self-induced vomiting, or use of cathartics or diuretics
- frequent weight fluctuations of more than 9.9 pounds caused by alternating binges and fasts

Other criteria include:

- the patient's awareness that the eating pattern is abnormal and fear of being unable to stop eating voluntarily
- the onset of a depressed mood and self-deprecating thoughts after eating binges
- the exclusion of anorexia or other known physical disorders as a cause of the bulimic episodes

Education about proper nutrition is important in the management of these serious eating disorders. Our society's preoccupation with slimness needs to be counterbalanced by sensible information about nourishment and eating habits. There is a lot we do not know about how eating disorders start. Both anorexia and bulimia bring anguish and pain to those who have them and to their families. The early recognition and treatment of both disorders are important and pose a challenge to families and physicians.

DIET AND CHRONIC DISEASES IN WOMEN

As we have noted, the most important nutrition-related condition that contributes to chronic diseases in women is obesity. But chronic diseases are also associated with genetic predisposition and with the interaction of genes and nutrients.

HOW GENES AFFECT
OUR SUSCEPTIBILITY TO DISEASE

Variations in the DNA sequence that exist throughout the human species produce individual differences. It is these common variants at a single location (alleles) or inherited variations (polymorphisms) that form the basis of human diversity. These variations extend from differences among humans in traits such as height, skin color, intelligence, and blood pressure, to our ability to respond to environmental insults such as bacteria, viruses, chemical carcinogens, and the excessive consumption of saturated fat and cholesterol.

During the course of evolution, the people who possessed traits that were beneficial to the human species in periods of famine survived and multiplied—a process known as positive selection. These variants were advantageous in the heterozygous state (an "abnormal" gene inherited from one parent and a "normal" one from the other parent). However, when environmental conditions changed, these variants were no longer beneficial. For example, the variants that benefited our hunter-gatherer ancestors by maintaining blood cholesterol concentration, blood pressure, and blood glucose now respond to our present diet rich in fats and sugar by predisposing people to major diseases, including coronary heart disease, hypertension, and diabetes.

CARDIOVASCULAR DISEASE

The chief cause of death in the United States and other industrialized societies is cardiovascular disease. Atherosclerosis—the clogging of the arteries by fats—is the principal cause of heart attacks and accounts for the majority of these deaths. Smoking, hypertension, and elevated serum cholesterol are the three major correctable risk factors for coronary heart disease. The predominant clinical and public health approach to this problem has been to try to modify these risk factors through changes in life-style by encouraging people to stop smoking and to lower their blood pressure and cholesterol.

Coronary heart disease is clearly a disease of many components, and researchers believe that nutrition and genetic factors are major contributors to it. Its tendency to cluster in families is rarely caused by a single gene defect but rather from the cumulative interaction of a number of genes with environmental factors, including diet. Coronary heart disease is a complex disorder that involves abnormalities in plasma lipoproteins, protein-coated packages that carry fat and cholesterol through the blood. They include high-density lipoproteins (HDL), sometimes referred to as "good" cholesterol; low-density lipoproteins (LDL), sometimes referred to as "bad" cholesterol; apolipoprotein A (ApoA); apolipoprotein B (ApoB); apolipoprotein E (ApoE); and lipoprotein (a) (Lp[a]). Also, the clotting system, the cellular elements of the blood, the cells that line the cavities of the heart and blood vessels, and the arterial walls all play a part in the development of coronary heart disease (CHD). Because of this, the number of genes involved is large.

Modern genetic techniques have identified an extensive array of genes involved in the normal regulation and function of the cardiovascular system (see Table 6.8). These new genetic markers contribute to our ability to predict the risk of heart disease. Identifying individuals at high genetic risk early in their lives is a very powerful health-care strategy for the prevention of heart disease.

Researchers have studied three disorders extensively and consider them to be due to single-gene defects: familial combined hyperlipidemia, familial hypercholesterolemia, and familial hypertriglyceridemia. In fact, it was the research findings from these conditions, particularly familial hypercholesterolemia, that led to the emphasis on serum cholesterol as an important risk factor in coronary heart disease. The dietary components that have been studied and found to be associated with elevated serum cholesterol levels have mainly been saturated fats and cholesterol. This approach has led to the emphasis on these dietary lipids in the development of heart disease.

Recently, however, research has been generating information on both genetic and other nutritional factors involved in coagulation defects that thicken the blood and increase platelet clumping leading to the formation of clots and subsequent heart attacks. Today we know that the risk for the multifactorial-multigenic form of CHD is 8 percent higher for men but only 3 percent higher for women with a family history of heart disease. We also know that 50 percent of the difference in the level of blood cholesterol is genetic.

Another risk factor is the amount of fibrinogen in the blood. Fibrinogen is a protein that is part of the coagulation system. Investigators have recently shown that genetic variation at the fibrin-

Table 6.8 Genetic Determinants and Environmental Risk Factors for CHD

Genetic Determinants

family history of CHD at an early age
total serum cholesterol, LDL, and ApoB levels
HDL cholesterol, ApoA-I, and ApoA-II levels
Lp(a) lipoprotein
LDL receptor activity
thrombosis/coagulation parameters
triglycerides and VLDL concentrations
RFLPs in DNA at the ApoA-I/ApoC-III, and ApoB loci
other DNA markers
blood pressure
diabetes
obesity
insulin level and insulin response
heterozygosity for homocystinuria

Environmental Risk Factors

smoking
sedentary life-style (lack of aerobic exercise)
diet (excess energy intake)
   high-saturated-fat intake
   low ω-3 fatty acids intake
psychosocial factors
   Type A personality
   social class

Source: A. P. Simopoulos, "Nutrition Policies for the Prevention of Atherosclerosis in Industrialized Societies," *Diet and Life Style*, edited by M. F. Moyal (John Libbey Eurotext, 1988), p. 377.

ogen level accounts for 15 percent of the total plasma fibrinogen concentration and, therefore, genetic predisposition affects clotting and the risk of heart attacks.

Researchers now recognize that genetic factors play a role in most of the hyperlipidemias, the diseases that increase the risk of heart trouble, because they all involve abnormalities in the way the body handles fat. In fact, an individual's lipid level is determined by both genetic heritage and environmental influences, such as diet, exercise, and smoking.

Three common genetic lipoprotein disorders are associated with premature coronary heart disease. Familial combined hyperlipidemia accounts for 15 percent of persons who develop heart attacks; familial hypertriglyceridemia accounts for 5 percent; and familial hypercholesterolemia accounts for another 5 percent of all persons with CHD who develop heart attacks. In familial combined hyperlipidemia, both triglycerides and serum cholesterol are raised; in familial hypertriglyceridemia, only the triglycerides are increased; and in familial hypercholesterolemia, only the serum cholesterol is elevated. These diseases affect both genders, but men develop symptoms 10 years earlier than women.

Researchers have studied familial hypercholesterolemia thoroughly. Over the years, they have noted that not everyone with high serum cholesterol developed heart disease and had a heart attack. A recent study that investigated the relatives of persons with the genetic form of hypercholesterolemia shed new light when it found another lipoprotein, called lipoprotein (a)—Lp(a). When elevated, Lp(a) increases the risk of heart disease in individuals who have received the gene for hypercholesterolemia from one parent. Among the patients in this study, most of the men and women who developed CHD had increased amounts of Lp(a) in their blood. This is an important finding, because genes determine the level of Lp(a), which causes blood clots and plaque accumulation.

Up to now, the treatment of hypercholesterolemia has been dominated by efforts to lower only serum cholesterol levels, and the drugs that have been developed do this by interfering with cholesterol metabolism. This new study makes it clear that doctors must consider lowering Lp(a) as well.

Two other lipoproteins influence the development of heart disease. Decreased amounts of both high-density, or "good," lipoprotein (HDL) and apolipoprotein A-I (ApoA-I) in blood have been associated with the premature development of coronary heart disease. Recent studies indicate that the genetic HDL deficiency may be the most common genetic lipoprotein disorder in patients with CHD in the United States.

Many factors affect HDL-cholesterol levels in addition to genetics. Obesity, a sedentary life-style, elevated triglycerides, diabetes mellitus, cigarette smoking, and being a male are all associated with decreased levels of HDL.

Current U.S. nutrition policies are based on screening for total serum cholesterol. This is not a *comprehensive* approach for the control of atherosclerosis, because it ignores the role of blood clots (thrombosis) as a risk for CHD. Of course, a high level of serum cholesterol is a major risk factor for heart disease and correlates with the low-density lipoprotein (LDL), or "bad," cholesterol. However, HDL is also significant, because the higher the HDL reading, the lower the risk of heart disease. HDL is particularly important for women, since studies have shown that, in women, it is the low HDL that correlates with heart attack (myocardial infarction) and not the total cholesterol.

There is general agreement that ideal total blood cholesterol values should be below 200 milligrams per deciliter (mg/dl) of blood plasma and that individuals whose cholesterol exceeds 250 mg/dl should be treated to reduce it. On the other hand, no such definite guidelines exist for levels of HDL cholesterol, which are so important for determining cardiovascular risk in women.

The study group of the European Atherosclerosis Society (1987) provisionally set a cutoff point of 35 mg/dl for the lower limit of HDL cholesterol. Prospective epidemiologic studies have indicated that the level of HDL is an independent inverse risk factor for heart disease and that each rise in HDL cholesterol of 1 mg/dl is associated with a 2 to 4 percent decrease in the incidence of heart disease.

In fact, the emphasis on decreasing dietary cholesterol to reduce serum cholesterol levels completely disregards individual differences in handling the metabolism of dietary cholesterol. For example, a recent study of 50 men 43 to 50 years of age who were free of cardiovascular disease found that, even with a fourfold increase in dietary cholesterol, two-thirds of the subjects did not exhibit an increase in blood cholesterol concentration. These men appeared to compensate for increased dietary intake by either decreasing absorption or reducing their bodies' cholesterol production.

In the near future, it should be possible to identify *all* individuals at risk and determine their susceptibility to developing coronary heart disease and heart attacks. At present, using family and genetic studies, physicians can determine susceptibility to heart attacks more specifically than by the serum cholesterol level alone. The cardiologist should take a family history and order the necessary tests, such as total cholesterol, LDL, HDL, ApoB, ApoA-I, Lp(a), ApoE, and so forth.

DIETARY RECOMMENDATIONS TO REDUCE
CORONARY HEART DISEASE RISK IN WOMEN

The most important protective action you can take to reduce your risk of heart attack is to achieve your desirable body weight by reducing calories and increasing exercise. Switch from saturated (hydrogenated) oils such as butter and margarines to olive oil to avoid lowering your HDL and, perhaps, to maintain or increase it. (Be aware, however, that *all* fats are high in calories.) Substantially reduce your consumption of red meat and substitute poultry and fish, and decrease the amount of saturated fat in your diet from other high-fat meats and dairy products. Read the labels when you shop for groceries so you can avoid hydrogenated oils (margarines) and vegetable oils in prepared foods. Be sure to eat at least 60 grams of protein a day, which you can get from nonfat milk, poultry, lean meat, fish, and beans. Some of the low-fat cookbooks contain wonderful menus and recipes: get one, and resist the high-fat alternatives. Limit your calories to about 1,900 to 2,000 daily.

If members of your family under 45 years of age have a history of heart disease or any of the hyperlipidemias, seek medical care to determine how great your genetic risk is and what other dietary and life-style strategies you can adopt to prevent or delay the development of these diseases.

HYPERTENSION

Hypertension—high blood pressure—is a risk factor for CHD as well as for other life-threatening conditions, such as kidney failure, stroke, and congestive heart failure. It is more common in women than in men. A recent government study defined hypertension as a systolic measurement of at least 160 millimeters of mercury or a diastolic measurement above 95. Using that criterion, 24 million Americans had high blood pressure uncontrolled by diet or medication; 30 percent of African American adults and 17 percent of Caucasian adults suffered from this disease. Substantially more African American women experienced high blood pressure than did Caucasian women between 18 and 74 years of age; the same was true for African American men compared to Caucasian men in the 25-to-64 age bracket.

Weight gain in adult life increases blood pressure, and weight reduction lowers it. This effect is apparent in both sexes and at all ages. Losing weight lowers blood pressure independently of sodium intake in obese patients with both normal and high blood pressure.

Hypertension, which is our most common disease and is also responsible for a great amount of disability and death, is difficult to control. Little wonder that it is now the leading reason for office visits to physicians and responsible for the largest portion of pharmaceutical sales.

Despite a tremendous increase in the number of patients identified as hypertensive and started on antihypertensive therapy, and despite a significant drop in illness and death from cardiovascular disease in the United States that almost certainly reflects the greater identification and treatment of high blood pressure, major problems remain in our management of hypertension.

The problems arise mainly from our lack of understanding of the *causes* of elevated blood pressure in more than 95 percent of hypertensive patients. Whether we refer to it as primary or idiopathic, hypertension is almost always of unknown cause. Researchers hypothesize that heredity must be involved, although the genetic connection has yet to be established.

The role of sodium in hypertension has received a great deal of attention. Excessive sodium intake raises blood pressure in sodium-sensitive individuals, but whether moderate sodium intake will prevent the onset of hypertension is still unclear. Since it is not possible to identify those who are salt-sensitive, lowering your salt intake makes sense if you or others in your family have high blood pressure.

Although obesity in women is the most serious risk factor for hypertension, alcohol, low dietary potassium, low dietary calcium, and high dietary sodium intake all raise the blood pressure. If there is hypertension in your family, or if your blood pressure is already elevated, you should work hard to maintain your weight within the range of the Desirable Body Weight table (see Table 6.1). Limit your alcohol intake to two drinks per day or less. Make sure that there is an adequate amount of calcium in your diet, since studies have shown that consuming fewer than 800 milligrams of calcium daily is associated with an increase in blood pressure. Eat plenty of vegetables and fruits, particularly bananas, an excellent source of potassium, and decrease the amount of salt in your diet. When you raise potassium intake, you elevate the potassium-to-sodium ratio. A low ratio is associated with high blood pressure.

CANCER

Dietary patterns influence most major cancers. Nevertheless, researchers lack sufficient data to evaluate the contribution of diet to overall cancer risk, or to determine the percent reduction in risk that might be achieved by dietary modifications.

In general, observation and research have shown that populations with relatively low-fat, low-caloric diets have less cancer and coronary heart disease than those who consume greater amounts of fat, particularly meat.

Cancer researchers are also investigating other nutrients, such as beta carotene and vitamin C—because of their role as antioxidants—as well as fiber. In epidemiologic and some experimental studies, fiber intake of more than 20 grams daily is associated with lower rates of colon cancer. Again, eating more fish and poultry and less meat; increasing your intake of green, yellow, and orange fruits and vegetables; eating more fiber; and limiting calories to about 1,900 to 2,000 daily will help you maintain a healthy nutritional life.

Breast cancer is the most common cause of death from cancer among women between the ages of 40 and 44. We know that hormones affect breast cancer, but diet also plays a role, especially high-fat diets. Excess fat intake also seems to be a factor in uterine cancer, but in both of these cancers, researchers have not distinguished between the impact of high total fat as opposed to high caloric intake. The evidence for an association between uterine cancer and diet is indirect, based on similar rates of the incidence of this disease and cancers of the breast and colon. Cancer of the uterus does not appear to be related to any one factor in the diet, but there is an association between this type of cancer and obesity as well as higher socioeconomic status.

The same pattern is true of ovarian cancer: There is indirect evidence of a relationship between the incidence of ovarian cancer and other diet-associated cancers, especially cancers of the breast and colon. Both high-fat and high-caloric consumption correlate with the incidence of and mortality from ovarian cancer.

Epidemiologic studies have provided strong evidence that cervical dysplasia, a precancerous condition, is sexually transmitted, and that the use of oral contraceptives as well as low folate levels influence a woman's risk of developing this condition. Although researchers do not know if it is the oral contraceptives or the low folate at work, you might want to eat more foods containing folate (see Table 6.5), or take a multivitamin that contains folate as a precaution.

OSTEOPOROSIS

One of the most serious health threats to postmenopausal women is the decrease in bone mass termed *osteoporosis*, the major underlying cause of bone fractures. (See Chapter 15.)

Doctors diagnose primary osteoporosis by documenting reduced bone density in a patient who has a typical fracture yet shows no other cause of excessive bone loss. A fall, a blow, or a lifting action that would not bruise or strain the average person can easily precipitate one or more broken bones in a person with severe osteoporosis.

Osteoporosis affects women in their 50s or 60s and continues to increase as women age. These who have passed menopause are especially vulnerable to it, because changes in the body's hormone levels accelerate the loss of bone tissue. As estrogen levels decrease, the body does not absorb calcium as easily as before and draws on calcium from the bones for other metabolic needs. However, the news is not all bleak. A recent study of 301 women with low calcium intake conducted by the Human Nutrition Research Center on Aging at Tufts University found that women over 55 can keep their bones strong by consuming 800 milligrams of calcium daily—the amount in three glasses of milk. While adding calcium to the diet did nothing to prevent bone loss in the first five years after menopause, ingestion of sufficient calcium stopped further erosion in the hips, wrists, and spine.

The Role of Vitamin D in Osteoporosis

The body requires vitamin D to absorb calcium and phosphorus from food, and milk fortified with vitamin D is one of the major sources of this vitamin. We also get it from the sun. People who live in climates with decreased winter sunlight often don't receive adequate amounts of vitamin D unless they drink fortified milk. One of the negative effects of a drop in vitamin D is an increase of parathyroid hormone secretions, which accelerates bone loss.

Estimates of the dietary requirement of vitamin D in elderly people differ widely and reflect the lack of information about their vitamin D requirements. Doctors can test the blood for vitamin D

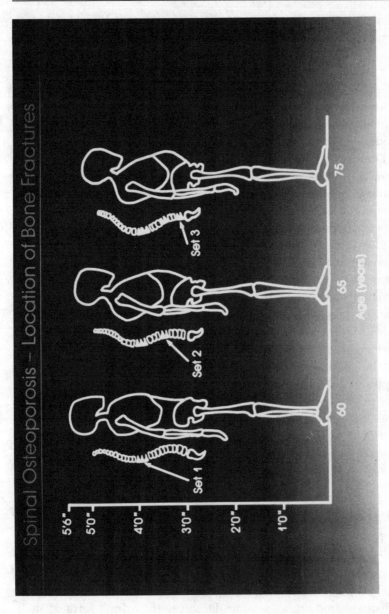

Fig. 6.3　Bone Loss in Osteoporosis

levels, but concentrations in normal subjects vary widely, which reflects the influence of both dietary intake and seasonal differences on vitamin D blood levels—high values occur in summer and lower ones in winter. A study of 333 healthy postmenopausal Caucasian women living in eastern Massachusetts found that they needed 220 international units (IU) of vitamin D daily to prevent a seasonal variation of vitamin D and parathyroid levels in their blood.

In terms of the treatment of osteoporosis, recent studies of the biologically active metabolites of vitamin D have led to new concepts of calcium balance. One of these metabolites, the 1,25-dihydroxycholecalciferol form, has been identified as the major hormone that controls calcium absorption. Because of this, derivatives of vitamin D may be an effective preventive treatment for postmenopausal osteoporosis.

Treatment

No safe and effective treatment is currently available to replace bone lost after menopause and during aging; women, therefore, need to adopt preventive strategies so that those at risk can be identified before bone loss occurs. Risk factors for hip fracture include:

1. Family history: Studies of identical and fraternal twins indicate that genetic factors may play an important role in determining bone mass loss.
2. Reduced bone mass: A recent study of the daughters of women with osteoporosis found that these women have reduced bone mass in the lower (lumbar) spine and, perhaps, in the neck of the thigh bone (femur), and that postmenopausal osteoporosis may result partly from a relatively low peak bone mass rather than from the excessive loss of bone.
3. Age-related elements: Poor vision, muscle weakness, fear of falling, and unsteady gait put older women at greatly increased risk for hip fractures. Specialists in orthopedics recommend that women have measurements made of their bone density before menopause, so that they can be compared to postmenopausal measurements.

Until research produces better data about precisely who is at risk for fracture, if your mother or grandmother had or has osteoporosis and/or hip fractures, you should have your bone mass measured, since you are at increased risk for hip fractures. Consume 1,200–1,500 milligrams of calcium daily and adequate vitamin D; a quart of fortified milk takes care of both requirements. If you cannot get this much calcium from your diet, use calcium supplements. Consult your doctor about the possibility and advisability of treatment with vitamin D derivatives. Start a regular program of modest exercise, either walking, biking, or jogging. At your own menopause, you should carefully consider the possibility of estrogen-replacement therapy (ERT). (See Chapter 15 for more on the pros and cons of ERT.)

DIETARY RECOMMENDATIONS FOR THE PREVENTION OF CHRONIC DISEASES

There is no evidence that, for the general population, a single or individual nutrient will prevent the major chronic killer diseases—coronary heart disease, high blood pressure, and cancer. In affluent societies health messages that a single food or nutrient might prevent disease are inappropriate and not consistent with the scientific evidence. The most relevant health advice should be formulated by considering your own *individual* history and should include the following considerations:

- Know your family history.
- Make appropriate dietary and life-style changes to promote your health based on your genetic background.
- Maintain desirable body weight.
- Eat a variety of foods.
- Balance your energy intake with your energy expenditure; if you are overweight, decrease your food intake and increase your energy expenditure.
- Decrease your total fat intake
  (1) Decrease your consumption of saturated fats.
  (2) Decrease your consumption of polyunsaturated fats.
  (3) Balance omega-3 fatty acids with omega-6 fatty acids by eating fish 2 to 3 times a week.
- Don't be influenced by fad diets or the claims of inappropriate supplements or additives

7

Birth Control

Florence Haseltine, M.D.

The ability of women to regulate their fertility is an important factor
in their physical and mental health. The search for adequate methods of birth control goes far back in history. Women in primitive
societies wore amulets made from a child's tooth or a weasel's
testicles to ward off unwanted pregnancies. Some early societies
recognized the cyclical nature of a woman's reproductive cycle and
knew about the "safe period," when conception was unlikely.
Egyptian women made a vaginal paste of honey, sodium carbonate,
and crocodile dung to prevent conception, and women during the
Middle Ages actually put salt in their vaginas. Douches date back
to 2000 B.C., and condoms made from materials as varied as linen
and animal intestines were described as early as the sixteenth century. For centuries, women have soaked sea sponges in lemon juice
or vinegar and put them in the vagina as barriers. The cervical cap
appeared in 1823, and the diaphragm was invented in the late
nineteenth century. And couples have practiced one of the oldest
methods of birth control, coitus interruptus—removing the penis
from the vagina before ejaculation—for hundreds of years.

Despite our high level of technological achievement in other
areas, relatively few contraceptive methods are available in the

United States. This fact takes on special significance when we consider that recent studies from the 1988 National Survey of Family Growth show that more than half (53 percent) of the pregnancies in the United States are unplanned—that is, occur before a woman feels ready to have a child, or after she has completed her family and does not want any more children. Moreover, the studies showed that of the couples who conceived, 30 percent reported having used a contraceptive. In other words, almost 20 percent of all U.S. pregnancies occur while a couple employs some method of birth control, indicating that the available contraceptives are not very reliable for the population as a whole. What this means is that, even if a man and woman who do not want a child use contraceptives diligently and carefully throughout their reproductive life spans, they still have close to a 70 percent chance of experiencing at least one unplanned pregnancy.

The cost we pay as a nation for this inadequate birth control is high. Fifty percent of all unintended pregnancies end in abortion. For young people under the age of 20, the rate is much higher; they terminate 80 percent of their pregnancies voluntarily. Abortion has become the chief method of birth control for this population, a practice that more and better contraceptive methods would greatly reduce.

WHY ARE SO FEW CONTRACEPTIVE METHODS AVAILABLE?

One reason for contraceptive failure is the absence of adequate contraception for both sexes.

INADEQUATE MALE CONTRACEPTION

Men have access to only two methods of contraception: the condom and sterilization. Many males dislike condoms, partly because putting one on and taking it off interrupts the sexual scenario and may diminish feeling during penetration; and sterilization is hardly an answer for the man who wants to prevent conception now but hopes to have a family later, as it is usually irreversible.

Attempts have been made to develop a male contraceptive that prevents sperm formation by the injection of certain substances, such as testosterone alone or in conjunction with gonadotropin-releasing factor antagonists. One of the major concerns that plagues this sort of research is that such medications are not 100 percent effective. Another is that men who are to use them with any success must do so daily, or at least on a regular basis.

Men also worry that such hormone-altering preparations may negatively affect their sexual drive, and a primary consideration of researchers and policymakers has been not to interfere with male arousal and sexual capacity. The effect of contraceptives on women's libido has never received equal concern, despite the fact that some women have reported a decreased sexual desire with hormonal therapy.

THE LACK OF RESEARCH

Not only is there an absence of adequate methods of contraception for both sexes, but drug companies that traditionally engage in medical research refuse to develop new methods because they fear they will be held financially liable if their products fail or cause harm. In fact, only one major U.S. pharmaceutical company does any contraceptive research at all. The fear is not unfounded. A. H. Robins was forced to remove its Dalkon Shield intrauterine device (IUD) from the market in 1975 because it was associated with deaths, severe pelvic infections, and perforation of the uterus. Ten years later the company went into bankruptcy after more than 10,000 lawsuits had been filed against it. Fear of similar litigation and financial loss have kept other drug companies from conducting contraceptive research, leaving only two IUDs on the market. Frequent reports of the side effects associated with other contraceptive methods have rendered drug companies even more fearful and unwilling to venture into new areas of research.

CHOOSING A CONTRACEPTIVE METHOD

When deciding about contraceptives, couples must consider safety, efficacy, cost, convenience, availability, protection against sexually transmitted diseases (STDs), their emotional responses to various methods, and the benefits and risks involved. No one method of

Table 7.1 Characteristics and Effectiveness of Contraceptive Methods
Generally Available in the United States

Method	Estimated % Use Among Contraceptors	% Accidental Pregnancy in the 1st Year of Use	What It Is and How It Works	Advantages	Disadvantages
Male sterilization (vasectomy)	14	0.15	Permanent method in which the vas deferens, through which the sperm travel from the testes to the penis, is cut and blocked so that sperm can no longer enter the semen.	Single procedure; no subsequent health or safety risks; failure of procedure is very rare.	Requires skilled medical practitioner; minor complications including swelling and pain are common; blood clots, infection, and epididymitis occur in 1–2% of patients; death from infection can occur but is very rare; procedure should be considered permanent, although with skilled micro-surgical techniques it can be reversed in about 50% of cases.
Female sterilization	19	0.4	Permanent method of contraception in which the fallopian tubes are occluded so that the	Single procedure; little health or safety risk; failure of procedure is rare.	Requires skilled medical practitioner; complications are rare (bleeding, infection,

Method			Description	Advantages	Disadvantages
			egg and sperm cannot meet. The tubes are surgically closed with bands, clips, electrocautery, or by cutting and tying. Laparoscopy, minilaparotomy, and postpartum laparotomy are the surgical procedures used.		injury to other organs, anesthesia complications); death can occur but is very rare; reversibility is limited and requires abdominal microsurgical procedure in skilled hands.
Combined (estrogen and progestin) oral contraceptive pill (OCP)	32	3	The oral contraceptive pill combines synthetic forms of the hormones progesterone and estrogen. Stops ovulation by interfering with cyclical hormonal changes required for ovulation. Pills are taken every day in 21-day cycles (or 28-day cycles, with 7 placebo tablets).	Easily used; reduces about 50% of the risk of certain pelvic infections; decreases risk of ovarian and uterine cancer by approximately 50% compared with nonusers of OCPs; causes regular painless menstrual periods with decreased blood loss (may help or correct anemia); protects against ectopic pregnancy, benign cystic breast disease, and ovarian cysts.	OCPs have an inhibiting effect on lactation. Failure rate increases if the pill is not taken regularly; common side effects include breast tenderness, nausea, depression, headache, vomiting, weight gain or loss, spotting between periods. Earlier high-dose OCPs were associated with a greater risk of cardiovascular diseases such as blood clots, heart attacks, and strokes; risk of heart attack and stroke increases for users over

Method	Estimated % Use Among Contraceptors	% Accidental Pregnancy in the 1st Year of Use	What It Is and How It Works	Advantages	Disadvantages
					age 35 who smoke, and/or have high blood pressure. OCP users have a greater risk than nonusers of developing gallbladder symptoms, but only during first year of use.
Oral contraceptive pill (OCP), progestin-only (minipill)	(unavailable for minipill)	5	The minipill contains progestin only. It is taken continuously and causes thickening of the cervical mucus, decreasing its penetrability to spermatozoa. It produces atrophy of the endometrium, interfering with implantation. It also may inhibit ovulation.	The minipill does not affect lactation; does not cause the OCP-related side effects, high blood pressure, and headaches.	The minipill has a higher pregnancy rate than combined OCPs; is more likely to cause menstrual irregularity and vaginal bleeding.

Intrauterine device (IUD)	3	6	Small plastic device placed in the uterus that is believed to induce an unsuitable environment for both eggs and sperm, but the process is still unclear. The two available IUDs in the United States include Progestasert, which releases progesterone and is replaced yearly, and Cu-T 380A, which contains copper and is replaced every 4 years.	Single procedure provides effective long-term protection; progesterone-releasing IUDs decrease bleeding in contrast to other IUDs.	Insertion requires trained health-care practitioner; common side effects include increased bleeding or spotting, cramping, and pain; perforation occurs in about 1/2,500 insertions; pregnancy while an IUD is in place may be ectopic or result in a septic spontaneous abortion—both potentially life-threatening; pelvic inflammatory disease (PID) is a rare but serious complication, seen most commonly as a result of an STD. PID rarer among women in monogamous relationships.
Condom	17	12	Sheath of thin rubber (latex) that is placed on the erect penis to collect semen and to prevent sperm from entering the vagina.	Easy to use; inexpensive; does not require a prescription; protects against STDs, including AIDS.	Condoms deteriorate and are ineffective when stored in too much heat, humidity, or sunlight and may tear if roughly handled.

Method	Estimated % Use Among Contraceptors	% Accidental Pregnancy in the 1st Year of Use	What It Is and How It Works	Advantages	Disadvantages
Diaphragm	4–6	2–23*	Soft rubber cup that covers the cervix. Contraceptive cream or jelly is placed in the diaphragm before intercourse.	Protects against certain STDs and cervical cancer; can be used safely by nursing mothers.	Women who use the diaphragm may be more prone to bladder infections; allergic reaction to rubber or cream or jelly is possible; diaphragm may dislodge during sexual intercourse; diaphragm must be cleaned and checked for weak spots and holes; requires fitting by a trained health-care worker; not recommended for women with poor vaginal muscle tone.
Contraceptive sponge	3	18	Synthetic substance that is soft, round, and impregnated with spermicide. The sponge is inserted into the vagina before sexual intercourse, where it	Does not require prescription; may protect against certain STDs.	Removal problems may occur; may cause an allergic reaction; risk of pregnancy is higher than with other reversible

Method					
	4		releases spermicide. The sponge is for one-time use only over a 24-hour period and should never be reused.	Requires no drugs.	methods; possible risk of toxic shock reported.
Natural fertility control (forms of periodic abstinence)	4	20	Requires the couple to refrain from sexual intercourse during the fertile period of a woman's menstrual cycle. The most common ways used to determine the approximate time of ovulation and the fertile period include the calendar, temperature, and cervical mucus methods.	Requires no drugs.	Risk of pregnancy is high; requires high motivation of both sexual partners.
Vaginal contraceptives	2	21	Foams, creams, jellies, tablets, and suppositories that contain spermicides and are inserted into the vagina before intercourse. They inactivate sperm and mechanically prevent sperm from entering the uterus.	Do not require prescription; may protect against certain STDs; may be used by any woman unless she is allergic to the product.	Relatively unreliable and must be inserted 5–10 minutes before each act of intercourse; may produce slight genital irritation.

*Training and proper use are critical; see text.

Source: Luigi Mastroianni, Jr., Peter J. Donaldson, and Thomas T. Kane, eds., *Developing New Contraceptives: Obstacles and Opportunities* (Washington, DC: National Academy Press, 1990).

contraception is ideal or totally reliable, and choice is a matter of balancing advantages and disadvantages (see Table 7.1).

EFFICACY

If you intend never to have children, or if you have finished having a family, sterilization is the most effective method of birth control available today. If pregnancy would spell disaster now, but you want children later, you might choose the oral contraception pill or Norplant, the newly approved hormonal implant system in which several small tubes are inserted under the skin and provide contraceptive protection for five years. Norplant's rate of failure is 1/10 to 1/20 that of oral contraceptives, which have a failure rate of only 3 percent for average users. Barrier methods fail between 12 and 21 percent of the time. Or you might want to use double protection, such as a diaphragm in combination with a condom.

Failure rates should be considered with care. What is referred to as the best reported rate represents the least degree of failure ever reported in a reputable clinical trial, while the typical rate of failure is exactly what it implies—the rate that is typical of most users. If you are more careful than the standard user, you will have less risk of failure, while if you take chances—even if only one—you may find yourself pregnant (see Table 7.2).

Older women have better success with contraception than younger women do. Beyond the method they choose and how careful they are at following directions, many other factors probably account for this. Young women may be more fertile, or have sex more often, or be less fearful of becoming pregnant because they plan to have a child "later" anyway. Older women who have completed their families may have more at stake, pregnancy may be more difficult and more dangerous for them, and they may not want to interrupt their careers. They may also be more adept and consistent at using birth control than younger women.

CHANGING CONTRACEPTIVE METHODS

Different contraceptives may be appropriate at various times in your life, and having the flexibility to change from one to another is valuable. For example, if you are currently very active sexually, you may prefer the birth control pill because it provides continuous

Table 7.2 Contraceptive Method Failures in the United States*

Method	% Users	No. (millions)	% Accidental Pregnancies	No. Accidental Pregnancies (1st year)
Male sterilization	14	4.2	0.15	6,300
Female sterilization	19	5.7	0.40	22,800
OCPs	32	9.6	3	288,000
IUD	3	0.9	6	54,000
Condom	17	5.1	12	612,000
Diaphragm	5	1.5	5	75,000
Sponge	3	0.9	18	162,000
Natural	4	1.2	20	240,000
Vaginal contraceptive	2	0.6	21	126,000
				Total: 1,586,100

*Based on estimated 30 million contraceptors in the United States.
Adapted from National Academy of Sciences, *Developing New Contraceptives: Obstacles and Opportunities* (National Academy Press: Washington, D.C., 1990).

protection (as long as you remember to take it) and doesn't interrupt lovemaking. At another time in your life, when you may not be having sex as often, a diaphragm may be a good choice.

COST AND CONVENIENCE

Condoms, sponges, and foam are all inexpensive methods of birth control that are available without prescription at a drugstore. Although cost and convenience probably do not affect a woman's initial choice, they certainly play a role in whether she will continue to use a given product.

INDIVIDUAL NEEDS

How a type of contraception will fit into your life-style is important. If you don't want children now but plan to have them in the future, be sure to consider the effect of the method you choose on your fertility. If you have several lovers, or if your only partner has other lovers, your chance of contracting an STD is high, and you might want to use a barrier method—for example, the diaphragm—which cuts in half your risk of contracting such a disease. All barrier methods require the accompanying use of spermicidal jellies, which not only kill the sperm but also destroy other microorganisms. (See Chapter 11.)

Talking about your own sexual history, or asking a new lover about his, can be a touchy and difficult subject, but unless you discuss it, you have no way of knowing whether your new partner currently has, or recently has had, multiple sexual partners. If you are interested in establishing a mutually monogamous relationship, it is wise to bring this issue up at the beginning of the relationship, because it has significant bearing on the birth control method you choose. Until you establish that your partner does not have other lovers and is not at risk for sexually transmitted diseases from any recent partners he has had, you should use a barrier contraceptive to protect yourself from infection.

Fear also plays a part in the birth control decision; many people choose a contraceptive method by weighing their fears rather than the benefits. Although this is unfortunate because it regards choice as a negative decision rather than one that can produce greater control, fears are nevertheless very real and must be taken into account. If, after informing yourself about the facts, you are still uneasy about employing a particular method, it is best not to use it, because your tension about it may interfere with the pleasure of your sex life.

SAFETY

The prevailing philosophy is that a medication or device given to a healthy person should present no medical risks. Doctors who practice in clinics and offices throughout the country are aware of the frustration women feel when they realize that they may not be happy with any available method of birth control. Clinicians often hear women say they don't want to use a diaphragm because it is messy, or that their partners refuse to use condoms, or that they don't feel at ease about using oral contraceptives. All contraceptive methods are, at best, a compromise. Until more contraceptive choices are made available in the United States, the trick is finding the method that requires the fewest concessions on your part while conferring the greatest protection and safety.

Safety is probably the most important consideration in the selection of a method of birth control. How high is the risk that a given birth control method will cause illness or infertility? For example, although it is true that women who use the birth control pill have an increased risk of liver tumors, the risk is so small (five in 100,000) that this should not be a factor in your considering the Pill. On the other hand, you should be concerned about the incidence of thrombophlebitis (inflammation of a vein because of the formation of blood clots) among women who use the Pill, because it is far more common. The risk, traditionally given as one in 1,000 users, is now less than that with the new, low-dose pill; for cigarette smokers, however, the risk of thrombophlebitis is much higher. You might want to ask your doctor whether or not the Pill would increase your individual chance of triggering this condition, considering your family history and the current state of your health. Similarly, if breast cancer is a concern, it will comfort you to know that, as of the 1991 statistics, epidemiologists have not seen an increase in the incidence of breast cancer among women who have used the Pill. Again, however, this information must be considered in terms of your individual risk. Thirty years of studying the epidemiology of this cancer have turned up five risk factors that account for 20 percent of all breast cancers. They include having had breast cancer, having a mother or sister with breast cancer, not having had children, starting to menstruate at a young age, and experiencing a late menopause. Although contraception will not be an issue if you are postmenopausal, if any of the other four risk factors apply to you, you should be sure to discuss the advisability of using the Pill with your physician.

If you are contemplating an IUD, you should understand that the risk of its perforating the uterus is small (one in 2,500 insertions), as is the increased risk it presents of developing pelvic inflammatory disease (PID). Though rare, both of these events can be serious indeed. (See Chapter 11.)

Another way to assess safety is to compare the particular birth control method with the risk of pregnancy. Although very few women die either as a result of pregnancy or from using a specific method of birth control, some do. For example, the risk of death from pregnancy is one in 10,000, while a nonsmoker's risk of death from taking the Pill is one in 63,000, and for a woman who smokes, it is one in 16,000. There is no risk of death involved in using the barrier contraceptives (except the risk of death from pregnancy if they fail), and the death rate from abortion before the ninth week of pregnancy is one in 400,000.

BIRTH CONTROL METHODS

Contraception works either by frustrating fertilization, preventing contact between sperm and egg, or interfering with implantation.

One way to interfere with the ability of sperm and egg to fuse is to put a barrier either in the vagina or over the penis to prevent the sperm from entering the uterus. In considering all the barrier methods described here, take into account whether you may have a medical problem that could prevent you from safely using a particular device or its accompanying product. For example, if you're allergic to latex, you should not use a diaphragm, cervical cap, or condom made from this material. And if you're allergic or sensitive to spermicides, you obviously cannot use them. If you have had repeated urinary tract infections, using a diaphragm might not be wise. If you've had a bout of toxic shock syndrome, you need to be very careful when using the contraceptive sponge, and most physicians will advise against using a diaphragm.

DIAPHRAGM

The diaphragm is a widely used barrier method. You insert it up through your vagina, slip it securely over your cervix, and lodge it behind your pubic bone so that, when the penis ejaculates semen into the vagina, the sperm do not penetrate the barrier. The diaphragm must *always* be used with a spermicidal cream or gel, which kills sperm. The diaphragm alone does not prevent the sperm from advancing into the cervical canal, but it does hold the spermicidal cream or gel in place against the cervix, creating a contraceptive barrier. These contraceptive jellies are relatively expensive. A careful review of research studies has found no evidence that contraceptive spermicides can damage the fetus should you become pregnant.

The traditional diaphragm, a dome-shaped circle of latex with a flexible rim, covers the upper end of the vagina. Diaphragm rims have three types of springs: flat, coil, and arcing. The rim helps you insert and remove the diaphragm and keeps it in place during use.

Diaphragms come in various sizes and must be fitted after a pelvic examination by a medical practitioner, who will recommend the size you need by determining the width and depth of your vagina and how strong your vaginal muscle is. Since vaginal depth increases during sexual excitement, your clinician will fit you with the largest size that is comfortable, so that the diaphragm can stay securely in place during intercourse.

To insert the diaphragm, hold it with the dome down and fill it with about a tablespoon of spermicidal cream or gel; then spread some over the rim. Insertion will be easier if you stand with one foot raised, squat, or lie down on your back. First bend the diaphragm so that the cream or gel is compressed inside the dome; then, gripping both sides of the rim securely with one hand, slip it firmly up the back of your vagina as far as it will go, so that the rear rim is behind the cervix and the front of the rim is tucked behind the pubic bone. Test it with your finger to be certain you can feel the tip of your cervix through the rubber dome, and do this every time you insert it.

Make sure the clinician who fits you shows you how to apply the spermicide and to insert the diaphragm, and spends the time you need to practice once or twice during the fitting so that you can feel the interior of your vagina, the cervix, and the pubic bone and are comfortable with the device. If the diaphragm has been properly fitted and if you insert it correctly, you should not be aware of it during intercourse. If you are, check to make sure you have placed it properly, and if you or your partner are still bothered by it or if it causes discomfort, use another type of birth control until your doctor checks the fit.

Don't use your old diaphragm after you have given birth or after having had surgery of your reproductive tract until you have been examined for refitting. *A diaphragm that does not fit correctly will not protect you.*

After inserting your diaphragm, leave it in place for at least six hours after intercourse, which will give the gel or cream time to kill the sperm (after six hours, spermicides leak out of the vagina). If you have intercourse a second time during the six hours your diaphragm is in place, insert additional gel or cream with an applicator without removing the diaphragm, and leave the diaphragm in place for another six hours. (Remember this six-hour spermicide rule if you insert the diaphragm some time before having intercourse.)

To remove the diaphragm, place one finger up your vagina, grasp the rim, and pull gently; the diaphragm will bend easily and slip out. Be sure to wash it carefully, dry it well, put it in its container, and store it away from heat. Inspect it periodically for possible tears. Never use petroleum jelly (Vaseline) on the diaphragm; it makes latex deteriorate. *Never leave a diaphragm in place for more than 24 hours, as this increases the danger of toxic shock syndrome.* (See Chapter 11.)

The major advantage of the diaphragm and spermicidal agent is that the side effects and contraindications are few. The diaphragm also greatly reduces the risk of common infections, and anyone who is concerned about STDs should strongly consider this benefit.

The major disadvantage of the diaphragm is lack of efficacy. Its effectiveness depends totally on the user; it will not work if left on the shelf while you have intercourse, or if used without the necessary contraceptive cream or jelly, which is, after all, the actual spermicide. Because interrupting foreplay to insert the diaphragm has provided an obstacle to its use, it's best to put your diaphragm in place regularly even if you don't think it's likely that you will use it. This way, if you want to have sex, you can do so without stopping for birth control protection. Just remember that the spermicide works for only six hours. Having the diaphragm there when you need it can be ensured by owning more than one at a time—for home and office, for example, or home and travel.

The diaphragm's efficacy is also dependent on how well it fits. The main problem here is that the size of the vagina changes so much during intercourse that it is sometimes difficult to obtain an accurate fit that will accommodate a vagina that is one size when not aroused and expands to a much larger dimension during intercourse. Thus the diaphragm's range of effectiveness is between 65 and 95 percent.

Side effects, though infrequent, include occasional irritation to the point of causing bladder infection. (See Chapter 11.) Allergies to the contraceptive creams or jellies required are rare, but they do occur. Using the diaphragm also increases the risk of toxic shock syndrome, although the overall risk of this condition to a single individual remains very small. In fact, the risk-benefit analysis of using a diaphragm comes down sharply in favor of its use when you compare the heightened chance of contracting toxic shock syndrome to the increased protection against sexually transmitted diseases that it provides. This is because STDs are rampant, while the incidence of toxic shock syndrome is very low.

A woman who has had toxic shock syndrome or repeated urinary tract infections, is being treated for a cervical lesion, has recently had cervical surgery, or has just given birth should use any of the barrier devices—except condoms—with special care, and only after consulting a doctor.

CERVICAL CAP

Another barrier, the cervical cap, covers only the cervix and relies partially on suction to hold it in place. Its advantage is that it is smaller and therefore not as apt as the diaphragm to press against the vaginal wall. Of the three varieties of caps, which differ in size and shape, only Prentif has received approval from the Food and Drug Administration (FDA).

The cap must be fitted by a clinician after a pelvic examination, and you must use it with a spermicidal cream or gel. Fill the cap with spermicide, slide it up through your vagina and onto your cervix, and feel for the cervical tip through the cap's dome. Insertion is more difficult than with the diaphragm. You can insert the cap up to six hours before having intercourse, and it must be left in place for six hours afterward. You take it out the same way as you remove a diaphragm, but the process is more difficult because the cap is smaller, and the suction on the cervix is stronger. Clean and store the cap the same as you would a diaphragm.

Some practitioners are concerned that the cap may cause cervical and pelvic infections and precancerous changes, but no research to date supports this. The main problem with the cap is its lack of efficacy. One study conducted at the University of North Carolina in the early 1980s found that 15 percent of college-age cap users became pregnant.

VAGINAL SPONGE

A third barrier method is the vaginal polyurethane sponge that contains the spermicidal agent nonoxynol 9. You can buy the sponge without a prescription and throw it away after use. To use the sponge, first moisten it well with water, then compress it prior to placing it in the vagina. It will expand in the area around the cervix. Because the sponge absorbs a great deal of water, the vagina can become very dry after you insert it, and the lack of normal lubrication can cause discomfort during intercourse. If this happens, use extra spermicidal jelly to replace the lost fluid. The sponge should not be used during your period, because its use then increases the risk of toxic shock syndrome; however, like the diaphragm, it provides substantial protection against STDs. Side effects, though infrequent, are the same as with the diaphragm. You can leave the sponge in your vagina for up to 24 hours and do not have to add more spermicide. It should remain in place for at least six hours after intercourse and is removed by pulling the string attached to it.

FOAMS, GELS, CREAMS, SUPPOSITORIES, AND FILM

Each of these products contain chemicals that kill sperm. Inserted deeply into the vagina, they spread over the vagina and cervix.

Although the foams, gels, and creams are ready to work instantly after you apply them, suppositories and film require time to melt before they become effective. Each of the products gives you one hour of protection; if you have intercourse again, you require another application. For contraception to be effective, proper timing is vital.

Foams, gels, and creams require an applicator for insertion. Although douching is never necessary and in fact may kill normal body cells and thus reduce your protection against infection, if you do douche, wait at least six hours after intercourse. It is particularly important to read and follow the instructions that come with each of these products. If you experience burning, itching, bleeding, spotting, odor, or unusual discharge after using one of them, you should discontinue use, see your doctor to make sure you have no infection, and try another product next time, if your doctor agrees.

These methods of contraception are not as reliable as the diaphragm, the cervical cap, and the sponge; their typical failure rate is 21 percent. Still, some studies show they can be very effective, with a lowest reported failure rate of 3 percent. This means that if you follow the instructions, you should have reasonably good protection.

CONDOMS

Condoms are the only form of barrier contraception for the male, and 10 to 15 percent of couples use them. The most effective condom is made of latex and is sold stored in a rolled form. Condoms can be applied only after a man has an erection. The condom is the best method to prevent the spread of AIDS and other sexually transmitted diseases, but it is not a very effective method of birth control. This is because it must be put on at the time of intercourse and removed as soon as ejaculation has taken place. The condom's efficacy is also poor because it can slip off if the penis becomes flaccid when still within the vagina.

For proper use, the condom must be rolled correctly onto the erect penis. Even then, it can break during intercourse, and if it does or if leakage otherwise takes place, you have no protection against pregnancy or the spread of sexually transmitted diseases.

Condoms have a failure rate among typical users that is slightly greater than 12 percent, but if they are used with contraceptive foam, the combination is very effective. This approach has the added advantage of both partners' sharing the contraceptive responsibility. The use of condoms has apparently doubled since the public has become aware of the AIDS epidemic.

Condoms are available in a great variety of materials, including natural-membrane condoms made from lamb intestine. Beware of these, however: Although they transmit heat, they do not survive the rigors of intercourse as well as those made of latex, nor do they prevent the spread of viral infections as effectively. Since many people find the condom uncomfortable because of the sensation of dryness associated with it, it is best to use a vaginal contraceptive jelly as a lubricant. This gives you the added advantage of spermicidal and antimicrobial protection.

The greatest advantage of condoms is that they are relatively accessible and inexpensive. But condoms need to be improved. A condom that could go on a flaccid penis and stay in place throughout intercourse, that would grip the penis even while the erection disappeared, and that could then be removed by the man at will would be a major advancement over those on the market today.

ORAL CONTRACEPTIVES—THE PILL

Oral contraceptives were first tested in a large clinical trial in Puerto Rico in 1956, and by 1960 the FDA approved them for use in the United States. Since then, 80 percent of American women have tried the Pill—as it became known in the early 1960s—during their reproductive years, making it the single most popular method of contraceptive employed by nonsterile couples. By 1991, 10 million American women were using the Pill.

The introduction of the Pill changed women's thinking about contraceptives. The first generation of birth control pills were "high-dose" substances; the quantities of active compounds in them were far larger than the amounts actually needed to prevent conception, and many complications ensued as a result. Research showed, for example, that women who used the Pill were at elevated risk for cardiovascular disease and that many of the side effects were related to the dosage of the hormones in the medication. As a result, lower-dose pills replaced the earlier versions. Decreasing the dosage has lessened the formation and number of clots in blood vessels noted among users of the higher-dosage pill, but it is not clear whether the very low dose pills on the market today will not turn out to cause some other long-range problem.

How the Pill Works

Birth control pills work by replacing the normal menstrual cycle with a pill cycle. Taken as prescribed, the Pill interferes with the normal functioning of the reproductive tract in at least three sites needed to promote ovulation, fertilization, and implantation of a fertilized egg. It thus provides a triplex of chances to frustrate conception. First, the Pill changes the pituitary pattern governing the release of hormones that stimulate the ovaries to produce eggs, so that ovulation usually does not occur. Second, it makes the cervical mucus inhospitable to the sperm traveling through the cervix and into the uterus, impeding their ability to reach the fallopian tubes, where conception takes place. Third, it acts on the lining of the uterus so that, even if a follicle releases an egg and a sperm fertilizes it, the uterine lining is not receptive to implantation. (See Chapter 9.)

Chemically, the Pill consists of synthetic hormones—either one or two steroidal compounds that imitate the hormones that the body produces normally during the menstrual cycle: estrogen and progesterone. These synthetic hormones are administered in relatively small dosages as compared with their naturally occurring counterparts; for example, only about 30 micrograms (mcg) of ethinyl estradiol go into a birth control pill, while a pill using biological estrogen would require 625 mcg to be equally effective.

U.S. drug companies use only two estrogen compounds in producing birth control pills today, ethinyl estradiol and mestranol. However, six different types of progesterone are used. (Progesterones protect the uterine lining from uncontrolled bleeding. Menstruation occurs when a woman stops taking the progesterone-containing pill.) Some progesterones, such as norethynodrel, promote estrogenic activity and cause increased breast swelling and fluid retention. Others, like norethindrone acetate, are androgenic; because androgen is the male hormone, the pills containing it may cause acne and increased body hair growth (hirsutism) and promote changes in the blood lipid pattern that are more characteristic of men than of women. The level of estrogenic or androgenic reaction occurs both because of the drug itself and the extent to which it suppresses a woman's ovarian production, as well as how fat (adipose) tissue and the adrenal glands interact with the Pill hormones.

Using the Pill

Depending on which kind of Pill is being used, women take birth control pills for either 21 or 28 days out of a four-week cycle. If you use a 21-day brand, you will take one pill a day and then stop for seven days each month. The 28-day variety uses two different kinds of pills, 21 of which contain hormones, which you take sequentially first, and then seven filled with an inert powder or a powder combined with iron. With both types, you will menstruate during the seven hormone-free days—that is, have a Pill-induced period.

It is a good idea to take your pill at the same time each day and to connect this to a regular daily event, such as brushing your teeth or with your morning orange juice, because this makes it easier to remember. Some women mark their calendars every day when they take the Pill; if you do this, you will have a written record. Always have a backup method of birth control handy, such as a diaphragm, condoms, or sponges, because you will have to use one until you have taken the first 14 pills in your first package, if you stop taking the Pill, or if you miss taking more than one pill.

If you miss one pill, double up the next day. Take the first pill as soon as you realize you have forgotten to take it, and take the second one at the regular time.

If you miss two pills in a row, take two for the next two days: take the first one when you realize you have missed two days and the second one at the regular time. On the second day, take two at the regular time. Be sure to use your backup method until you have your next period.

If you miss three or more pills consecutively, stop taking them altogether, use your backup method of birth control, and wait for your next period; then start taking a new pack as you would normally after your period begins. Be sure to continue to use your backup birth control until you have taken the first 14 pills in the new pack.

Another type of Pill, the triphasic, uses three different quantities of progestin for different phases of each pill cycle. Overall, the amount of progestin is lower than in previous pills, and researchers hoped this would reduce possible negative blood lipid effects, but investigation has yet to document this benefit. Triphasics "mimic" the normal hormonal changes of a woman's natural cycle. However, since women take birth control pills to change the cycle, not to replicate it, such pills provide no particular benefit.

The Advantages of Oral Contraceptives

The Pill is 99 percent effective when used as directed, and its overall efficacy ranges from 95 to 99 percent. It does not interrupt lovemaking and provides continuous protection against pregnancy. It decreases whatever heavy menstrual bleeding and severe menstrual cramps may have been present, substituting instead a light, regular, and relatively painless period. It also protects you from several illnesses, providing a high degree of lifetime reduction in ovarian and endometrial cancer. Pill-takers are also less likely to develop

- iron deficiency anemia, because they bleed less
- benign breast disease (and the need for breast lump biopsies), because of the steady supply of hormones provided
- ovarian cysts, because they do not ovulate
- pelvic inflammatory disease (PID), possibly because less blood is present in the vagina to nourish bacteria and the thick mucus in the cervical canal keeps bacteria from getting to the uterus and tubes

The Disadvantages of Oral Contraceptives

The insert in a package of birth control pills contains a long list of side effects, but determining how common or how rare any of them are is difficult. The synthetic estrogen in the Pill classically causes minor complications, such as nausea, breast tenderness (with an increase in size), fluid retention, and headaches. More serious are the rare complications that occur when blood clots travel in the bloodstream from their site of origin to plug another blood vessel. This is particularly dangerous when the clot lands in the pulmonary artery or in one of the blood vessels in the head, robbing the heart and brain of their needed blood supply and oxygen and causing heart attack or stroke. The Pill also generates a slightly increased risk of benign and cancerous liver tumors, vascular lesions in small blood vessels, and the growth of fibroids. Using the Pill also produces a heightened chance of chlamydia infections, yeast infections, cervical gonorrhea, gallbladder disease, and cervical ectropion, which occurs when the glands lining the cervical canal grow out onto the surface of cervix, giving it a reddish appearance. Ectropion, which is more common in younger women, does not require treatment because it is not a dangerous condition. It sometimes confuses clinicians, however, who think what they are seeing is a change in cervical tissue.

The progesterone used in the Pill may cause other complications, including increased appetite and weight gain, depression, fatigue, decreased libido, acne, oily skin, increased breast size, decreased ability to tolerate carbohydrates, symptoms related to diabetes, headaches, and itching. Progesterone also may increase the level of low-density lipoproteins (LDL), the so-called bad cholesterol that promotes fatty accumulations in the blood vessels, while decreasing the beneficial high-density lipoproteins (HDL) that remove cholesterol from blood vessel walls. However, it is not clear that the progesterones used in the birth control pills prescribed in the United States today cause any of these side effects. The overall balance of estrogen and progesterone may neutralize the side effects of either hormone.

In combination, synthetic hormones used in the Pill can aggravate diabetic symptoms. They may also cause hypertension and cervical dysplasia, a precancerous condition of the cervix, and dark spots on the forehead, cheekbones, and upper lip called chloasma. Reducing the amount of estrogen in the Pill has lessened the risk of heart attacks but not of stroke. Stroke is a rare occurrence and is seen almost exclusively in smokers. Smoking, of course, increases the chance of developing cardiovascular disease, and many physicians will not prescribe the Pill to any woman over 35 who smokes.

Some women continue to take estrogen and progesterone beyond their reproductive years. This occurs when a gynecologist prescribes the birth control pill until a woman reaches menopause and then recommends hormone-replacement therapy for the same woman. The risks of taking the Pill until menopause have not been determined but seem low in healthy nonsmokers.

There is no evidence at present to indicate that taking the Pill will produce long-range side effects. However, we still have minimal information about such long-range consequences because the first group of women to use the Pill are only now entering menopause. In addition, the birth control pills that were available 20 to 30 years ago are not the ones women use today. Even if the first group of long-term users developed complications, researchers would still have to study the future lives of the women who have taken the lower-dose pills for many years.

There is no indication that "going off" the Pill periodically prevents undesirable side effects, but there is a great deal of evidence that vacations from the Pill result in a significant increase in pregnancy rates. It should also be noted that oral contraceptives provide no protection from sexually transmitted diseases. Some doctors feel that this may be the cause of the increased incidence of chlamydia and gonorrhea among Pill takers.

The Contraceptive and Reproductive Evaluation branch of the Center for Population Research at the National Institute of Child Health and Human Development monitors the health of women who have taken the Pill. They follow the complications among Pill users carefully and hope to be able to conduct studies that will determine long-term benefits and risks to women who have used them.

The main contraindications to using the Pill refer to the formation and movement of blood clots. *Do not use the Pill if you have thrombophlebitis, often manifested as blood clots in the leg veins; pulmonary embolism, a clot that may have lodged in the lung; or any clot that might plug a blood vessel, such as the retinal vein, the mesenteric vein, or the pelvic vein; cerebrovascular disease; or heart disease. In addition, if you smoke, have breast cancer, liver tumors, or are pregnant, you should not use birth control pills. Using the Pill while nursing will expose the newborn to the hormones the Pill contains, which can enter the breast milk.*

Other contraindications include high blood pressure, diabetes, and gallbladder disease. These contraindications and others are listed in the oral contraceptive package insert. Although they are well known to clinicians, you should consider them carefully.

Even assuming that you are free of any of the conditions that might make taking the Pill dangerous to you, there still is no way to know in advance whether a particular version of the Pill will cause specific side effects in individual women. If you decide you are a good candidate for this kind of contraception, you and your doctor will have to evaluate how you react to a specific brand, and keep trying combinations of hormones until you find an acceptable one.

MINIPILLS

This birth control pill provides a continuous low dose of progestin but no estrogen and is thus particularly useful to those women who want to use oral contraceptives but cannot tolerate estrogen. Progesterone works by affecting the uterine lining and causing the cervical mucus to be inhospitable to sperm. When a woman takes a progesterone-only Pill, she probably ovulates 50 percent of the time, but the sperm cannot get through the thick cervical mucus to fertilize the egg. Even if sperm do penetrate the cervical mucus, progestin may alter the normal rhythmic contractions in the fallopian tubes, hampering the passage of the fertilized egg through the tube. The continuous supply of progestin also inhibits endometrial development, making implantation of a fertilized egg unlikely. You should ask your doctor for the brand that has the lowest progestin dose.

Minipills, taken daily, have a low failure rate, about 3 percent. However, the chance of pregnancy increases if you fail to take one for even one or two days, and you lose protection almost completely if you skip as few as three days in a row. If you use this kind of birth control pill and forget to take one, use another contraceptive method until your next period. If you are ill and vomit or have diarrhea, call your doctor to find out whether you should continue to take pills or use another type of contraceptive for the rest of the month. Always call your doctor if you do not have a period within 45 days.

Like combined oral contraceptives, minipills provide continuous protection when used properly. Since you take a pill daily, you don't have to remember where you are in the cycle, as you do with the 21-day pills. Your periods may be irregular, but you will probably experience lighter bleeding, less severe premenstrual symptoms, and no menstrual cramps as compared with your experience before using an oral contraceptive. Because minipills have not been used widely, what other benefits they confer are still unclear, but doctors consider the following hypothetical advantages:

- the absence of estrogen and its side effects
- a lower dose of progestin than in Pills using estrogen and progestin in combination
- the fact that using minipills does not totally suppress the normal hormonal cycle

The major problem with minipills is that the "periods" of the women who use them are irregular and unpredictable. In fact, the original research on contraception with hormones started with progestin, and researchers added estrogen to achieve a regular bleeding pattern. While irregular bleeding is not in itself dangerous, if a woman mistakes bleeding that indicates a serious infection or other medical problem for merely an irregular period, she may delay seeking the proper diagnosis and treatment. Nevertheless, the minipill is a good choice for women who cannot take estrogen.

The risk of ectopic pregnancy, in which a fertilized egg implants in a fallopian tube, is higher for minipill users. (See Chapter 9.)

HORMONAL IMPLANT

In late 1990, the FDA approved the hormonal implant Norplant for use in the United States. Heralded in the media as the first new contraceptive in 25 years, this system uses a set of small, soft tubes made of a blend of silicone and plastic (Silastic) and filled with levonorgestrel, a synthetic progestin that is released at a slow, steady rate. The tubes are placed under the skin, usually in the upper arm, and provide a smaller hormone dose than the Pill but do so around the clock rather than once a day. Using local anesthesia, a doctor can place the implant just under the skin through a quarter-inch incision, closing it with one stitch or a bandage. This office procedure takes 15 minutes. The hormone leaches out of the tube and enters the bloodstream.

The two primary advantages of Norplant are that it is extremely effective—with a 99 percent success rate in women who weigh less than 155 pounds and 92 percent protection for those who weigh more—and that it can remain in place for five years—giving a woman long-term protection without having to remember to take a pill daily. Its effects are completely reversible; after the implant is removed, fertility returns by the next menstrual cycle. Norplant has been extensively tested on 50,000 women in 44 countries and is on the market in 14 nations. More than 350,000 women have used it, and researchers report that the vast majority like the method whatever their religious belief or socioeconomic status.

Norplant's main side effects are longer menstrual periods and irregular spotting between periods. Half of all users experience a change in bleeding patterns, and about 2 to 7 percent of women had the implant removed during the first year because of bleeding irregularities. The FDA warns women who have breast cancer; blood clots in the legs, lungs, or eyes; acute liver disease; and unexplained vaginal bleeding not to use Norplant.

Although this product will probably be less expensive than the cost of purchasing five years' supply of birth control pills (about $900), the entire projected cost of approximately $500 must be paid at the time of the initial insertion, and this expense may discourage many women from considering it further. Norplant is also less expensive than sterilization for women, which costs $1,100 or more, but it is more costly than male sterilization, which averages around $300.

INTRAUTERINE DEVICE (IUD)

A small device with a string attached, an IUD is inserted in the uterus by a doctor; it causes a minor inflammation that results in a series of altered bodily reactions that act to inhibit pregnancy. Studies have shown that although ovulation occurs, fertilization usually does not. Specialists are not sure of the reason. It may be because the sperm have a poor chance of getting past the cervical mucus that is more hostile to them because of the minor inflammation in the uterus, or because the uterine environment, responding to the presence of the IUD, may produce spermicidal toxins. Even if a sperm does manage to fertilize the egg, it may not be able to implant because the lining of the uterus is inhospitable.

The use of the intrauterine device has been severely restricted in this country as a result of product liability lawsuits, specifically those against the A. H. Robins Company. These suits resulted in the company's bankruptcy after its IUD, the Dalkon Shield, was found to be associated with several deaths, miscarriages, and serious illnesses. As a result, almost all IUDs have been removed from the U.S. market, including those that were not associated with major problems, leaving only two (medicated) IUDs still available. One, which must be replaced annually, has small quantities of progesterone embedded in it. The other is a copper-containing IUD that can remain in the uterus for as long as seven years. Both these agents make the IUD more effective than the earlier, nonmedicated varieties and reduce the increased amount of heavy menstrual bleeding that was characteristic of the first generation of IUDs. However, IUD users today may still experience bleeding patterns that are heavier than normal.

The advantage of the IUD is that, once it is inserted and the first three months of using a backup contraceptive method have passed, no additional action is necessary—no pills to take or other paraphernalia to buy or insert. The IUD is extremely effective as a birth control technique, with a best possible reported failure rate during the first year of use as low as .5 percent and a typical failure rate of 6 percent.

The main disadvantage of the IUD is that its use increases the risk of pelvic infection, which can cause infertility. Moreover, women who plan to have children at a later date should not use it because of this greater-than-average risk of infertility. There have been 17 documented deaths from IUD use. The IUD is not a suitable form of birth control for anyone with multiple sexual partners because it does not decrease the high risk of sexually transmitted diseases.

The IUD's lesser problems include causing heavier-than-normal menstrual bleeding, irregular bleeding, and cramps. You may find it hard to distinguish between the cramps and bleeding that commonly accompany IUD insertion and those that indicate possible infection; if such cramps and bleeding continue for more than 12 to 24 hours, you should see your doctor.

Anemia is not usually a problem for a healthy woman, but if you were anemic before IUD insertion, you may need supplemental iron thereafter. Discuss this with your doctor, who can check your blood count to determine anemia.

The litigation surrounding the IUD as a result of its association with pelvic infection and other severe damage has made the pharmaceutical industry very cautious about its production. A U.S. doctor cannot obtain an IUD without signing a long form explaining that the user understands the risk of infection and bleeding and their possible consequences. An accompanying "informed consent" document places the responsibility for the IUD's correct use in the hands of the patient, and the list of contraindications is long. Essentially, to limit their liability in the event of litigation, the drug companies wish to restrict IUD use to women who have already had children and who are in mutually monogamous relationships. The consent forms have clearly become unrealistic, not only in intent but also in terms of the information they require from potential users. Despite these extensive screening attempts, as well as the voluminous package inserts with their warnings and descriptions of side effects, women who use the IUD still have great difficulty in assessing how the data apply to them individually. Although the forms and the inserts can make a couple aware that they are responsible for their own protection from pregnancy, they certainly are not very helpful to patients.

Complications

If you use an IUD and you suspect you are pregnant, it should be removed immediately; you can become gravely ill very quickly. The risk of miscarriage is also much higher if you become pregnant with an IUD in place, and IUD users are at heightened risk for an ectopic pregnancy, in which a fertilized egg implants and begins to grow in a fallopian tube as opposed to the uterus.

In addition, if you have an unexplained fever and symptoms of the flu, you should see your doctor at once and have your IUD checked. If an infection is suspected, the doctor will remove the IUD and prescribe antibiotics to clear it up. Sometimes physicians prescribe antibiotics when they first insert the IUD to reduce the chance of infection during the procedure. However, if you take antibiotics to prevent or treat infections at other times, they can reduce the effectiveness of an IUD because they may decrease the low-grade uterine inflammation the IUD intentionally produces, compromising its protection.

If you feel pain during intercourse while wearing an IUD, or have a discharge with an unpleasant odor, your doctor should examine your uterus. Always make sure that you can feel the string that is attached to the IUD; if you cannot, have your health-care provider see if the IUD is still in place. One common problem with the IUD is spontaneous expulsion, which happens in 5 to 20 percent of users. You may not be aware that the IUD has come out, or you may experience bleeding, spotting, unusual vaginal discharge, cramps, or abdominal pain. In any event, this kind of spontaneous expulsion can result in pregnancy unless it is detected quickly, so IUD users should frequently take care to confirm that the device is in place, particularly during the first few months after its insertion and during menstrual periods.

Another problem is that the IUD can enter the body by perforating the uterus and moving into the abdominal cavity. This serious complication takes place most often during insertion, but it can occur at other times as well. Frequently, the doctor can correct this by removing the IUD through a laparoscope.

You should not use an IUD if any of the following conditions are present:

- current pregnancy, confirmed or suspected

- previous ectopic pregnancy

- previous episodes of PID, STDs, or infection after delivery or abortion

- an abnormal uterus

- uterine or cervical cancer

- multiple sex partners, or a partner who might have multiple sex partners

- abnormal bleeding or Pap smear

"MORNING AFTER" BIRTH CONTROL

RU-486, while not specifically a contraceptive, is an antiprogestin that can be used to produce an abortion when other contraceptive methods fail, or when a couple has had unprotected intercourse. RU-486 was developed by the French pharmaceutical firm Roussel-UCLAF. The compound terminates an early pregnancy if a woman takes it between the nineteenth and twenty-fifth day after her last menstrual period. Success with RU-486 diminishes and prostaglandins become more necessary to produce an abortion as the pregnancy progresses. When used in combination with various prostaglandins, it has a 95 percent success rate and minimal side effects, the main one being bleeding. The only problem is that RU-486 is not available in the United States. Although it is currently marketed in France and China, the prospects for its use in other countries is not clear. In the United States the news of its existence has caused loud and acrimonious debate.

Some physicians prescribe four birth control pills, usually Ovral, two each to be taken 12 hours apart the day after unprotected intercourse has taken place, which gives the uterine lining a large enough hormonal load so that it becomes inhospitable to any possible developing egg. Nevertheless, despite this already available morning-after procedure, there is no FDA-approved morning-after pill developed specifically to provide this function.

"NATURAL" FAMILY PLANNING (RHYTHM)

Natural family planning involves couples identifying the time in a woman's cycle when she is ovulating and when it is, therefore, not safe to have intercourse if they want to avoid pregnancy. The procedure requires dedication, an intimate knowledge of the woman's menstrual cycle, and the willingness to be diligent about periodic abstinence. Those who use natural family planning must be highly motivated. The efficacy is generally in the same range as the barrier methods—that is, 65 to 90 percent.

Charting the Menstrual Cycle

In order to decrease your chance of becoming pregnant, keep track of the alterations in your body caused by the different hormonal levels that characterize the various stages of your cycle. First, enter the changes you observe on a chart. For example, ovulation makes your body temperature rise slightly during the second half of the cycle and alters the quality of cervical mucus and vaginal discharge that you normally excrete. Accurate charting takes effort, for you must keep track of cyclical changes on a daily basis. The charting counselors on the staffs of many family planning clinics can help women learn charting skills. Forms that make charting easier are available from Planned Parenthood and other family planning clinics (see Table 7.3).

Charting Calendar Days

The simplest part of charting involves keeping track of when each period begins and ends on your calendar to document the number of days in your cycle and whether it stays regular month after month. If you establish that you are regular, this can help determine when you ovulate, since ovulation usually occurs 14 days before bleeding starts; this knowledge is enormously useful in either planning or avoiding pregnancy. Never forget that while the egg lives for only 12 to 48 hours, sperm survive for two to three days, so you can have intercourse on Thursday, ovulate on Friday, and become pregnant on Saturday. You should consider yourself fertile for about a week on either side of the day you think you have ovulated. It is best to use a barrier method of contraception or abstain from intercourse entirely during this time if you do not want to become pregnant, because charting helps you determine when you have ovulated only after the fact. (Obviously, if you are using charting to conceive, you should have intercourse frequently during your fertile days.)

Charting Temperature

Basal body temperature (BBT) is your lowest body temperature when you are awake, and it will normally rise after ovulation in response to progesterone. To keep an accurate record, take your temperature for five minutes every morning before getting out of bed and record it on your chart. You can take your temperature orally, rectally, or vaginally, but you should decide on a location and stick with it because you must be consistent. Special BBT thermometers with large print to make temperature readings easier are available at your drugstore (see Table 7.4).

Charting Cervical Mucus

Some women try to chart differences in cervical mucus discharge during various times of their cycles—mucus becomes more abundant and creamy immediately before ovulation. This is a risky business at best for a number of reasons. Cervical mucus can be mistaken for semen. Its quality changes if you douche, use lubricants, or have an infection. You should not try to diagnose ovu-

Table 7.3 Sympto-Thermal Fertility Chart

Name _____ Year _____ Phone _____ No. Days of Last Cycle _____

Month _____

Day of Month																																				
Day of Week																																					
Day of Cycle	1	2	3	4	5	6	7	8	9	10	11	12	13	14	15	16	17	18	19	20	21	22	23	24	25	26	27	28	29	30	31	32	33	34	35	36	37
Headache																																					
Breast sensitivity																																					
Abdominal pain																																					
Mood changes																																					
Bleeding (S,M,H)																																					
Mucus sensation																																					
Intercourse																																					
Cervical opening																																					
Consistency																																					
Height																																					
Temperature 99.2 99.0																																					
Time taken ___ a.m. ___ p.m.																																					

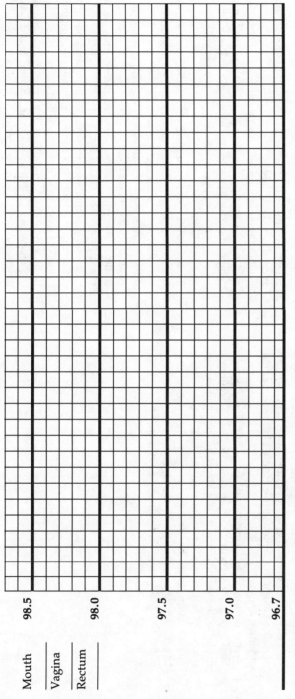

MUCUS

D — Dry sensation, absence of mucus
W — Wet sensation, white or cloudy mucus
(W) — Slippery & lubricative, stretchy & raw eggwhite (Peak)
T — Tacky, sticky, thick, opaque

CERVIX

Cervical opening — ▬ ○ ○
Consistency — S - Soft
— F - Firm
Height — Low - ↓
— High - ↑

Mouth
Vagina
Rectum

98.5
98.0
97.5
97.0
96.7

Source: Planned Parenthood of Northern New England

Table 7.4 Basal Temperature Record

Explanation

Knowledge that ovulation (discharge of an egg from the ovary) occurs and when it occurs are essential in your investigation and treatment. The time of ovulation may be estimated from a record of daily temperatures. The majority of normal women ovulate approximately 14 days *before* menstruation begins.

The normal *basal* temperature is below 98.6 degrees. Slight variations occur, and readings must be accurately made to the nearest tenth of a degree. The temperature normally is lower after menstruation and higher before menstruation, with the shift occurring at the time of ovulation. Ovulation is inferred when there is a sustained rise of 0.4 to 0.6 degrees. (See sample chart below.)

Instructions

1. Learn to read the thermometer accurately. If you do not know how to read the thermometer, ask the doctor or nurse.
2. Shake down the thermometer the night before! Place it on the bedside table.
3. The first waking moment, before stirring from the bed and before smoking, drinking, or eating, take your temperature for five minutes by the clock. Record this reading on the appropriate day on the graphic chart as a black dot.
4. Transform the dot indicating the reading into an asterisk (see sample chart) if the previous night's rest was fitful, less than eight hours, or if fever, cold, or other causes exist for alteration in temperature. Explain by notation on chart.
5. Indicate time of intercourse by an arrow pointing to the appropriate date on the temperature chart.
6. Chart days of menstrual flowing as illustrated on sample chart. Take your temperature during your period.
7. Bring the chart to your physician at each visit.
8. Begin a new chart on the first day of menstrual bleeding (cycle day 1). Fill in the year, month, and day as illustrated on the sample chart.

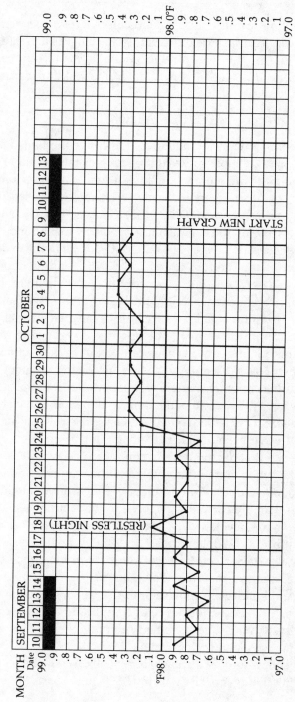

Source: Department of Obstetrics and Gynecology, Yale University School of Medicine

lation according to the kind of mucus discharge you experience; evaluating cervical mucus is best left to gynecologists and infertility specialists. If you still want to keep track of changes in cervical mucus, you need detailed instructions from a charting counselor.

STERILIZATION

Sterilization is one of the major contraceptive methods used in the United States; almost 30 percent of couples rely on either tubal ligation (tying off the woman's fallopian tubes) or vasectomy (ligating the vas deferens in the male). The methods used in the United States are highly effective. (See Chapter 14.) The surgical procedure to close off the fallopian tubes requires a small abdominal and/or pelvic incision (average cost: $1,500–2,000); in the male, the surgeon incises the scrotum to reach the tubes and tie them (average cost: $700–1,000). Both procedures can sometimes be reversed with subsequent surgery, with a success rate that can be as high as 80 percent for women if very little of the tube was damaged by the sterilization procedure. The successful reversal of a tubal ligation implies only that the tubes can be put back together, creating an open passage from end to end. Becoming pregnant after this procedure is another matter; pregnancy after reversal surgery occurs only about 15 percent of the time, and there is a much higher rate of tubal pregnancies in women who have had reversal surgery.

The reason that such a high percentage of U.S. couples request tubal ligation is that the methods of contraception available are still so limited and the failure rates so high. Other countries offer a far wider range of contraceptive products as well as more methods of sterilization than are currently available in the United States. Doctors abroad have developed nonsurgical methods of closing (occluding) both the fallopian tubes and the vas deferens; these techniques also have a better potential for reversibility than do the current U.S. surgical methods. For example, Chinese researchers have injected liquid polyurethane into the vas deferens of 12,000 men to form a plug. The incidence of complications has been low, and 51 of the 86 men who have had the plug removed have subsequently impregnated their partners.

The oral contraceptives available abroad also offer a wider range of progestational agents than their U.S. counterparts. Injectable forms of contraceptive steroids are also available. In addition, intrauterine devices come in many more forms than are now offered in the United States, and a much wider range of spermicidal agents are also available.

Both ethical and practical considerations indicate that U.S. policymakers should put a high priority on allowing into this country the additional and more effective contraceptive methods that are already in use elsewhere. Our government should also support generous funding for contraceptive research that will explore additional devices and medications, so that the greatest number of women and men will be offered the widest possible contraceptive choice (see Table 7.5).

Table 7.5 Pregnancy Rates* (shown as a percentage of the U.S. rate) Among Women Aged 15–44 in Six Western Nations, by Age Group, 1985

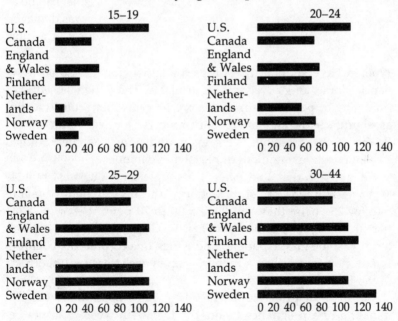

*The sum of abortions and live births per 1,000 women.

8

Abortion

Mary Jane Gray, M.D.

Women have sought abortion as a solution for unwanted pregnancies for as long as records are available. The ancients used aloe, iron, ginger, pepper, saffron, black ivy berries, fern root, and rice as abortifacients and menstrual inducers, together with magic. (Many of these potions were toxic, and none has been studied systematically using modern research techniques.)

We noted earlier that even if a couple uses the most reliable available methods of contraception with only a 2 percent failure rate for 25 years, they still have a 50 to 70 percent chance of experiencing an unplanned pregnancy. Given the degree of their fertility, some may experience more than one contraceptive failure. In any case, more than a million women each year seek abortions in the United States.

The medical profession generally defines abortion as the termination of a pregnancy before the twentieth week from the beginning of the last menstrual period. Abortion can be either "spontaneous"—that is, happening naturally without any intervention—or "induced"—brought on by medical or surgical means. *Spontaneous abortion* is the medical term for miscarriage.

Spontaneous abortions, nature's way of ending imperfect pregnancies, are extremely common. Recent studies involving highly sensitive pregnancy tests indicate that 50 to 60 percent of very early pregnancies of between one and six weeks are lost, a rate that turns out to be much higher than was previously assumed. We have no way of knowing, of course, just how many fertilized eggs fail to implant in the uterine wall, but chromosomal studies of tissue from spontaneously aborted fetuses show that about half of them have grossly abnormal numbers and types of chromosomes. It is important to understand that this high rate of spontaneous abortion is absolutely normal, inevitable, and desirable. This means that if you lose a pregnancy, you need not feel concerned or guilty that you might unwittingly have done something to bring on the miscarriage.

Once the process of spontaneous abortion has begun, it is referred to as "inevitable" abortion, which usually indicates that the fetus was not developing normally and that there was no way to prevent the loss of the pregnancy. When the fetus has died but has not been expelled and must be removed by one of the interventions described below, this is referred to as a "missed," or incomplete, abortion.

The terms *first, second,* and *third-trimester abortion* reflect the U.S. Supreme Court's attempt to grapple with medical terminology. Since doctors define a full-term pregnancy as lasting 40 weeks on average, each trimester covers about 13 weeks. (See Chapter 9.) Thus, a first-trimester abortion is an *early abortion,* while *mid-trimester, second trimester,* and *late abortion* are terms that cover roughly the period from 14 to 26 weeks of pregnancy. The latter part of the second trimester extends well beyond the time of most abortions. The term *third-trimester abortion* is a misnomer, as this portion of pregnancy is never subject to abortion. Indeed, if it becomes necessary to induce labor for reasons of fetal or maternal survival, doctors expect to deliver a live, although possibly premature, infant.

The term *therapeutic abortion* dates from the era before abortion was legal in the United States. At that time, doctors were required to present to medical committees the case histories of women who needed abortions. These committees would then approve—or disapprove—and justify the procedure on the basis of their perception of medical need. Within this restrictive system, the medical conditions where pregnancy was considered to pose a risk to a woman's life included the presence of heart and kidney disease, suicidal depression, diabetes, and high blood pressure; the abortion was granted on the basis of medical need and it became a part of the woman's medical therapy. Later medical committees added "fetal indications"—warnings that the fetus had a high risk of developing into an abnormal infant—to the standards that would allow therapeutic abortion. In some circumstances, these committees considered the mental health of the woman, including her response to rape or incest.

Therapeutic abortion is not entirely history. In 1989, doctors caring for a comatose pregnant woman, the victim of an auto accident, believed an abortion might save her life. Her husband approved the procedure, only to have it prevented by a local antiabortion group, which obtained a legal injunction against its taking place. The husband became his wife's legal guardian, fighting the case all the way to the Supreme Court in order to secure the abortion. Eleven months later, this woman emerged from her coma and has since been making a remarkable recovery, visiting her husband and four-year-old daughter at home while still living and working on her recovery at a rehabilitation center.

DECIDING TO HAVE AN ABORTION

In the past, husbands, lovers, parents, physicians, and even judges and hospital committees played important roles in determining whether or not a woman should obtain an abortion. Today we know that although support and consultation can be extremely helpful, the woman who will carry, bear, and raise the child must make the ultimate decision.

Because the safety of an abortion is directly related to how far the pregnancy has progressed at the time it is terminated, the longer you wait, the greater the risk of complications. The decision to abort, therefore, should be made as soon as possible after pregnancy is determined (see Table 8.1).

If you suspect you might be pregnant, you can start to confirm the pregnancy as soon as you have missed a menstrual period. Either visit a doctor or clinic, or use a home pregnancy test, available at most drugstores. These tests are approximately 95 percent accurate when you follow the directions carefully; however, this degree of accuracy is reliable only for positive results. If the results

Table 8.1 The Earlier an Abortion Is Performed, the Safer It Is

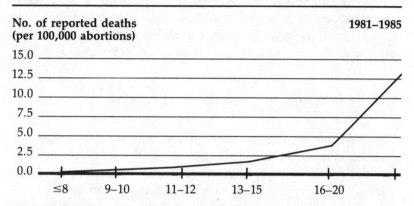

No. of reported deaths (per 100,000 abortions) — 1981–1985

Sources: **Deaths from legal abortion**—S. K. Henshaw, special tabulations of 1981–85 data from the Centers for Disease Control (CDC). **Number of abortions by gestational age**—S. K. Henshaw and J. Van Vort, eds., *Abortion Services in the United States, Each State and Metropolitan Area, 1984–1985* (New York: The Alan Guttmacher Institute [AGI], 1990), p. 90, updated for 1985 from CDC and AGI data. Reprinted from *Abortion and Women's Health.*

are negative, this may mean only that it is still too early to detect the pregnancy, and you should repeat the test weekly for the next three weeks if you don't get your period. At this point, if results are still negative, you should see a doctor to find out if you are pregnant or not. If you are taking oral contraceptives, your period may simply be late, for women frequently skip periods when on the Pill. Nevertheless, it's best to get medical confirmation one way or the other.

Women who are considering abortion have an easier time with the procedure and feel more positive about themselves afterward if they have received thoughtful and supportive counseling beforehand. If you are considering an abortion, it's wise to seek such counseling—at a family planning clinic or a woman's health counseling service. Some advertisements for pregnancy or abortion counseling are placed by antiabortion activists who try to discourage women from making choices; be forewarned of this as you seek counseling.

An experienced counselor will also be able to describe the abortion procedure, how and where it can be done, what anesthesia is used, whether you will experience pain or discomfort, whether you can have your partner or another close relative or friend with you, how long it will take, when you can go home, what possible complications might occur, and how long it will be until you can resume your everyday life. You can also explore with your counselor why the pregnancy occurred and how to avoid repeating it.

WHERE TO HAVE THE ABORTION

The three most common sites for abortion are doctors' offices, abortion clinics, and hospitals. The earlier the abortion, the more choices you have regarding where it may be performed. Many gynecologists perform very early abortions as routine office procedures. Depending on the extent of their own experience, physicians observe deadlines for office abortions of anywhere between six to 16 weeks. Because abortions performed after six weeks require special surgical instruments and emergency equipment, not all doctors are able to perform abortions as office procedures after this time. This is another important reason to confirm the pregnancy early if you want to consider abortion.

Abortion clinics regularly terminate pregnancies until 12 weeks, and many go beyond this cutoff date. Any office or clinic should be able to tell you over the phone what their policies are. After 16 weeks, the procedure requires special skill, and often doctors admit women who need these late abortions to a hospital. Both expense and safety relate directly to the duration of the pregnancy at the time of the abortion and to the gynecologist's skill.

PREOPERATIVE PROCEDURES

Before the procedure itself, a preoperative medical workup will take place. This includes a medical history and a complete physical examination, including a pelvic exam. (See Chapter 1.) The doctor will also order tests to confirm the pregnancy, determine if you are anemic, and check your blood type and Rh factor. It is important to determine anemia beforehand because of any possible heavy blood loss during the abortion; if you are anemic, you will receive iron supplements. The same is true of blood type; if unusually heavy bleeding occurs, you may need a blood transfusion. And Rh typing is vital because, if you are Rh negative and your fetus is Rh-positive, blood from the fetus entering your circulation can cause you to produce antibodies against the Rh-positive factor now, which, in your next pregnancy, can cross the placenta and attack the red blood cells of a future Rh-positive fetus and destroy or damage it. This condition is called erythroblastosis, or Rh disease. Therefore, as a precaution, an Rh-negative woman carrying a potentially Rh-positive fetus will receive a shot of immunoglobulin (Rhogam) to prevent this sensitization from taking place.

The doctor will also test for sexually transmitted diseases (STDs), since the organisms that cause STDs are among those that provoke postabortion infections. For example, taking preprocedure cultures for chlamydia and gonorrhea, two common STDs, and providing immediate treatment of these cervical infections, if necessary, reduce the risk of serious postabortion infection, as does the common practice of giving three to four days of antibiotic treatment to all women after abortion. (See Chapter 11.) If you are overweight, unusually tense, or otherwise difficult to examine, or if there is any doubt about the duration of the pregnancy, the doctor will order an ultrasound image of the uterus and its contents to determine accurately how far along you are.

ABORTION METHODS

The most common surgical methods of abortion use dilatation—stretching of the cervix—and either curettage, which involves the scraping out of the contents of the uterus, or suction, which uses a method called vacuum extraction to empty the uterus. These procedures are known as dilatation and curettage (D&C), suction currettage, and dilatation and evacuation (D&E). If the abortion takes place very early in the pregnancy, the gynecologist can often introduce a small, flexible catheter into the uterus through the vagina without stretching open the cervix, and the fetus can be removed through the catheter by suction. The clinician can use this technique—called miniabortion, menstrual extraction, or endometrial aspiration—up to about six weeks of pregnancy. Although it is very safe and often less painful than procedures performed later in pregnancy, the chief complication is a failure to abort the pregnancy because the fetus is so tiny that the doctor can miss it. Therefore, if you have a very early abortion, you must be sure to visit your doctor for repeat pregnancy tests until the test becomes negative. If the test remains positive for more than two weeks after the procedure, you may require another suction procedure to be sure that the fetus has indeed been removed.

For many years the D&C was the standard operation for terminating pregnancies up to 12 weeks after the last menstrual period. In this procedure, a metal measuring rod called a sound is placed inside the uterus to determine its size. The doctor then introduces rounded, closed metal tubes of gradually increasing size, called dilators, through the vagina into the cervix to stretch it open; this usually produces the sensation of mild menstrual cramps. Once the dilating is complete, the doctor uses a sharp curette to scrape the fetus and placental tissue off the wall of the uterus. In the past, doctors performed D&Cs under general anesthesia to obliterate all pain. But because general anesthesia relaxes the blood vessels and the uterine muscle, increasing blood loss, it is now rarely used for early abortions. Instead, practitioners inject a local anesthetic, such as Novocain, around the cervix to minimize pain—a sensation that is experienced as a pinch or slight pressure, if at all.

Currently, the favored method for performing early abortions is suction curettage, or evacuation of the uterus. After opening the cervix with dilators, as in a D&C, the doctor places a plastic tube or curette into the uterus and attaches this to a vacuum pump. The uterus is then emptied of the fetal and placental tissue by a gentle vacuum suction process. The more advanced the pregnancy, the more the cervix must be opened to admit a suction tube wide enough for the tissue to pass through. The cervix can be injured in this process, requiring a stitch or two. After the procedure, the doctor collects the tissue in a jar and examines it to make sure it is complete and that no tissue has been left behind to cause increased bleeding or infection later.

After the abortion, a nurse or other medical caregiver will stay with you for an hour or more to monitor your condition, depending on the type of procedure, the amount of bleeding, and how you feel. If your blood type is Rh negative, this is when you receive a shot to prevent Rh problems in future pregnancies. Often the doctor will order antibiotics to prevent infection. Your physician will also tell you how to get help if you start to bleed heavily after you go home, when it is safe to resume having intercourse, and how

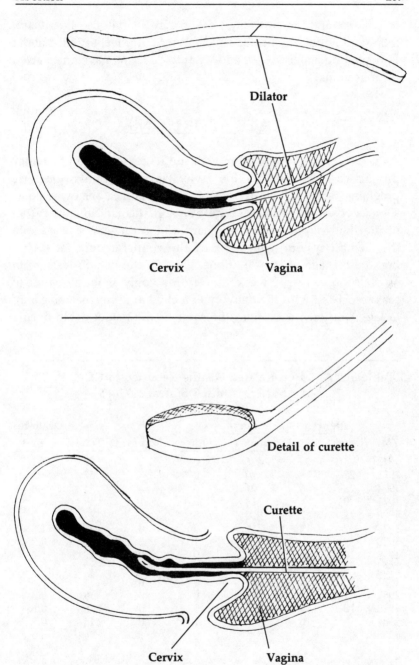

Fig. 8.1   Dilator and Curette, Instruments for a D&C

to prevent another unwanted pregnancy. You'll also be given a follow-up appointment. Don't leave until you feel satisfied about how you can expect to feel and what to do if you have unexpected complications.

LATE ABORTIONS

As noted, complications from abortion increase as the pregnancy progresses (see Table 8.1). This is why it is so important to diagnose pregnancy early so that, if desired, an abortion can be obtained as soon as possible. Young teenagers have particular difficulty recognizing that they might be pregnant and getting themselves into the medical system, which is why the young account for such a high percentage of late abortions. Overall, the risk of death from an abortion before 12 weeks is very low, only about a quarter of that associated with the delivery of a child at term (see Table 8.2); in late abortions, it is about the same as the risk of death during

Table 8.2 Abortion-Related Deaths Reported to CDC, by Type of Abortion, United States, 1972–85

Year	Induced Legal	Illegal	Sponta- neous	Other	Unknown	Total	Death-to- case rate
1972	24	39	25	0	2	90	4.1
1973	25	19	10	0	3	57	4.1
1974	26	6	21	0	1	54	3.4
1975	29	4	14	0	1	48	3.4
1976	11	2	13	0	1	27	1.1
1977	17	4	16	0	0	37	1.6
1978	9	7	9	1	0	26	0.8
1979	18	0	9	0	0	27	1.4
1980	9	1	6	0	1	17	0.7
1981	7	1	3	0	0	11	0.5
1982	11	1	6	0	0	18	0.8
1983	10	1	7	0	0	18	0.8
1984	11	0	6	1	0	18	0.8
1985	6	1	6	0	1	14	0.5

Source: Morbidity and Mortality Weekly Report, CDC Surveillance Summaries, September 1989 (Volume 38/No. SS-2). Washington, D.C.: U.S. Department of Health and Human Services.

delivery. (Currently, there are about eight maternal deaths per 100,000 births in this country.)

There is little difference in either the type of procedure used or the rate of complications that result in abortions performed from the thirteenth through the sixteenth week of pregnancy. Late abortions, those done after 16 weeks, are more difficult surgical procedures; after 17 weeks, when a woman can feel the baby move, the abortion decision can be much more difficult as the fetus becomes more of a reality.

From about the sixteenth week of pregnancy until the arbitrary cutoff, usually 20 to 24 weeks, several methods of abortion are available, but none is quick or easy. Pregnancy terminations after the possibility of fetal survival usually occur only because of major, life-threatening medical problems or because of a misjudgment of fetal size, and are extremely rare.

Beyond 16 weeks, no matter which procedure is used, the doctor dilates the cervix by inserting plugs, called laminaria, which gradually absorb fluid and expand, slowly opening the cervix. These laminaria substitute for the forcible dilation of the cervix with metal dilators employed in earlier abortions. They are not used in early abortions because the cervix needs less dilation; although they are gentler than metal dilators, they take several hours to work.

After the cervix is dilated, an abortion can be performed in two ways. In the first, the doctor induces labor by injecting an irritating substance, such as a concentrated salt solution, into the amniotic fluid inside the uterus; the salt solution irritates the uterus and is fatal to the fetus. Or, the doctor may administer prostaglandins, those naturally occurring compounds in the body that induce labor when full-term birth takes place. These prostaglandins can be administered either as suppositories in the vagina or by injection into the uterus. Sometimes the physician uses both saline and prostaglandins. The prostaglandins stimulate the onset of labor, decreasing the time until delivery. Labor may last up to 24 hours, is uncomfortable, and ends with the vaginal delivery of the fetus.

The second late-abortion procedure is called a dilatation and evacuation (D and E). It involves the surgical removal of the pregnancy and requires great skill and expertise. The doctor removes the fetus by using instruments introduced through the cervix into the uterus. This procedure is quicker and less emotionally trying for the woman than injecting a salt solution and/or prostaglandins and subsequent labor, and in experienced hands, it is safer. If you must obtain a second-trimester abortion, be sure to consider the doctor's or clinic's experience—that is, which procedure they have performed the most often—in deciding which method to choose.

COMPLICATIONS OF ABORTION

The possible complications following abortion include bleeding, perforation of the uterus with the additional risk of damage to the intestines, and infection—especially likely if fragments of placental tissue have been left inside the uterus. If the uterus is perforated, the surgeon can make an abdominal incision and stitch the cut closed, but the size and location of the defect will affect whether or not the repair will hold during a subsequent vaginal delivery, or if the woman will need a cesarean section in ensuing pregnancies. There can also be complications from local or general anesthesia.

The two most common immediate problems complicating abortion are bleeding and infection. Some bleeding begins the moment the doctor places an instrument inside the uterus, and it may continue until the next menstrual period. Bleeding is usually moderately heavy for the brief duration of the procedure. Therefore, anything that increases the difficulty of the operation and the time it requires will increase blood loss.

Practitioners control bleeding by getting the muscles of the uterus to contract, clamping down around blood vessels and compressing them. The drugs Ergotrate and Pitocin are often used to cause uterine contraction and control bleeding, and doctors administer them either intravenously or intramuscularly at the time of the procedure; Ergotrate can also be administered orally later, if needed. Since any retained fetal or placental tissue can impede the ability of the uterus to contract, if there is greater-than-normal postoperative bleeding, the gynecologist may place an instrument inside the uterus again to be certain that all the fetal and placental tissue has been removed. It is very rare (in fewer than one out of 1,000 procedures) for postoperative bleeding to be heavy enough to cause shock. Should this occur, you must be hospitalized immediately and receive a blood transfusion, and the doctor must determine if an instrument may have perforated the uterine wall.

Such injuries can often be successfully repaired, but, occasionally, the medical team may have to perform a hysterectomy to stop massive bleeding.

If infection occurs, it will be indicated by a fever of more than 100° or by an increase in painful cramping. Infection usually is caused either by the presence of a preexisting sexually transmitted disease or by tissue that has not been completely removed at the time of the abortion. Antibiotics are the treatment of choice for postabortion infection, and they are usually effective if given orally in adequate doses. However, if the infection continues unabated, you will need to be hospitalized so that you can receive intravenous antibiotics, and there is then a risk of tubal damage and even death. Any surgical procedure that requires general anesthesia always presents a slight risk of death. There is also the possibility of an allergic reaction to local anesthetics.

These complications are rare. In general, your experience after an early abortion might include moderate bleeding for several days to as long as a month, cramps for one or two weeks, a let-down feeling or, conversely, a feeling of relief. You can bathe and resume intercourse after two days.

DOES ABORTION HAVE LONG-TERM EFFECTS?

Medical reports based on retrospective studies of women who had late, illegal abortions by methods no longer used gave rise to the myth that abortion caused premature labor and infertility (see Table 8.3). Similarly, when abortions were performed in operating rooms under general anesthesia on women with severe heart and kidney disease or, alternatively, were performed by untrained personnel in unsuitable circumstances, the complications were frequent and serious and abortion was justifiably feared. Today we know that medical evidence of serious physical or emotional consequences of abortion is rare. The Center for Disease Control and many other organizations have studied elective abortions over the last 20 years and found them to be among the safest surgical procedures performed. The overwhelming emotion reported by women once the abortion is over is relief. If women feel ambivalent about having had the abortion, have not looked carefuly at their options before-

Table 8.3 Deaths from Abortion Have Declined Dramatically Since Legalization

No of
Abortion-
Related Deaths

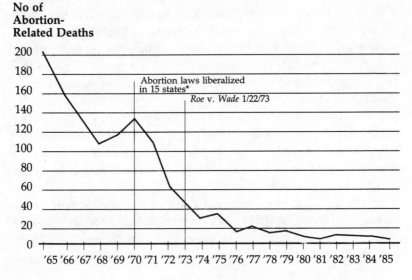

*By the end of 1970, four states had repealed their antiabortion laws and 11 states had reformed them.

Note: Numbers include deaths from both legal and illegal abortion, but exclude those from spontaneous abortion.

Sources: 1965–67—National Center for Health Statistics, *Vital Statistics of the United States, 1965; Vol. II—Mortality, Part A* (Washington, D.C.: GPO, 1967); ———, *Vital Statistics of the United States, 1966; Vol. II—Mortality, Part A* (GPO, Washington, D.C., 1968); ———, *Vital Statistics of the United States, 1967: Vol. II—Mortality, Part A* (GPO, Washington, D.C., 1969). To distribute deaths categorized as "spontaneous or unspecified," it was assumed that the ratio of spontaneous abortion deaths to pregnancy and childbearing deaths (excluding abortion and ectopic pregnancy) during 1965–1967 was the same as during the years 1968–1972, and the remaining "unspecified" deaths were induced abortion deaths. **1968–1971**—C. Tietze, "The Effect of Legalization of Abortion on Population Growth and Public Health," in C. Tietze et al., *Abortion 1974–1975; Need and Services in the United States, Each State & Metropolitan Area* (New York: The Alan Guttmacher Institute, 1976), pp. 110–113. **1972–1985**—H. W. Lawson et al., "Abortion Surveillance, United States, 1984–1985," *CDC Surveillance Summaries, Morbidity and Mortality Weekly Report* 38, no. SS–2 (September 1989), p. 11.

hand, or have not made the abortion decision of their own free will, they may indeed be left with issues that they need to work through with competent counselors, but the decision and the experience of the abortion itself produce no long-term, medically adverse effects.

Some reports suggest that there might be an increased incidence of premature delivery after repeated early abortion, but a recent study failed to corroborate these earlier findings. One issue that remains unclear and needs further research is whether or not there is a slightly increased risk of future premature deliveries after late abortions. The Johns Hopkins School of Hygiene and Public Health released a study early in 1990 that showed teenagers who had had abortions did better educationally and economically than pregnant adolescents who had their babies and better than teenagers who had not been pregnant. There is no question that abortion is safer than delivery at term. Nonetheless, like all other surgery, abortion is better prevented than performed.

THE MEDICAL INDUCTION OF ABORTION

Since the beginning of recorded time, women have taken potions to induce abortion, but it is only in the last decade that there has been a safe and effective medical means of ending an unwanted pregnancy. Progesterone is a hormone that enables the embryo to implant on the uterine wall during a normal pregnancy. RU-486 is an antiprogesterone, a compound that attaches to the sites of action of progesterone within the cells of the reproductive tract, prevents progesterone's normal activity, and, therefore, thwarts implantation. Researchers are investigating other antiprogesterone agents, but RU-486, also known as Mefepristone, is the agent we know most about because it has been extensively studied. It was developed by the distinguished French research physician Étienne-Émile Baulieu, who refers to it as a contragestational pill.

If a woman takes RU-486 between the nineteenth to the twenty-fifth day after her last period, its actions will keep the fertilized egg from implanting and bring on a menstrual period. Combining RU-486 with orally administered prostaglandins, those naturally occurring compounds that cause the uterus to contract, will produce a complete abortion at home in 95 percent of women who take these two drugs to terminate pregnancies up to seven weeks after the last period. The other 5 percent require the standard surgical procedure.

RU-486 is not available in the United States, and the prospects for its introduction here are unclear. However, more than 2,000 women in any month are receiving it and prostaglandins in France. When questioned, the majority of those who have had both a suction abortion and an RU-486 abortion greatly prefer the medical over the surgical procedure. In the Third World, where, according to estimates by the World Health Organization (WHO), more than 200,000 women die annually from the combination of improperly performed abortions and inadequate medical facilities to treat complications, the potential for saving lives with RU-486 is enormous. In addition to its preventing pregnancy and inducing abortion, RU-486 may also be of value in inducing labor and in the treatment of ectopic pregnancy, adrenal tumors, and cancers of the breast, ovary, and uterus.

RU-486 and other antiprogestational compounds have wide-ranging therapeutic use with the potential for saving lives. Research in the United States and some other countries has been hampered by political pressure from the antiabortion lobby. If such antiprogesterone drugs are not released for research and use in this country, the practice of medicine will be hindered substantially. The possibility also exists that the prohibition will produce a black market in these potent drugs that, if unsupervised, may cause serious problems for women.

9

Pregnancy

Florence Haseltine, M.D.

Pregnancy, or gestation, can be one of the most exciting events in a woman's life. It is also a thoroughly transforming experience for a couple, changing their twosome into a family and bringing with it new concerns and questions as well as feelings of well-being and joy.

Conception, seemingly the simple result of sexual intercourse, is actually a complex physiological process. The female reproductive organs include the uterus, with the lower end or cervix extending into the vagina; the ovaries, attached to a fold of the lining of the abdomen (or peritoneum) and lying next to the uterus; and the fallopian tubes, which extend from the corners of the uterus to the ovaries.

A woman is born with a total complement of eggs in her ovaries, 1 to 2 million of them, that remain inactive until puberty releases the necessary hormones for their development. Every month from then until menopause, her pituitary gland releases the luteinizing hormone (LH), which, in turn, allows one of her ovaries to discharge an egg, also called an ovum or oocyte. The egg enters one of the fallopian tubes, where it can be fertilized for a period that ranges from 12 to 24 hours.

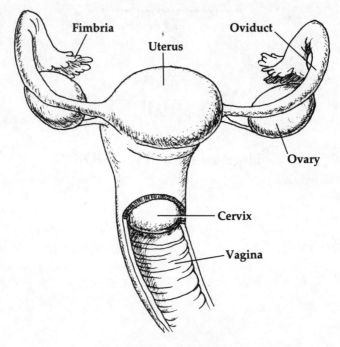

Fig. 9.1   Female Reproductive System

The male testicles, on the other hand, manufacture millions of sperm daily, which are carried in the seminal fluid produced by the prostate gland and the seminal vesicles. Each time a man ejaculates during intercourse he deposits a huge number of sperm, perhaps 100 million, in the woman's vagina, but because they must travel through the cervix and uterus to the fallopian tubes, where conception takes place, only about 200 complete the arduous journey. Sperm live for between 48 and 72 hours. After a single sperm enters the egg, a chemical reaction under the egg's surface prevents any additional sperm from penetrating it. The fertilized egg, or embryo, then travels back through one of the tubes to the uterus, where, if it finds a nurturing environment, it implants in the uterine wall and continues to grow.

Once the fertilized egg implants in the uterine wall, doctors call it a blastocyst; at two weeks it is considered an embryo; at eight weeks, a fetus; and, at birth, a baby.

The most obvious sign of pregnancy is a missed menstrual period. You can confirm pregnancy very early—actually a few days before the expected onset of your menstrual period—with a blood test for the pregnancy hormone called human chorionic gonadotropin (hCG). This test can provide accurate results 22 days after the start of your last menstrual period. Alternately, a urinary test will diagnose pregnancy shortly after the expected date of your next period. Inexpensive home pregnancy tests, available at drugstores without a doctor's prescription, can also be used 28 to 37 days from your last menstrual period; if you follow the directions carefully, these are 95 percent accurate.

Early diagnosis is important for many reasons. The fetus is most susceptible to harmful agents—such as alcohol, a wide range of drugs, tobacco, and environmental toxins—during the first three months. If you know you are pregnant immediately, you can be sure of avoiding these harmful substances. Good prenatal care and adequate nutrition can begin at once. In addition, early diagnosis of an ectopic pregnancy—one that takes place outside the uterus, usually in the fallopian tubes—can be life-saving. And if you do not feel emotionally or physically able to have a baby at this time, you can obtain a safe, early abortion. (See Chapter 8.)

Many doctors now advocate preconception care to make sure a woman is in optimum health before becoming pregnant. Although such a degree of preplanning is probably beneficial for women who are markedly under- or overweight, so that they can secure medical help to lose or gain weight before attempting a pregnancy, as well as for women with chronic medical problems, the average, healthy, well-nourished woman does not need to consult a doctor prior to pregnancy.

DATING THE PREGNANCY

One of the confusing areas of pregnancy is the way obstetricians use dates. They calculate that pregnancy lasts for 40 weeks, or 280 days, but women are not actually pregnant for that long. Doctors start counting from the first day of the last menstrual period, two weeks before fertilization, and three weeks before implantation. They use this method because, before they knew when a woman actually conceived, the only date available was the date at her last menstrual period; they subtracted three months from the beginning of her last period, and then added seven days to come up with the expected date of delivery. In using this dating system, doctors have added three extra weeks to pregnancy—a practice that is particularly perplexing to those women who have kept a diary and know precisely when they conceived. This historic gestational age terminology hangs on in medical practice simply because obstetricians are used to it. All medical decisions about pregnancy are based on this method of dating, even though it is only an estimated figure, since women do not all have regular menstrual periods and their fertilized eggs do not always implant at the same time. This is why babies seem to have a way of arriving both before and after what doctors refer to as the expected date of confinement or delivery.

FETAL AND PLACENTAL DEVELOPMENT

The role of the fetus in pregnancy is interactive in a dynamic way, producing biological agents that are essential to the pregnancy; the role of the mother is to provide it with food and oxygen and to dispose of the waste products that it generates during gestation.

Once the egg arrives in the uterus, it breaks through the zona pellucida, its outer coat. From the time of the egg's fertilization to its appearance in the uterus, it has already divided many times; after it reaches the uterus, it continues to split until it has formed two major types of cells, termed *trophoblast cells* and *inner mass cells*. Trophoblast cells develop into the placenta, while the inner mass cells become the fetus.

The placenta is a critical organ that the fetus needs to develop. When the trophoblast hatches from the zona pellucida, it tries to interact with the tissue that lines the uterus, which has been maturing during the menstrual cycle so that it will be ready for this interaction—the moment when pregnancy actually begins. At this point, the lining of the uterus (endometrium) changes to become the decidua, which separates the developing fetus from the maternal circulation and may play a vital (though not yet understood) role in initiating labor.

After the fertilized egg implants in the lining of the uterus, the placenta develops rapidly and, by 12 days after fertilization, produces distinguishable and characteristic small protruding hairlike structures. At 14 days, the maternal and arterial blood enters the spaces between these structures that have formed within the placenta, and by 17 days blood starts circulating. The human placenta is a two-way street, transferring materials between the mother and the fetus, bringing the fetus oxygen and nutrients and removing its waste products. The placenta does not provide a perfect barrier to separate the fetal circulation from the maternal circulation, however; some fetal red blood cells escape into the maternal circulation, and it is this process by which a mother with an Rh-negative blood type can adversely affect her Rh-positive fetus. (See Chapter 8.) The maternal cells also cross into the fetus, but in fairly small numbers.

While the placenta is growing, the inner cell mass develops rapidly and forms layers of fetal tissue called the ectoderm, endoderm, and mesoderm. The ectoderm becomes the skin (epidermis) and the nervous system. The mesoderm turns into the vascular system, the skeletal system, and the inner layer of skin (dermis). The endoderm will form the lining of the gastrointestinal tract and the liver. This differentiation of function starts at the embryo's head and goes to its rump. The nervous system and the sensory organs begin to function by the eighth week of pregnancy (see Fig. 9.2). The fetal digestive system develops so that, by the eleventh week, the small intestine has rhythmic movements (peristalsis), the same action that aids digestion after birth. Although the sex of the fetus is established at fertilization, determined by whether a sperm bearing an X (female) or a Y (male) chromosome unites with the egg, the actual process of sex differentiation does not begin until seven weeks, when, in a fetus with a Y chromosome, the early testes produce matter called the Müllerian-inhibiting substance, which disrupts the Müllerian system needed for normal female development. At 10 weeks, the fetal testes can synthesize testosterone, assuring a male fetus, and by 16 weeks they produce other androgens (male hormones), which form the external genitalia and penis. In the female, where the X chromosome has prevailed, the ovaries form around the twelfth week. The fetus can hear by the twenty-fourth week (see Fig. 9.3).

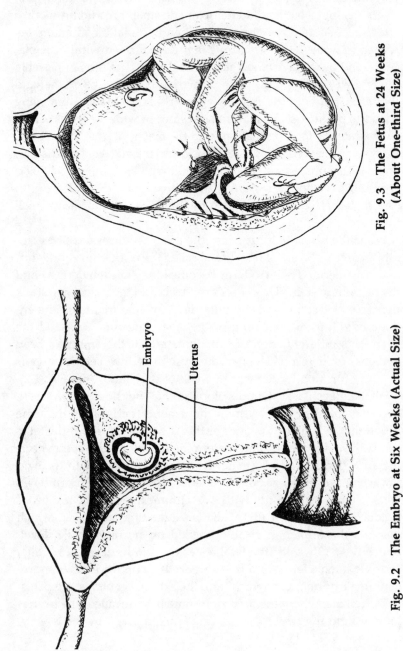

Fig. 9.3 The Fetus at 24 Weeks (About One-third Size)

Embryo

Uterus

Fig. 9.2 The Embryo at Six Weeks (Actual Size)

ECTOPIC PREGNANCY

Ectopic means "out of place." Sometimes the fertilized egg implants elsewhere in the reproductive tract, most often in one of the fallopian tubes. (Ectopic pregnancies can also occur in the ovary, in the cervix, or in the abdominal cavity, with the placenta implanting on the back of the uterus or on the lining of the abdominal cavity or bowel.) At the present time, almost two out of every 100 pregnancies is ectopic, and the rate is rising. Although the elements that lead to tubal pregnancies are still to be firmly established, previous tubal infection is known to be a precipitating factor. Thus researchers correctly anticipated that the increase in tubal infections would play a role in boosting the number of ectopic pregnancies. (See Chapter 10.)

In a tubal pregnancy, the fallopian tube cannot stretch enough to accommodate the growing fetus. Eventually it ruptures, usually within the first six weeks, sometimes accompanied by enough bleeding to be life-threatening. Currently, ectopic pregnancy and its complications are one of the two most common causes of death in pregnant women. However, death rates from ectopic pregnancy have declined substantially since 1970, presumably because of early detection and intervention (see Fig. 9.4).

Because the tube does not offer a favorable environment for a fetus, the pregnancy sometimes simply dies and is reabsorbed. Sometimes the pregnancy aborts and is expelled out of the end of the tube, reimplanting wherever it lands. Doctors believe this is the route abdominal pregnancies take.

The symptoms of an early ectopic pregnancy are much like those of a uterine pregnancy: the absence of menstrual periods, nausea, and breast tenderness, with the exception that a woman usually experiences discomfort on one side of the lower abdomen, around the rectum, or in the lower back. Often there is some irregular bleeding. If the tube ruptures, there is almost always a sudden onset of very severe abdominal pain, usually followed by weakness and fainting. This rupturing is a true emergency. A doctor must examine the woman immediately, make the diagnosis, and initiate surgical intervention at once, or she may die.

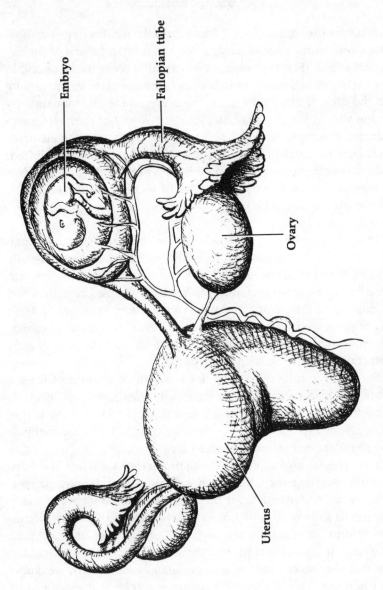

Embryo

Fallopian tube

Ovary

Uterus

Fig. 9.4 Ectopic Pregnancy

DIAGNOSIS

Physicians suspect an ectopic pregnancy if a woman has the symptoms of pregnancy but they are accompanied by pain and bleeding. The kind of sensitive pregnancy tests currently in use are usually positive, although such a test does not differentiate between a pregnancy in the uterus and one in the fallopian tube or elsewhere. Further diagnostic steps include ultrasound examination, serial blood pregnancy tests, and laparoscopy, a procedure that uses a surgical periscope inserted into the abdomen to enable the physician to see the uterus, tubes, and ovaries. Because of the seriousness of the condition, doctors perform a laparoscopy whenever they suspect that an ectopic pregnancy is a real possibility. (See Chapter 14.)

TREATMENT

The treatment for ectopic pregnancy is surgery in which the surgeon removes the misplaced embryo and placenta. Often the fallopian tube must be removed as well. If the tube has already ruptured, this may be the operation of choice, because bleeding can be controlled immediately by placing one clamp across the tube. If the tube has not ruptured, the surgeon can make a small incision in the tube through which the fetal sac can be removed. Although this saves the tube, it leaves the possibility that a subsequent ectopic pregnancy can occur there. Any woman who has had one ectopic pregnancy has a 12 to 15 percent chance of another. Increasing surgical skill with the laparoscope has made it possible for some gynecologists to excise ectopic pregnancies with the use of miniature instruments. (See Chapter 14.) Some cancer-treating drugs, which are capable of destroying placental tissue, may prove to be useful in treating this condition without surgery.

In addition to those who have had one or more ectopic pregnancies, women who use an IUD are also at relatively higher risk of experiencing an ectopic pregnancy. The IUD prevents implantation of the fetus in the uterus, but it has no such preventive effect in the tube.

CANCER AND PREGNANCY

Obstetricians sometimes diagnose cancers of the reproductive system, especially when caring for young pregnant women. Premalignant growth and malignancies of the cervix are not rare during pregnancy. Often treatment of a potential cancer can wait until after the baby's birth, but only if the physician carefully evaluates the patient and determines the true extent of the disease process. Most chemotherapeutic medications are harmful to the developing fetus, and most surgical procedures for cancer of the uterus or ovaries involve removing the pregnancy. But waiting to treat the cancer until the fetus has developed enough to survive outside the uterus may mean that the tumor has advanced too far for a cure. The choices here are very difficult ones. If you are in this situation, you must make the final decision, but you should do so only after obtaining as much information as possible. You need to know what your chances of survival are with optimal treatment for the type of cancer you have and whether the proposed therapy can maintain your fertility so that you can look forward to another pregnancy.

CHORIOCARCINOMA

There is a family of illnesses called gestational trophoblastic disease, which originate in pregnancy. Gestational trophoblastic disease can be benign, in which case it takes the form of a hydatidiform mole or a molar pregnancy; or malignant, in which it takes the form of choriocarcinoma. It begins in placental tissue, starting in those cells (trophoblasts) that normally burrow into the lining of the uterus in early pregnancy, attaching the fetus to its supply of oxygen and nutrients. This normal tissue (of fetal origin) shares so many of the characteristics of malignancy that it is remarkable that it becomes malignant so rarely.

In the benign form of the disease, which occurs in about one in 1,000 pregnancies in this country (but much more frequently in the Far East), a portion of placental tissue disintegrates into small cysts, which can then grow, usually ending in bleeding and spontaneous abortion of the pregnancy. Sometimes no trace of the fetus can be found. The obstetrician makes this diagnosis when bleeding is present along with rapid growth of the uterus or a high titer—the lab test showing high levels of the hormone hCG, human chorionic gonadotropin—on a pregnancy test. The practitioner then removes the mole or cystic tissue along with all the tissue inside the uterus by suction curettage, controlling heavy bleeding by emptying the uterus rapidly. (See Chapter 14.)

Approximately 20 percent of women with hydatidiform moles will have or will develop the malignant changes of choriocarcinoma. Other choriocarcinomas apparently can develop from normal pregnancy. Any woman who has had a mole must be followed with serial pregnancy tests until at least two tests are negative. If positive test results persist, the obstetrician must presume that malignant tissue remains in the uterus, which can often be confirmed with a D&C. If you have this condition, it is extremely important that you avoid another pregnancy until the issue has been settled. To do so, you should use the oral contraceptive pill, the most reliable method of preventing pregnancy.

Once the diagnosis of malignant mole or choriocarcinoma has been made, the obstetrician will order a chest X ray or CAT scan of the chest cavity, because this malignancy frequently spreads to the lungs. The treatment of choice after the uterus has been emptied is single-agent chemotherapy, usually Methotrexate.

Even with the spread of cancerous tissue, or metastasis, the outlook for this tumor, which was fatal before the development of chemotherapy, is now good. Perhaps the fact that the tumor is of fetal origin and therefore different in genetic makeup from the woman herself makes it easier for the body, with a little help, to mount defenses against this very aggressive malignancy. If you have this condition, your doctor must follow it carefully by ordering quantitative serial pregnancy tests (serum hCG) until the results become *and remain* negative. Most patients do not require a hysterectomy, and some women have become pregnant after they were cured. After adequate treatment, there is a long-term survival in about 90 percent of women.

HOW YOUR BODY CHANGES
DURING PREGNANCY

As your body starts to accommodate the growing fetus, a wide range of changes begins to take place, some of them immediately more evident than others.

UTERUS

The first change is that the muscle (myometrium) of the uterus enlarges as fibrous tissue accumulates, particularly in the external muscle layer. The amount of the uterus's elastic tissue also increases. The size and number of blood vessels in the uterus continue to expand until, at term, when the baby is about to be born, the blood flow between the uterus and the placenta has become more than one pint every minute so that the fetus can receive the nourishment it needs. The uterus enlarges most in its upper part (the fundus). By term, it weighs 18 times more than it did before conception.

CERVIX AND VAGINA

The cervix also changes substantially; in fact, its swelling (edema) and additional blood flow bring on two of the very earliest signs of pregnancy, the softening of the cervix and its bluish discoloration (cyanosis). The vaginal tissue alters as well. Here, additional blood flow gives a violet color to the mucosa that makes up the lining of the vagina, while the smooth muscle of the vagina enlarges and the length of the vaginal wall increases. The vagina becomes more acidic as well.

URINARY TRACT

Another early sign of pregnancy is frequent urination, as the kidneys enlarge to accommodate the body's increased blood flow. The tubes from the kidneys to the bladder (ureters) dilate and sometimes become blocked at the brim of the pelvis after the uterus has emerged from the pelvis into the abdomen. This can happen between 10 and 14 weeks after conception, depending on the size of the uterus and how many pregnancies you have experienced before the current one. As the kidneys enlarge, they can process fluids faster, but there is an increasing probability that they will not retain and reabsorb glucose (sugar) as they normally do. This is the reason for the regular urine tests at monthly checkups: to see if there is glucose in the urine. Although some glucose may normally escape into the urine, it can still be an early warning sign of diabetes mellitus. Protein in the urine is also a trouble signal, indicating possible kidney damage from toxemia, a serious disease of pregnancy.

ABDOMEN

As pregnancy progresses, the abdominal wall expands and the abdominal wall muscles stretch, causing a noticeable separation at the midline; in some women this area takes on extra pigment to form a brown or black stripe, called the linea nigra. The growing uterus forces the contents of the abdomen to change their anatomic location. For example, your appendix, usually in the lower right side of the abdomen, may move upward and sideways so that it is closer to the diaphragm. The enlarging uterus compresses your stomach, and this can cause reflux, where the contents of the stomach cavity rebound into the esophagus, bringing on the well-known heartburn of pregnancy.

CHEST

The lower rib cage expands and, as the abdominal cavity enlarges, it forces up the diaphragm, which separates the abdomen from the chest cavity. This rib cage extension usually lasts beyond pregnancy, so that, even if you attain your prepregnancy weight, you may still find that your chest size is larger. The side-to-side width and the circumference of the rib cage increase, moving your heart upward and to the right and rotating it slightly along its long axis. This is only one of the changes that take place in your cardiovascular system. Your blood volume increases an average of 50 percent above the nonpregnant level, because 33 percent more red cells and more plasma, the fluid portion of the blood, are present during pregnancy. Your cardiac volume accelerates to accommodate both the increase in blood volume and the additional metabolic requirements of your body and the fetus. The heart swells the mass of its ventricular wall and puts out more blood per minute by raising both the amount of blood pumped and the number of beats. This additional cardiac output begins in the first trimester and continues throughout pregnancy. Cardiac output will also increase progressively during the first and second stages of labor. Because the volume of blood flow to the skin increases during pregnancy, women usually feel warmer when they are pregnant.

You may experience swelling of the ankles and legs (dependent edema), varicose veins, and hemorrhoids (varicose veins of the rectum). If the swelling accumulates during the day, it will often decrease at night after you have been off your feet for several hours.

The extra progesterone and, to a lesser extent, estrogen your body produces send messages to the respiratory center in the brain, which increases your respiration rate. This raises the volume of air you exchange with the fetus, and the amount of oxygen removed from your blood expands to accommodate the fetus's growth.

BREASTS

Your breasts enlarge and become tender during the first three months and sometimes tingle. Meanwhile, the nipples become bigger and darken, displaying more erectile capacity and stria. Often, they swell again prior to delivery. If you have already delivered and nursed a child, your breasts may express milk spontaneously before the birth. If this is your first pregnancy, your breasts may also leak colostrum, the first form of breast milk.

OTHER CHANGES

Some women develop brownish patches of varying size on their faces and necks, similar to those that occur in some women who use oral contraceptives. The high level of estrogen causes little blood lines that look like vascular spiders, and in some women the palms of the hands take on a red color. Another common complaint is acne. And thanks to the weight gain of pregnancy, sometimes women say that their skin feels softer. All of these changes usually disappear after the birth.

Stretch marks, however, do not vanish, although they become much less noticeable after delivery. These pink or brownish red streaks can appear on the abdomen, buttocks, thighs, and breasts.

As the pregnancy progresses and your body enlarges, elastic fibers in the skin break down, causing these striations. They take on color because there is an increase in the pituitary hormone that stimulates pigment-containing cells throughout your body. There is no way to prevent them, but rubbing with a moisturizing cream, which keeps the skin supple, minimizes them. Maintaining an erect posture and providing good support for your enlarging abdomen and breasts also help.

You may notice a change in your posture as your pregnancy advances, which is often referred to as saddle back or swayback or, more gallantly, as "the pride of pregnancy." A progressive increased curvature of the spine sometimes takes place, which doctors call maternal lordosis. Your joints become looser and more mobile. You may experience back pain due to additional stress on several nerves, the realignment of the pelvic ligaments, and the motion of joints in the mid- to lower-back region of the spine.

During pregnancy there is a change in the bacteria and/or organisms that grow in the vagina, and you may develop repeated yeast infections (candidiasis). These can cause a substantial vaginal discharge and be quite uncomfortable because of inflammation of the perineal tissue, the area between the vagina and anus. However, they are not usually dangerous to the fetus. Some women have other problems, including gallstones and swollen, bleeding gums.

FEELING FETAL LIFE

You will usually feel movement from the fetus somewhere between the sixteenth and twentieth week of gestation, experiencing this stirring first as a flutter and later as definite movement or kicks. Be aware that the absolute number of fetal movements per day is less important than the degree of change in their frequency. A sudden decrease can be a sign of possible trouble for the fetus. Movement or kicks of the fetus is one of the great moments of pregnancy that your partner can share by putting his hand on your stomach. You will feel these movements regularly with increasing strength until immediately before delivery, when the baby's head descends into the pelvis, which has a constricting effect and decreases fetal activity slightly. This descent, long referred to in lay terms as the "baby dropping," is medically known as the "engagement of the head."

Several factors affect how you will recognize fetal motion. Experience is one: First-time mothers are never quite sure if the initial fluttering they feel is gas or the baby. As the fetus grows, the kicking gets stronger and is unmistakable. The time at which you first detect fetal movement also depends on the location of the placenta; if it is on the part of the uterus directly beneath the abdominal wall, called an anterior placenta, you might not be aware of fetal movement as early as when the placenta is located in the back of the uterus.

FATIGUE

One early sign of pregnancy is drowsiness, because the placenta produces additional progesterone, which causes fatigue in non-pregnant women as well. Although progesterone is present in the circulation throughout the gestation, you will usually stop feeling sleepy sometime between the twelfth and sixteenth week. However, you may feel tired again at the end of the pregnancy as a result of your size and the increased energy you need simply to move around.

PREGNANCY SICKNESS

You may have problems with nausea and vomiting during the first trimester, a condition that is frequently and erroneously called morning sickness, since pregnant women are often nauseated at other times of the day as well; a more accurate name is pregnancy sickness. This nausea is probably caused by the changes that occur in the gastrointestinal tract and by the exposure of the gut to the increased level of hormones that pregnancy produces. The stomach empties less frequently because both gastric tone and the rhythmic mobility of the gut decrease. Nausea usually abates by the twelfth to fourteenth week. Be aware that some foods and vitamin supplements will make you feel worse; predicting who will have difficulty, and with what substances, is difficult, but doctors usually do not prescribe supplements during this period, particularly iron, as it can upset the stomach.

Although there is no good evidence on how beneficial some

common remedies for pregnancy sickness are, they seem to work for many women. Adding complex carbohydrates, such as whole-wheat bread, whole-grain cereals, wheat germ, and pasta and green leafy vegetables, to the diet tends to help, perhaps because these foods contain substantial amounts of vitamin B_6. Eating several smaller meals a day instead of three big ones is also a good idea, because your stomach empties more slowly and can handle less food during pregnancy. Drinking plenty of fluids neutralizes acids in the stomach and prevents dehydration from vomiting. If you do wake up feeling nauseated, try having a snack at bedtime; the next morning, eating crackers before getting up may ease the discomfort. Although the early nausea of pregnancy can be very trying, remember that it is temporary.

Don't worry if you cannot eat much during the first trimester because of nausea and do not gain weight. If you are generally well nourished, this is not a problem; the fetus will not be deprived, and you can still put on enough weight during the last two trimesters by consuming an extra 300 calories daily. Even if you don't experience nausea, you may find you are not as hungry as usual during the first trimester. Appetite usually returns to normal and then decreases again at the end of pregnancy.

DIET AND WEIGHT GAIN

The total caloric intake during pregnancy and the amount of weight a woman gains influences the birth weight of the infant. Although the National Academy of Sciences (NAS) recommends a weight gain of 25 to 30 pounds, we believe a range of 22 to 24.5 pounds is probably sufficient, particularly if you were overweight before you became pregnant. However, if you were underweight at the start of your pregnancy, you should add the number of pounds you were underweight to your pregnancy weight gain. The weight you gain during pregnancy will often include 13 pounds of retained water. (See Chapter 6 for more on nutrition during pregnancy.)

GESTATIONAL DIABETES

During pregnancy, carbohydrates and fats (lipids) are metabolized differently. The placenta produces a protein called human placental lactogen, which promotes the breakup of fat and may also oppose insulin action, increasing insulin levels in blood plasma to maintain the proper amount of glucose in the blood. The increase in estrogen and progesterone also triggers an expanded plasma insulin response to glucose. Obstetricians refer to the switch from glucose to lipids in pregnancy as "accelerated starvation," because the pregnant body utilizes glucose more quickly than in the non-pregnant state. As a result of these effects and the greater sensitivity of the pancreatic islet cells to a glucose challenge, 2 to 5 percent of all pregnant women develop gestational diabetes late in the second trimester or early in the third, which disappears after delivery. Because this condition carries with it a greater risk of complications, such as preeclampsia, delivery problems, abnormally large babies, and an increased chance of prematurity, it requires close medical supervision.

EMOTIONAL CHANGES

Anxiety and fear about the condition of being pregnant and the outcome of pregnancy are normal, and pregnant women often have nightmares. Worry about all aspects of pregnancy often precipitates questions to the midwife, doctor, or other caregiver, and you should be sure to ask any that occur to you naturally, no matter how farfetched they may seem to you, including questions about all aspects of your behavior and how it may affect your fetus. Don't stifle any query because you think your doctor or midwife is too busy; they should make time to talk with you about your concerns. Fear is a common part of pregnancy, and it is something you should deal with before you go into labor, because fear can make labor longer and more painful.

BENEFICIAL LIFE-STYLE CHANGES

STOP SMOKING AND DRINKING

Most responsible medical personnel encourage women to change their smoking and drinking habits during pregnancy, and many women are able to do this, encouraged by a desire to protect the fetus. Women who smoke when pregnant tend to have infants who are an average of 300 grams lighter than the babies of non-smokers, and any loss in birth weight is potentially harmful to the fetus. Low-birth-weight babies (under 2,500 grams or five and a half pounds) account for the largest proportion of infants who are sick and who die during the period just before, during, and after birth. The effect of smoking is probably due to carbon monoxide poisoning of the red blood cells; maternal plasma volume decreases and blood vessels constrict so that they cannot bring enough oxygen to the placenta and fetus. Smoking can also reduce appetite and rob both mother and fetus of needed nutrients.

Drinking alcohol can cause fetal alcohol syndrome, which generates defects in many organ systems, ranging from facial and limb abnormalities to cardiovascular defects and growth retardation. Lifetime neurological deficits result in impaired gross and fine coordination, abnormal speech, and mental retardation. Since doctors do not know the minimum amount of alcohol that triggers fetal alcohol syndrome, the only sensible advice is for women not to drink alcohol when pregnant.

AVOID DRUGS

While opium derivatives such as heroin and cocaine, as well as barbiturates, can cause severe intrauterine distress, low-birth-weight, and drug-addicted babies, *you should also stay away from other medicines, even nonprescription drugs, unless your medical caregiver directs you to take them.* Some medications are absolutely necessary to your health even during pregnancy; don't stop taking them without consulting your physician.

AVOID ENVIRONMENTAL HAZARDS

It is wise under any circumstance to avoid known environmental toxins, but the necessity to do so is especially acute during pregnancy. Lead is a major danger to the reproductive system of both men and women; avoid lead paint and lead-containing gasoline, and let your tap water run for a few minutes before drinking it in case there is lead in your drinking water.

Always be sure to tell any doctor you consult for any reason that you are pregnant, because a number of medical therapies can pose a danger to the fetus. X rays can cause birth defects as well as an increased incidence of leukemia in children, but the dose required to cause these problems is not known. If you must have a mammogram or an X ray of your chest, extremities, or teeth while you are pregnant, make sure to cover your abdomen and pelvis with a lead apron. Avoid thyroid and lung scans and radioactive drugs. However, if you experience a life-threatening emergency during pregnancy, a needed X ray will present a small risk to the fetus.

Questions have been raised about the effects of low-level radiation from video display terminals (VDTs) because of reported clusters of increased miscarriages and birth defects. So far, no study has proved a connection between the emissions from VDTs and subsequent reproductive problems. However, high levels of radiofrequency/microwave radiation (RF) from equipment used in metal manufacture can damage the male reproductive organs and, in animal studies, have produced fetal malformation.

Although animal studies have implicated numerous chemicals as possible reproductive hazards, not much research has been conducted on human exposure. Higher rates of miscarriage have been documented among women exposed to ethylene oxide (EtO), a clear, colorless gas used to make antifreeze, polyester fiber and films, and detergents, and also used in hospital sterilization equipment, and as a fumigant. Anesthetic gases also have been associated with spontaneous abortion; if you work in a hospital operating room, make certain the anesthesia machines have scavenging hoses that gather up to 90 percent of waste anesthetic gases. Many solvents, such as the carbon disulfide used to clean electronic components, have been implicated in reduced male fertility and increased rates of spontaneous abortion. Other suspect agents include carbon tetrachloride, styrene, xylene, toluene, and benzine used in the electronics and other industries. If you regularly come into contact with any of these chemicals at work, you should request a pregnancy transfer, preferably before you conceive. If you need more information, contact the National Institute for Occupational Safety & Health, Hazard Evaluation & Technical Assistance Branch, 4676 Columbia Parkway, Cincinnati, OH 45226 (513-841-4386), your local health department, or the Teratogen Information Service nearest you (see Appendix).

If you are pregnant or intend to become pregnant, avoid renovation jobs that require using lead paint and products containing solvents. Don't use oven cleaners that contain methylene chloride;

look instead for those made with baking soda. Keep away from pesticides; if your home must be treated with them, stay out of the house until after they have been applied, and ventilate well before you return. Don't use kerosene burners in winter, because they give off carbon monoxide. *And if you own a cat, don't clean out the cat box;* find someone to do it for you. Cat feces carry the organism that causes toxoplasmosis. If you garden, wear gloves to avoid another possible contact with cat feces.

EXERCISE

If you have been active beforehand, there is no reason to limit exercise during pregnancy, but expect a greater cardiac output during the last trimester. This means that your heart beats faster and with greater volume because of the increased fluid your body produces when pregnant. You can swim (and take baths) unless your membranes have ruptured. In fact, swimming often relieves the stress and pulling that some women experience in their back and is a comfortable form of exercise when pregnant. Runners can continue jogging, although one study indicates that their babies will weigh less at birth. Other suitable forms of exercise include walking, stationary cycling, and modified forms of dancing and calisthenics. Cycling on a bicycle is dangerous because of the possibility of falls; the same is true of snow and water skiing. Racquet sports or any activity that requires jumping or rapid changes in direction may be even more hazardous, because the looseness of a pregnant woman's joints make them more susceptible to injury. Some women do not use automobile safety belts during pregnancy because they fear they will harm the fetus; this is not true, and it is much safer to be restrained than not when riding in a car.

You should stop exercising and consult your physician immediately if you suspect that the fetus is not growing properly, or if you experience any complications, such as pain or bleeding. The American College of Obstetricians and Gynecologists has published general guidelines for exercise during pregnancy (see Table 9.1).

In general, you should not push yourself physically beyond your usual activity level. If your work requires physical exertion, you should avoid severe physical strain and undue fatigue. You also should be able to rest adequately during the working day. If you

Table 9.1 Heart Rate Guidelines for Postpartum Exercise
Beats per Minute

Age	Limit*	Maximum
20	150	200
25	146	195
30	142	190
35	138	185
40	135	180
45	131	175

*Each figure represents 75 percent of the maximum heart rate that would be predicted for the corresponding age group. Under proper medical supervision, more strenuous activity and higher heart rates may be appropriate.

have a history of prior pregnancy problems, you should minimize physical work. You can continue to travel without ill effect; the major risk of travel is that you might need medical care in an area that has no adequate treatment facility. It is a good idea to find out what care is available before starting on a trip.

Exercise Guidelines*

The following guidelines are based on the unique physical and physiological conditions that exist during pregnancy and the postpartum period. They outline general criteria for safety to provide direction to patients in the development of home exercise programs.

Pregnancy and Postpartum

1. Regular exercise (at least three times per week) is preferable to intermittent activity. Competitive activities should be discouraged.
2. Vigorous exercise should not be performed in hot, humid weather or during a period of febrile illness.
3. Ballistic movements (jerky, bouncy motions) should be avoided. Exercise should be done on a wooden floor or a

*American College of Obstetricians and Gynecologists, *Exercise During Pregnancy and the Post Natal Period* (Washington, D.C.: The College, 1985).

tightly carpeted surface to reduce shock and provide a sure footing.

4. Deep flexion or extension of joints should be avoided because of connective tissue laxity. Activities that require jumping, jarring motions or rapid changes in direction should be avoided because of joint instability.

5. Vigorous exercise should be preceded by a five-minute period of muscle warm-up. This can be accomplished by slow walking or stationary cycling with low resistance.

6. Vigorous exercise should be followed by a period of gradually declining activity that includes gentle stationary stretching. Because connective tissue laxity increases the risk of joint injury, stretches should not be taken to the point of maximum resistance.

7. Heart rate should be measured at times of peak activity. Target heart rates and limits established in consultation with the physician should not be exceeded (see Table 9.1 for recommended postpartum heart rate limits).

8. Care should be taken to rise from the floor gradually to avoid orthostatic hypotension. Some form of activity involving the legs should be continued for a brief period.

9. Liquids should be taken liberally before and after exercise to prevent dehydration. If necessary, activity should be interrupted to replenish fluids.

10. Women who have led sedentary life-styles should begin with physical activity of very low intensity and advance activity levels very gradually.

11. Activity should be stopped and the physician consulted if any unusual symptoms appear.

Pregnancy Only

1. Maternal heart rate should not exceed 140 beats per minute.

2. Strenuous activities should not exceed 15 minutes in duration.

3. No exercise should be performed in the supine position after the fourth month of gestation is completed.

4. Exercises that employ the Valsalva maneuver should be avoided.

5. Caloric intake should be adequate to meet not only the extra

energy needs of pregnancy, but also of the exercise performed.
6. Maternal core temperature should not exceed 38°C.

Special Exercises for Pregnancy and the Postpartum Period

Exercises for the Back

The back is subjected to significant stress during pregnancy and
the postpartum period. Many traditional back strengthening exercises are not recommended during pregnancy because they require the supine position of the Valsalva maneuver. One exercise
that can be done throughout pregnancy, however, is the "pelvic
tilt," which strengthens abdominal musculature and reduces lower
lumbar lordosis. The exercise is performed in this manner:

Stand with your feet shoulder width apart, knees bent slightly.
Contract the muscles of the buttocks and abdomen and thrust the
pelvis gently forward, rotating the pubic bone upward. Hold this
position for ten seconds and then release.

The pelvic tilt can also be performed while lying or sitting down.
Pregnant women should be encouraged to perform this maneuver
as many times as possible during the day.

After delivery, back pain and injury remain a significant problem
because of the repeated bending, lifting, and carrying associated
with childrearing. At this time, a full program of strengthening
and stretching exercises for the abdomen, back, and legs can be
incorporated into the daily routine. The pelvic tilt should still be
continued.

Exercises for the Pelvic Muscles (Kegel's Exercises)

The physical and hormonal changes of pregnancy cause relaxation
of the pelvic supporting tissues. Vaginal delivery stretches these
tissues even further. Most women are not troubled by these
changes, but some will complain of discomfort or stress inconti-
ence. Others may be concerned about looseness of the vagina during intercourse.

Exercise will not alter major anatomic defects. However, in patients with mild pelvic relaxation, the regular use of Kegel's ex-

ercises may be all that is necessary to provide symptomatic relief in the postpartum period. Symptomatic patients should be taught how to perform these exercises and encouraged to use them. (See Chapter 5.)

SEX DURING PREGNANCY

Unless you have vaginal bleeding, it is usually safe to have sexual intercourse throughout pregnancy until the cervix dilates. Once the cervical canal opens, there is a possibility of uterine infection.

When women stop having sex earlier in pregnancy, it is usually for a practical reason: Intercourse can become very uncomfortable if you are on top with your legs bent, which can cause painful cramping in the legs. Try a side-by-side position, or have your partner massage your clitoris manually, or use a low-level vibrator. The vaginal discharge following intercourse may also cause discomfort and, because of its volume, can make oral sex difficult. Don't be concerned that lovemaking might injure the fetus, or bring on premature labor—it won't.

PRENATAL CARE

Doctors today believe that prenatal care should be a continuation of comprehensive health care prior to pregnancy. This interaction between you and your medical caregiver can help determine if there are problems with the pregnancy and ensure that you see a specialist trained to give you the care you need, if necessary. For those who receive proper prenatal care, maternal and fetal outcome has greatly improved. It is no longer common to expect a woman or her infant to die during a pregnancy or a delivery. Among the many reasons for this fall in pregnancy- and birth-related mortality are the improved overall health and nutrition of most American women; the presence of family planning programs; the availability of selective therapeutic and elective abortion; better and more available care after delivery; greater attention to the evaluation of fetal well-being; the increased cesarean section rate that, when employed properly, saves fetuses that are truly at risk of injury or death; and the availability of high-quality care for newborn babies.

Many women wonder why they should seek medical care from

a midwife, family practitioner, or obstetrician when they are healthy and can diagnose their own pregnancies. The most important reason is that doctors and midwives have been trained to spot the ten danger signals requiring close medical supervision that may occur at any point in pregnancy. These are (1) vaginal bleeding, (2) swelling of the face or fingers, (3) severe or continuous headaches, (4) dimness or blurring of vision, (5) abdominal pain, (6) persistent vomiting, (7) chills or fever, (8) pain on urinating (dysuria), (9) escape of fluid from the vagina, and (10) marked changes in the frequency or intensity of fetal movements. Furthermore, you may have an undetected medical problem or develop one during pregnancy, and your health requires its evaluation and treatment. In addition to preexisting medical conditions such as diabetes, heart trouble, and hypertension, other reasons to classify a pregnancy as "high risk" include drug and alcohol addiction, maternal malnutrition, and previous poor pregnancy outcome. At this time it is difficult to determine what percentage of all U.S. pregnancies are at high risk, but at least 30 percent of them deserve some extra guidance and evaluation, if not therapy. In addition, your doctor or midwife can provide you with information and help answer questions regarding the medical and emotional changes that occur during pregnancy.

As we have noted, the first trimester of pregnancy extends from implantation until 12 weeks; the second spans 12 to 24 weeks; and the third runs from the twenty-fourth week until delivery. Pregnant women generally see their medical caregivers once each month for the first eight months, and then weekly until they give birth. At these prenatal visits, doctors and midwives evaluate your general health to see if there is a potential problem. Because good nutrition is a key ingredient of a healthy pregnancy, they should also survey your nutritional status and give you advice about diet. The practitioner will monitor your blood pressure, weight, the condition of your breasts, your uterine size, and the height of the top (fundus) of your uterus. The uterus resides fully within the pelvic cavity until approximately 12 weeks of gestation. When you are examined early in pregnancy, the practitioner can feel the uterus only by a bimanual exam—that is, placing two fingers in your vagina and one hand on your abdominal wall right above the pubic bone. (See Chapter 2.) The size of your uterus is then determined by measuring it between the examining fingers inside the vagina and the hand on your abdomen.

Practitioners also monitor fetal movement and note the part of the fetus, either the head or buttocks, that is presenting at the pelvis. They estimate the dimensions of the bony pelvis, the size of the fetus, and the amount of amniotic fluid; they listen to the fetal heart rate and date the pregnancy. On your first visit they order a urinalysis to check on protein and glucose, a blood count (hematocrit), a serologic test for syphilis, a blood test to determine hepatitis B carrier status, a cervical culture for gonorrhea, and, in some clinics, a screening test for antibodies to HIV, the AIDS virus.

With ultrasound, the doctor can see the fetal sac easily at seven weeks with the use of a vaginal probe, can frequently observe fetal trunk movement by eight weeks, and fetal limb movement at nine weeks of gestation. Around 10 weeks a small hand-held ultrasound device can pick up and magnify the sound of blood flowing through the fetal heart, right in the doctor's office. You will note that the normal fetal heartbeat is very fast, exceeding 150 beats per minute. In the third trimester, a sonogram can picture fetal lungs working and the fetal bladder filling and emptying.

The main uses of ultrasound are to determine the age of the fetus, its size, and the location of the placenta. A sonogram can verify that the pregnancy is properly in the uterus, and can determine the presence of multiple fetuses, abnormal amounts of amniotic fluid, some congenital abnormalities, and, sometimes, malfunctioning of the organs.

As your uterus rises out of your pelvis, it is easier for the doctor to feel and measure it within your abdomen. At 16 weeks of gestation, the top of your uterus (fundus) has reached a point midway between your pubic bone and your belly button (umbilicus). From then on, the distance between the fundus and the umbilicus serves as a measure of the number of weeks of gestation. For example, at 20 weeks, the fundus has reached the belly button. As it rises above the umbilicus, the doctor adds a week for every two centimeters, roughly the width of a finger, that the uterus shows above the umbilicus. This is yet another way to follow the progress of a normal pregnancy.

One of the reasons the clinician checks your blood pressure during each prenatal visit is that it usually decreases during the second trimester, or early in the third trimester, and then rises. As the uterus enlarges, it may partially close off veins in the pelvis and the inferior vena cava, the blood vessel that returns blood from the body to the heart. Lying on your left side will relieve this circulatory slowing, because it reduces the pressure on the vena cava and increases the blood flow from the veins in the legs, permitting your heart to increase its output. This is why doctors use what they call the rollover test for measuring blood pressure, taking it first while you are lying on your back, and then having you roll over onto your side, which gives a more accurate reading.

PRENATAL TESTING

AFP SCREENING

The fetal liver produces alpha-fetoprotein (AFP), which enters the maternal bloodstream. Because its level will often indicate if a fetal abnormality is present, one of the routine blood tests of early pregnancy, called maternal AFP screening, measures this protein. The most accurate time for this test is between 15½ and 18½ weeks of gestation. Because a fetus with a neural tube defect, where the spinal cord does not close completely, often produces high levels of this protein, the doctor orders further evaluation if the test indicates an elevated level. A low AFP sometimes indicates a chromosomally abnormal fetus, including one with Down's syndrome, characterized by particular facial features, mental retardation, and, sometimes, lung and respiratory disorders. Particularly high or low results may also indicate that the dates of the pregnancy may be wrong. This can easily be confirmed with an ultrasound exam, which will date the pregnancy correctly.

AFP is only a diagnostic test that indicates whether other studies are required. Because it is noninvasive, poses no danger to the mother or the fetus, detects possible serious problems that can be confirmed or denied by additional tests, and produces few false positive results, we believe all women should have AFP.

ULTRASOUND (SONOGRAPHY)

Ultrasound scans use pulsed sound waves vibrating at high frequencies to produce a visual image of the fetus on a screen. They detect severe abnormalities, confirming neural tube defects and other gross malformations of the brain, heart, kidneys, or bowel. Doctors employ them to date the pregnancy, diagnose twins, and determine the sex of the fetus. This is useful if a sex-related abnormality runs in your family. While advocates of alternative birth methods question the widespread use of sonography because of its unknown long-term effects, the medical community assumes the test is safe. The American College of Obstetricians and Gynecologists takes a middle road, recommending sonography only if the uterus is much larger or smaller than it should be at a particular stage of the pregnancy; if a woman has not received medical care throughout her pregnancy; if she has previously had a malformed child; if the AFP is abnormal; or if the mother has diabetes, high blood pressure, or other medical complications of pregnancy.

AMNIOCENTESIS AND CVS

Amniocentesis and chorionic villus sampling (CVS) are diagnostic tests that can identify an abnormal fetus. Researchers developed amniocentesis during the 1960s as a diagnostic tool to detect bilirubin in the amniotic fluid, which indicates if a baby is having difficulty with Rh disease. (See Chapter 8.) As soon as geneticists learned how to grow cells from the amniotic fluid, they could recognize certain chromosomal abnormalities.

In amniocentesis, the doctor inserts a thin needle covered by a sheath through the abdomen into the uterus to remove a sample of amniotic fluid; ultrasound visualization is used to guide the needle into the amniotic sac to avoid puncturing the placenta and the fetus. The needle is immediately removed, leaving the blunt sheath in place. A sample of amniotic fluid is drawn out through a syringe attached to the sheath. The sample then goes to the laboratory, where technicians separate from the fluid the cells that have been shed by the fetus and analyze them. Only by the fifteenth and sixteenth week of pregnancy is there enough amniotic fluid to perform this test successfully, and the results do not become available until the eighteenth or twentieth week, because it takes two to four weeks to culture and analyze the tissue samples. If they show an abnormality, such as Down's syndrome, and you decide to terminate the pregnancy, you must then have a second-trimester abortion. (See Chapter 8.)

The photographs of the chromosomes secured during amniocentesis also indicate the sex of the fetus, which you may or may not want to know. If you don't wish to learn the sex of your fetus, be sure to tell your doctor or midwife so that it is not inadvertently revealed to you.

Because of the heightened risks of second-trimester abortion, the development of CVS during the 1970s proved beneficial since it provided a way of growing cells after only eight weeks of gestation. As the placenta develops, it grows villi, short hairlike structures with the same chromosomal content as the fetus; analysis of cells in the villi is equivalent, then, to examining fetal chromosomes. To obtain samples of the villi, doctors use a thin catheter to enter the uterus through the cervix, or they insert a needle through the abdominal wall into the uterine cavity, and remove placental cells. Both amniocentesis and CVS have a very slight rate of increased spontaneous abortion. Recent large-scale studies comparing their safety and efficacy have found the risk and accuracy about equal if specialists are able to obtain sufficient tissue during CVS on the first attempt; second and third passes increase the risk of pregnancy loss. However, it is difficult to limit your doctor to one pass, and if you are very concerned about possible miscarriage, you may prefer waiting until you can have amniocentesis.

Most women prefer CVS because they can have the test early, ideally between the ninth and eleventh weeks, and can elect a first-trimester abortion if the fetus carries an abnormality. CVS has become a widely accepted alternative to amniocentesis in assessing fetal chromosomal abnormalities. It is, however, not offered by all hospitals. If you decide to have CVS, make sure the clinician at the hospital you choose has sufficient experience, and has done at least 500 procedures.

Because abnormalities increase with maternal age, these prenatal tests find more abnormalities among older women. For example, after age 37, one in 250 fetuses will have some problem, and by age 48 the number skyrockets to one in 10.

Obstetricians can also obtain a sample of fetal blood with direct puncturing of the fetal umbilical cord under ultrasound guidance.

Now that it is possible to diagnose many genetic diseases, such as sickle cell anemia, with other methods, doctors tend not to do fetal blood sampling. However, fetal blood sampling is still used to manage blood disorders prior to the onset of labor. In addition, samples of fetal blood are analyzed during labor to evaluate whether the fetus is getting enough oxygen. However, during labor it is relatively easy to obtain fetal blood samples from the fetal scalp.

THE FINAL WEEKS

The fetal position changes during pregnancy; at 20 weeks, 33 percent of single pregnancies are breech—that is, with the fetus's buttocks presenting at the cervix—but by term, only 3 to 4 percent are in that position. Knowing the position of the fetus is vital in determining the best way to deliver the baby. Several conditions are associated with an increased incidence of breech presentation. They include many prior pregnancies; multifetal pregnancy; previous breech deliveries; uterine abnormalities; uterine tumors; a fetus with an enlarged head (hydrocephalus) or one lacking part of the head (anencephalus); abnormalities of the placenta, such as when the placenta lies across the cervix, preventing vaginal delivery (placenta previa); and either too much or too little amniotic fluid.

In the ninth month of pregnancy, the doctor or midwife examines the cervix to evaluate its softness, its position, how thin it has become, and how much it has opened (dilated). The doctor or midwife also determines how far the presenting part of the fetus (head or buttocks) has moved into the pelvis, how much the vagina will stretch, and the firmness of the perineum, the area between the inner vaginal lips and the anus. If the presenting part of the fetus is not the head, then the physician must determine how the fetus lies. Some doctors can turn the fetus by putting pressure on the fetal buttocks with one hand and using the other hand to rotate the baby into a head-down position. This is done on the mother's abdomen and can be quite uncomfortable for her. If turning the fetus is not possible, the physician must determine if vaginal delivery will be safe.

During the last four weeks of pregnancy, the uterus prepares itself for labor and delivery. By then, most fetuses are upside down with the head at the pelvis, in the position called a vertex presentation. Several weeks before the onset of labor, a change takes place in the shape of the abdomen as the head descends into the pelvis. The fetal descent is called lightening and results from the development of the lower uterine segment. Lightening decreases the height of the fundus. Frequently during the pregnancy the uterus has irregular contractions, referred to as Braxton-Hicks contractions. They are either imperceptible unless your hand is on the abdomen, or they may cause discomfort in your lower abdomen and groin. When these contractions become more intense, it is called false labor if it does not produce progressive dilation and thinning of the cervix and descent of the fetus. False labor may progress to true labor, in which the discomfort begins at the top of the uterus and radiates to the lower back. As the muscles of the lower segment of the uterus lengthen, the muscles of the upper uterus shorten. In normal labor, contractions in the lower uterine segment are shorter and less intense than those in the upper uterine segment because the whole process of labor is to expel the fetus out of the uterus and through the bony pelvis.

As you approach the end of pregnancy, your doctor will assess the well-being of the fetus. If you do not feel adequate fetal movements, if you do not gain weight, if you have gone beyond your estimated date of delivery, or if you show signs of medical problems, the medical team will use ultrasound to investigate; this procedure can pick up both the heart rate and the movements of the fetus and measure the general physical aspects of the fetus's condition. Additional tests that may be performed at this time are the stress test and the nonstress test. The first evaluates the relationship between the fetal heart rate and contractions by stimulating the uterus to contract with either the drug oxytocin or by nipple stimulation while monitoring the fetal heart rate during the contractions. The nonstress test monitors fetal activity and heart rate without using oxytocin or nipple stimulation. A satisfactory nonstress test requires three or more fetal movements while the fetal heart rate accelerates by 15 beats per minute or more. Other tests measure fetal motion. The fetus should move its body or limbs at least three times and extend and flex a limb one or more times within 30 minutes to demonstrate good fetal tone; it should also exhibit at least one episode of breathing movements within 30 seconds. Physicians may also use ultrasound to assess the maturity of the placenta.

LABOR AND DELIVERY

TESTING DURING LABOR

The membranes surrounding the fetus can rupture prior to, during, or at delivery. If they rupture before your labor has started, the obstetrician may manage your labor differently because of the possibility that the fetus might become infected. An amniocentesis may be performed at this point to determine if the fetus is infected and if it has developed enough lung maturity to be born; if so, the practitioner will induce labor.

During labor, uterine contractions become more and more frequent until they occur about two minutes apart and last for one minute. The uterus reduces blood flow to the placenta during a contraction. The interval between contractions is important because that's when the fetus can get oxygen from your body and also that's when you can rest.

The heart rate of a fetus is variable, with a normal range between 120 and 160 beats per minute. The heart rate will typically drop during contractions when the fetal head is compressed. Declines in the fetal heart rate after a contraction, however, may indicate that the fetus is not getting enough oxygen. A heart rate that does not commonly rise with activity is not normal, and one without variability in its rate can indicate problems requiring further evaluation. The obstetrician does additional tests at this point only if it appears that the fetus is in trouble, particularly since there are normal factors that inhibit a variable heart rate, including certain medications, prematurity, and fetal sleep.

If these evaluations are not normal, the doctor frequently orders a contraction stress test, using drugs to stimulate the uterus to contract three times in 10 minutes for at least 40 seconds per contraction. The test is normal if the fetal heartbeat does not slow down. If it does slow down, this means that the fetus is not getting enough oxygen from the placenta so that it has a sufficient oxygen reserve to tolerate the next contraction. Other possible fetal problems are a rapid heart rate, called fetal tachycardia, which can reflect the fact that the mother has a fever, or a severely slow heart (bradycardia). These tests are important so that the pediatrician who will care for the newborn can evaluate the infant and provide the necessary treatment at once.

If any of the tests indicate that the fetus may be at risk, or if the mother has medical complications, such as preeclampsia, a serious condition characterized by high blood pressure, edema, and protein in the urine, then the doctor may have to deliver the fetus immediately. If the fetus is at risk, the doctor may induce labor so that the mother can attempt a vaginal delivery rather than have a cesarean section.

It is important to monitor a woman whose labor is induced. Medication causes the uterus to contract more vigorously than with unaided labor, and she may need additional medication to modify these strong contractions so that they are effective but not so powerful that the uterus ruptures or the oxygen supply to the baby is cut off. Doctors also induce labor when a woman is overdue, usually if she is two weeks beyond her estimated date of delivery. But delivery of a baby before the onset of normal labor should occur for only two reasons: the mother's well-being or to improve the baby's chances of survival and health. Before rushing to delivery, doctors can sample amniotic fluid to determine fetal lung maturity and if the fetus will be able to breathe.

FIRST STAGE

The doctor or midwife usually tells the mother-to-be to time her contractions once she goes into labor until they are regular and occur every four minutes before calling her or him. You should be as comfortable as possible during labor. In early labor it's best to walk around, but once active labor has progressed to the point where contractions occur every two minutes, you will probably find it more comfortable to sit upright, squat, or lie on your side. The most uncomfortable position, and one that may slow labor, is lying flat on your back. (Long-delayed changes in hospital procedures and doctors' attitudes have made this position rare today. Most women labor in a bed or chair that has a tilted back, and lie flat only to be examined.)

After you are admitted to a delivery facility, the labor room staff will ask you how frequent and intense your contractions are and whether you have discharged either fluid or blood from your vagina, which means you have expelled the mucous plug that has sealed off the cervix during pregnancy.

The first stage of labor is the period during which the lower segment of the uterus thins and the cervix opens to allow the fetus through. The obstetrician can feel changes in the cervix during a vaginal examination. At the start of labor, the opening of the cervix is often in the posterior portion of the vagina and will admit only the fingertip of the examiner. As labor progresses, pressure from the fetal head dilates the cervix and the opening moves forward. Trained labor room personnel can usually gauge the intensity of uterine contractions manually without using fetal monitors. They monitor the fetal heart rate with a stethoscope and evaluate its response to contractions. If the fetal heart rate is less than 120 beats per minute, they might suspect fetal distress, particularly if it slows following a contraction.

Ideally, every laboring woman should have a nurse, midwife, or physician with her to monitor her progress closely, using hands and stethoscope, so that a fetal monitor is not required. Unfortunately, the tremendous shortage of nurses and midwives, and the heavy caseloads most doctors carry, make it very difficult to deliver the kind of hands-on care that most doctors would like to provide, and as a result, physicians still rely on fetal monitors. Another factor is practice style; many physicians are trained to use fetal monitors. Women's health advocates believe that the dependency on fetal monitors, with their high rate of false positives—that is, inaccurate indications of fetal distress—has contributed greatly to the substantial increase in unnecessary cesarean sections in recent years.

During the first stage of labor, the cervix opens until it is dilated to a diameter of 10 centimeters. Since the head of the fetus measures between nine and 10 centimeters at term, once the cervix has opened fully, the head can pass through the uterine opening. The final phase of first-stage labor, called transition, is the most intense, with contractions lasting 60 to 90 seconds, every one to three minutes. It is during transition that the cervix opens completely. Each labor has its own pace, and this first stage of labor can last anywhere from less than an hour to 18 to 26 hours, depending on how many children you have had and the size of the fetus. The short transition phase between first- and second-stage labor lasts for 45 minutes to an hour, but produces the strongest contractions.

SECOND STAGE

The second stage of labor (pushing) usually takes between two and four hours. It begins with the cervix fully dilated and the fetus's head pressing on the pelvis; this makes you want to bear down and push the fetus out. Now is the time for you to use all you have learned in childbirth preparation classes to shorten your labor and help deliver your baby. As you push, the head continues to mold to the shape of the birth canal until its presenting part becomes visible at the opening of the vagina. It is normal for the vaginal opening to appear smaller during the relaxation period between contractions as the fetus rocks back under the pubic bone. As the head slowly appears at the vaginal opening and you bear down and push the baby out, the perineum may begin to tear. The more rapidly the baby comes out, the greater is the chance of tearing.

EPISIOTOMY

The doctor or midwife can make an incision, called an episiotomy, to prevent tearing of the tissue in an uncontrolled manner. The episiotomy can be of the median type, on a direct line between the vagina and anus, or mediolateral, in which the incision is made off to the side (see Fig. 9.5). Episiotomies are preventive measures, and many women's health advocates maintain that they should never be performed routinely. Be sure to discuss episiotomy with your medical practitioner beforehand, so you can agree about the circumstances that would require it. When a woman can control the pace of pushing the baby out, there is time for the vaginal muscle and the skin to stretch. Massaging the perineum with warm oil during delivery helps it stretch and may prevent tearing and/ or the need for an episiotomy. Delivering in an upright position also helps to avoid tearing. Small tears that might occur during a slow, controlled delivery are not a problem and heal nicely. But if the fetus descends through the canal before stretching can occur, or if its shoulder pops out of the vagina immediately after the head, the vaginal tear may be large.

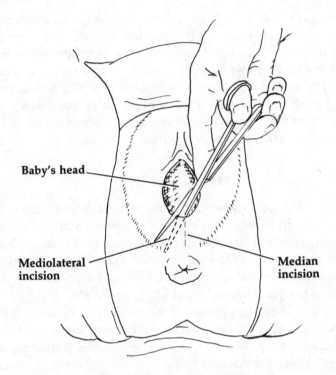

Fig. 9.5 Episiotomy Incisions

Two types of tears are serious. The first is one that occurs in the vulva tissue that goes to the urethra, tearing the small vessels around the urethra and causing substantial bleeding. This tear requires stitches that are quite painful. The second, and of greater concern, is a tear that rips into the rectum. A controlled cut, even one that goes through the rectal sphincter, can be fixed easily, while a tear into the rectum and through the sphincter is more difficult to correct. If the repair does not heal properly, a woman might be incontinent of stool and have a fistula (opening) between the rectum and the vagina. A delivery that damages the floor of the vagina can lead to a relaxed vaginal wall that needs repair. (See Chapter 14.)

As the head of the baby arrives, the doctor removes any mucus from the mouth and nose, wipes the baby's face, and checks to see if the umbilical cord is around its neck. If so, and if the cord cannot be slipped over the baby's head, the doctor will clamp and cut it, which means that the baby must be delivered promptly. In most cases, the shoulders come out spontaneously, but sometimes they need to be eased out gently. Once the shoulders are through, the rest of the baby slips out easily. When this happens, you will feel a tremendous surge of relief, and, if your partner is present, both of you can experience the excitement of finally seeing your infant. Breast-feeding soon after delivery helps control uterine bleeding because it stimulates the secretion of natural oxytocin, the hormone that makes the uterus contract.

THIRD STAGE

The third stage of labor, when the uterus must expel the placenta, follows the delivery of the baby. As the uterus contracts, the interface between the placenta and the uterine wall shrinks, and the placenta shears off from the uterine wall. When there is bleeding between the uterus and the placenta, the blood serves as a wedge to separate the placenta, forcing it out of the uterus. This usually occurs within five to 20 minutes of the delivery of the baby. If the placenta does not come out on its own, the practitioner performs a manual separation by placing a hand in the uterus, finding the cleavage between the placenta and the uterus, and manually shearing the placenta off the uterine wall.

Infrequently, an abnormality of the placenta, called an accreta, prevents it from developing properly and allows it to grow into the wall of the uterus. The doctor usually removes an accreta surgically. A placenta accreta or a postpartum hemorrhage that cannot be controlled are the two most common reasons for a hysterectomy immediately after delivery, but both are very rare events.

You will lose an average of 600 milliliters (2½ cups) of blood after a vaginal delivery. This blood loss usually presents no problem, because your blood volume will have increased by at least that amount during the pregnancy.

ANESTHESIA

Obstetrical anesthesia is a special field. Anesthesia is not administered in obstetrics the way it is in other areas because the issue of pain relief for the mother must be balanced against the necessity of not harming the fetus. The objective is to prevent exposing the fetus to the anesthetic agents that may help the mother through labor.

The anesthesia used during labor today consists of either short-acting narcotics or regional nerve blocks. Meperidine (Demerol) is the narcotic most commonly used during childbirth. It relaxes you and eases the pain of labor, allowing you to rest between contractions. If given too early, however, it can slow labor, and, if administered too close to the time of birth, it can seriously depress the fetal heart rate and respiration. Small doses, properly administered, should not have any deleterious effects. The effects of Demerol last for about four hours; other short-acting narcotics act for shorter time periods.

Nerve blocks numb the nerves from the uterus and the interior and exterior of the vagina. Anesthesiologists start to administer this type of anesthesia, called a peridural or epidural, when you are in active labor and your cervix has begun to dilate. The anesthesiologist places a needle through your back into the canal between the spine and the spinal column, injecting quick-acting Xylocaine or related drugs through a catheter attached to the needle.

The chief disadvantage of some epidural medications is that some women to whom they are given cannot feel any sensation and are consequently unable to help push the baby out, thus lengthening labor. On the other hand, women experiencing a great deal of pain sometimes become more tense and the consequent anxiety may increase the pain of labor as well as prevent the relaxation of the pelvic floor. The peridural removes this pain and relaxes the pelvic floor, allowing a woman to rest. Often, a woman can recover enough to push more effectively when it comes time to deliver.

Doctors also use local anesthesia to numb the tissue in the vaginal canal and lessen pain as the head comes out, or when performing an episiotomy. They rely on general anesthesia only for emergency cesarean sections, and, even then, take care to give a medicine that does not cross the placenta rapidly, so that the mother is asleep and the baby is out of her uterus before the medication succeeds in crossing the placenta.

The type of anesthesia is a matter of choice only if there is a trained anesthesiologist available. If not, the obstetrician usually can administer only limited amounts of fast-acting and short-lived narcotics and local anesthesia to relieve pain as the baby's head descends through the pelvis.

Although the health of the fetus makes it imperative that medication be administered conservatively, the reason women request pain medication is to relieve the real pain of labor, and it is unfair to women to suggest that they are not experiencing genuine pain by calling it "discomfort." All of us perceive and handle pain differently, and all laboring women should be asked if they need help handling their pain in a manner that will not make them feel as if they had failed by accepting medication.

NATURAL CHILDBIRTH

Natural childbirth is based on the assumption that pregnancy and birth are natural processes, not diseases, and that nothing should be done that interferes with the mother's choices about how she will manage her labor and deliver her baby. This approach has been summed up by the famous Dutch professor of obstetrics G. J. Kloosterman this way:

> Giving birth is mostly a normal physiological event that does not require any form of medical intervention . . . a natural phenomenon that only requires medical interference in pathological and rather exceptional situations. . . . [W]e cannot improve labor in a healthy woman. We can change the process, we can shorten it, we can speed it up, we can try to take away pain, but at best we will do this without doing any harm. This leads to the conclusion that the ideal obstetrical organization brings aid to women and children who need help (the pathological group) and protects the healthy ones against unnecessary interference and human meddlesomeness.

Advocates of natural childbirth, from its innovator, Dr. Grantly Dick Read, to today, maintain that intervention in the natural process of childbirth negatively interferes with a finely tuned and extremely efficient system to its detriment; that women, left to their own devices, know how to birth their babies, mostly with the help of other, experienced women; and that the pain of childbirth is vastly increased by the fear and tension generated by American obstetrical hospital departments employing unnecessary and possibly harmful technology. If a woman is in a quiet, secure, private, and safe environment, she will usually be able to experience labor and birth without the help of anesthetics; when both she and her newborn are awake, the natural process of bonding can begin at once. Bonding involves not only holding and cuddling the infant but immediate breast-feeding, which has the added advantage of increasing uterine contractions and helping to expel the placenta.

Natural childbirth recognizes the fact that all labors and laboring women are unique and individual and does not specify time constraints for the various stages of labor. Women are free to move around; to interact with their partners and other family members and friends whom they choose to have with them; if they choose, to eat lightly and drink fluids during labor, which is hard work and requires a major expenditure of energy; and to select the position in which they will deliver their babies. Some women prefer to squat; some to be upright, either holding on to or being held up by their partners; others use a birthing stool or chair, which has an opening so that the birth attendant can catch the baby; and still others prefer lying on their side. There are no fetal monitors; instead, birth attendants use a stethoscope to check the fetal heart rate and a blood pressure cuff to monitor the mother's vital signs.

Some hospitals have established birthing rooms so that low-risk mothers who choose natural childbirth can have it while still enjoying the security of backup medical care should the need arise. Many natural birth advocates, however, question whether a truly natural birth is possible in a hospital birthing room; they believe the very existence and proximity of obstetrical technology makes its use in such settings likely. Many freestanding birth centers, usually staffed by midwives, also practice natural childbirth for low-risk mothers.

HOME BIRTH

Throughout the world, most women give birth at home. This is not true, of course, in the United States, where only a small minority of women—less than 2 percent—choose home birth. Those who do cite the ability to have natural childbirth in a familiar setting surrounded by people they love, with only a midwife to attend them, as their primary reasons for favoring home birth.

Midwives who help women deliver at home say mothers are much more relaxed and, therefore, frequently have easy and relatively short labors. Midwives, however, are trained to assist the woman whose labor is long, identifying those actions the laboring mother takes that help the baby's progress down the birth canal, so that the mother can repeat them and move her labor along. Midwives are also trained to identify the danger signals—outlined earlier in this chapter—that indicate the need for transfer to a hospital. If a woman needs or requests a transfer, some hospitals allow the midwife to continue to act as the mother's advocate in the hospital.

SAFETY OF HOME BIRTH

The major issue surrounding home birth is, however, safety. Doctors believe hospital birth is safer because the two major complications of childbirth—maternal hemorrhage and true fetal distress requiring immediate delivery—can only be dealt with in a hospital. They cite as proof the decrease in maternal and fetal mortality, which occurred simultaneously with the move from home to hospital birth.

Home birth advocates say that there is no proof that the move to hospital birth is the reason for decreasing maternal and fetal mortality, and maintain that the improved health status of mothers is a major reason for the decline. While admitting that the rare cases of maternal hemorrhage and true fetal distress require rapid transfer to the hospital, they claim that, overall, home birth, and birth in maternity clinics that practice natural childbirth, is safer than hospital birth. They cite statistics that show maternal and fetal mortality rates well below the national average for the few midwifery services.

In addition, they point to a recently published analysis of birth statistics in England, whose obstetrical practices with respect to the use of technology are quite similar to those in the United States. Statistician Marjorie Tew compared maternal mortality of high-risk and older mothers delivered at home and in the hospital and found it higher in hospital births. In addition, she compared two different periods, 1964 to 1966 and 1973 to 1975, and discovered that, as more of these women had their babies in the hospital, their mortality rate rose; if hospitals were really safer, it should have fallen.

Tew also studied stillbirths and perinatal mortality—those deaths that occur in babies just before, during, and right after birth—before 1970, when one-third of British births were still taking place outside obstetric hospitals. Absolute comparisons would, of course, find a higher mortality in the hospital group because it was larger; therefore, Tew used relative comparisons and found that, for high-, moderate-, and low-risk mothers, more babies died in the hospital than at home. Although these results are interesting, cross-cultural comparisons are not necessarily valid.

THE ROLE OF YOUR PARTNER

Mothers who have given birth at home cite the increased involvement of their partners, who often "catch" the baby or cut the umbilical cord, as a primary reason for choosing home birth. Partners often train as labor coaches, taking courses in the Bradley method or other programs that prepare fathers for this role. If your partner does this, he can help you with breathing and relaxation exercises to make labor easier, can assist you as you move around, can hold you as you deliver, and can bond with the infant immediately, just as you do.

If your partner does not choose the coaching role, he can encourage and comfort you throughout your labor; can care for the older children, if they are there, as you need and desire more privacy; and can take care of domestic chores during and after the birth, when you will need to rest. Many women who have given birth at home say their partners were an enormous help in managing labor, and that having them as an integral part of the birth brought the couple closer together.

SURGICAL DELIVERY: CESAREAN SECTION

Cesarean section is major abdominal surgery during which the doctor makes an incision in the abdominal and uterine walls to deliver a baby and remove the placenta (see Fig. 9.6). Postoperative recovery is longer than with vaginal birth, and the rate of infection

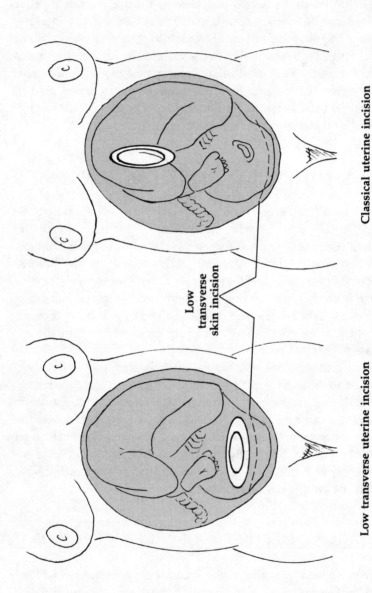

Classical uterine incision

Low transverse uterine incision

Low transverse skin incision

Fig. 9.6   Incisions for Cesarean Sections

is higher when the woman has been laboring for 24 hours or more. Infection rates are lower than for vaginal birth if the c-section is elective, without a previous trial of labor. Thus the crucial decision to make is whether a c-section is actually necessary. If it is necessary, it is essential not to wait too long to perform it. Cesarean section involves an increased risk to the mother because of the need for anesthesia.

The rate of cesarean section in the United States has increased enormously over the last 20 years, jumping from about 5 percent of all births in 1970 to approximately 25 percent today. The primary reasons for the rise are:

- a policy of performing repeat c-sections for all women who have once experienced a surgical birth
- failure to progress in labor (dystocia)
- fetal distress
- breech presentation
- all other complications and issues, including greater financial rewards to doctors and hospitals for surgical births, greater convenience to physicians, and physician fear of lawsuits charging malpractice during normal delivery

The fact that abdominal delivery is no longer as risky for the mother as it used to be, thanks to modern surgical techniques, antibiotics, anesthesia, and an emphasis on minimal trauma to the baby, has also contributed to the increase.

UNNECESSARY CESAREAN SECTIONS

In 1987, the Public Citizen Health Research Group reported that half of the estimated 900,000 cesarean sections done in 1985 and 1986 were unnecessary. It cited the medical policy of performing repeat cesareans as the main culprit, contributing to 48 percent of the increase between 1982 and 1987. Failure to progress in labor was reported to be the second largest cause (29 percent of the increase between 1980 and 1985), followed by fetal distress at 15 percent. While the report found no conclusive data that physician fear of lawsuits contributed to the decision to operate, it mentioned increased fees to doctors for cesarean sections and the longer hospital stays that run up higher bills as possible factors, citing recent studies that showed elevated c-section rates for women who had private physicians as opposed to the lower rates among clinic patients. But military hospitals that offer no financial rewards have cesarean rates similar to those of civilian hospitals where payment for them is higher.

In November 1988, the American College of Obstetricians and Gynecologists issued new guidelines urging that a trial of labor and vaginal birth after an earlier cesarean section become routine and noting that vaginal birth was safe for women who have had two or more surgical deliveries—particularly for those women whose previous cesarean was attributed to failure to progress in labor. It should be noted that this "failure" can be interpreted differently by the doctors who decide when it is present: Medical opinions about how long is too long range widely. One study found that physicians' practice style was a major influence in determining the frequency of c-sections, with a range in c-section rates from 19.1 to 42.3 percent among individual obstetricians. This study did not find any obvious differences in neonatal outcome associated with the variations in the rate of cesarean section. And a 1990 paper in the *Journal of the American Medical Association* that looked at different strategies for reducing surgical births reported that formal programs to lower rates at individual hospitals were the most effective, with declines up to 34 percent achieved at some teaching hospitals. But it is clear that there are either not enough hospitals instituting formal programs, or that this "most successful" strategy is not working, because of the 3,909,510 births that occurred in 1988, 966,000 (24.7 percent) were cesarean births, 615,000 for the first birth (primary) and 351,000 repeat procedures.

INDICATIONS FOR CESAREAN SECTION

Indications for cesarean section include evidence that the fetus is in danger of central nervous system damage as the result of a traumatic labor, or that the fetus is not tolerating labor well. The clinician determines this by measuring the mother's contractions and monitoring the fetus's heart pattern and rate. If the practitioner believes that the fetus is at risk, a blood sample is obtained by making a small nick in the part of the fetal scalp that can be seen presenting in the vagina. While this takes only a few minutes, you might feel that it is taking forever, because the fetal sampling is performed while you are in a very awkward position, with legs apart and a speculum in the vagina. If the fetal blood values indicate that the fetus is not getting enough oxygen or has a low pH, which places it in an acidic environment that is dangerous, the practitioner will perform a cesarean section. It is not possible to know before delivery how often a danger reading on a fetal scalp sample is a false positive, although afterward the doctor can determine whether the fetus was either safe or in distress.

It is important to remember that the purpose of monitoring labor or sampling blood is to prevent damage, not to wait until the practitioner must try to rescue an infant from certain harm. Although a vaginal delivery might have produced just as healthy a baby and mother, this does not classify a c-section as unnecessary, as it is always easier to have correct answers after the fact. If a doctor honestly believes there is a danger to mother or infant in waiting, most mothers prefer a surgical delivery to taking a chance that their infant will be harmed.

If your doctor suggests a cesarean because your labor is not progressing satisfactorily, there is usually plenty of time to consider whether it is really necessary. This gives you a choice, and if you agree to a surgical delivery, allows you to have regional anesthesia so that you are awake when your baby arrives. If, however, the fetal monitor indicates that the baby is in trouble, and this is confirmed by fetal scalp sampling, sometimes the surgery must be done so quickly that there is only time for general anesthesia.

Other reasons for c-section include a failure of the fetus to progress through the birth canal during labor and an abnormal fetal position, such as when the fetus is lying sideways across the opening of the birth canal. In addition, many physicians use c-section for all breech presentations, although some favor a trial of vaginal birth. The concern with a breech presentation is that trauma can occur during delivery. The head of a normal, full-term infant is its largest diameter; thus, if the head comes through first, the rest of the baby will follow relatively easily. However, if the baby is breech, with either the feet or buttocks presenting, the head may not get through the vagina. In an attempt to deliver the head, the baby might choke, or its head might become hyperextended, causing a spinal cord injury. When evaluating the breech, the obstetrician will usually decide to perform a cesarean section if the fetus is larger than 3,500 grams or 7.6 pounds, if the woman's pelvis is small or its shape presents difficulties, if the baby's head is hyperextended, if labor is not progressing smoothly, if the fetus is premature, if the mother has a history of delivery problems, or if the mother requests a cesarean section.

Previous vaginal injury is also an appropriate reason for a cesarean. For example, women who have had surgery to correct a fistula, or because the vagina and rectum failed to heal properly after a previous traumatic delivery, need surgical delivery to avoid further trauma to the vagina. Similarly, a woman who has had fibroids removed from her uterus, which involved entering the uterine cavity, requires a cesarean to avoid the risk of rupturing the uterus during a vaginal delivery. And some infertility patients have medical indications requiring cesarean sections.

The incidence of c-section for the first delivery increases with maternal age, and at some centers can approach 50 percent of all births to older women. However, for women who have had previous children vaginally, the rate of cesarean section is not much higher for older mothers than it is for younger ones.

CHOICE OF DELIVERY

Be sure that you become well informed about the methods used during labor and delivery so you can responsibly participate in deciding about the type of delivery you want. While the legitimate reasons for a c-section should be medical, your practitioner should be willing to consider your request for an elective c-section with care and respect. Many such requests come from women who fear vaginal deliveries, particularly if they have already had a traumatic delivery, or have been troubled by stories about difficult births from close family members or friends. As more women who have had one cesarean section are opting for vaginal birth, having one surgical delivery no longer means routine repeat cesarean sections in subsequent pregnancies, and this, too, must now be taken into consideration when determining the type of delivery you have.

CULTURAL ATTITUDES
TOWARD CESAREAN SECTION

Some cultures may prefer c-section to vaginal birth because the vagina is not dilated during delivery and the assumption is that the woman will be protected from losing vaginal tone and the loss of her partner's sexual pleasure. This is not a valid reason for a c-section; if a woman actually does lose vaginal tone that does not respond to pelvic exercises, and her sex life changes as a result, it is sometimes possible to repair her vagina surgically at a later time. (See Chapter 14.)

QUESTIONS YOU SHOULD ASK

Whether you prefer natural childbirth, the use of anesthesia to help with pain, or a surgical birth, be sure to discuss well in advance the attitude of your practitioner toward delivery, and the criteria of the hospital where you plan to give birth. What is the percentage of cesareans that the doctor's practice performs? (Higher than 20 percent is too high.) What is the doctor's opinion of it? Does the hospital have rigid standards in defining slow-moving labor and thus a high rate of cesareans? Don't be intimidated by social and economic factors that may make your own particular case a casualty of the needs of medical professionals. A cesarean section is major surgery and should be performed only when your own needs require it. The box on page 265 lists some of the other questions to ask your doctor and the hospital administrator.

AFTERWARD

THE APGAR SCORE

The Apgar score is a uniform system for rating the newborn's condition at one and five minutes after birth. It measures the infant's heart rate, respiration, muscle tone, reflexes, and color on a score of 0 to 2 respectively. The best score is 10, two for each of the five indicators. A one-minute Apgar between 7 and 10 means the newborn is in excellent shape; 5 to 7 indicates mild depression, and any score lower than 5 indicates the baby is in trouble and needs to be resuscitated. The five-minute score is more accurate in indicating a serious problem. A low one-minute score often improves on the five-minute score, meaning that the problem was temporary. For example, if the airway was obstructed by mucus, after the doctor clears it the infant's breathing will become normal (see Table 9.2).

Table 9.2 The Apgar Score

Criteria	0	1	2
Color	Body blue, pale	Body pink, extremities blue	Body all pink
Heart rate	Absent	Less than 100	More than 100
Respiration	Absent	Irregular, slow	Good, crying
Reflex response to nose catheter	None	Grimace	Sneeze, cough
Muscle tone	Limp	Some flexion of extremities	Active

LACTATION AND NURSING

Nursing is an integral part of pregnancy and birth. It has important advantages and few drawbacks. Breast-feeding promotes intimacy and bonding and is a remarkably satisfying emotional and sensual experience. Breast milk is ideally suited to your baby's needs, containing just the right nutrients. It strengthens the infant's ability to resist infection and the common diseases of childhood. Colostrum, the liquid produced in your breasts before the milk comes in, is particularly high in antibodies that protect the newborn from staphylococcus infections, polio, infant diarrhea, and other problems. Allergies and skin rashes are less common among breast-fed babies, as are tooth decay and misaligned teeth. One recent study found less need for orthodontic work to straighten teeth later

Questions to Ask an Obstetrician

1. What is your c-section rate? (Doctors with high-risk practices should be less than 17 percent. Doctors with low-risk practices should be under 10 percent.)
2. Do you offer a "trial of labor" to women who have had a previous c-section? If so, what percentage of them deliver vaginally? (The percentage should ideally be at least 60 to 70 percent.)
3. Do you use fetal blood sampling or fetal stimulation techniques if electronic fetal monitoring suggests fetal distress, prior to performing a c-section? (Ideally, both of these tests should be done.)
4. Do you consider an independent second opinion for elective c-sections good medical practice?
5. When confronted with a baby in breech position, do you routinely perform external cephalic version, or turning the baby, after 37 weeks?

Questions to Ask a Hospital Administrator

1. What is the c-section rate for this hospital? (If it is a community hospital, how close is it to 7 percent? If it is a referral hospital, with a neonatal intensive care unit, which sees more difficult cases, how close is it to 17 percent?)
2. Does this hospital offer a "trial of labor" to patients who have had a previous c-section? If so, what percentage of patients who have had a previous c-section do deliver vaginally? (The percentage should ideally be at least 60 to 70 percent.)
3. Is fetal blood sampled or a fetal stimulation test routinely done if electronic fetal monitoring suggests fetal distress, prior to doing a cesarean section? (At least one of these tests should be performed unless a serious emergency is noted.)
4. Is a second opinion required before a nonemergency c-section is performed? (A second opinion has been shown to lower c-section rates without affecting the quality or safety of care.)
5. Does this hospital have any other policies to help prevent unnecessary c-sections?

in life among babies who were breast-fed for one year or more. Breast-feeding is relatively easy because you don't have to make formula, sterilize bottles, or get up during the night to warm a bottle. It is relatively inexpensive, since you don't have to buy formula, bottles, and a sterilizer. And it should help you lose weight, because your body will burn more calories to make the milk than you consume even if you increase the amount you eat— unless you go way overboard. (See Chapter 6.)

The only major disadvantage of nursing is that it is sometimes restricting. Nevertheless, even a woman who returns to work shortly after birth can breast-feed by using a breast pump to extract enough milk into a bottle for one or two feedings during her absence. There are inexpensive battery or electrically operated small pumps on the market for this purpose, and you can rent larger, more efficient ones if you plan to prepare several bottles daily. This will allow your partner to take over some of the baby's feedings, particularly in the middle of the night, so that you can get extra rest. You will probably need a small pump even if you stay at home or take a substantial maternity leave, because you may have more milk in your breasts than the baby can take at first. This can lead to sore and engorged breasts, and pumping out the excess milk will provide relief. Sometimes holding a bottle over the other breast while nursing will collect enough milk to relieve discomfort. It's a good idea to massage your nipples with a few drops of colostrum and, when it comes in, breast milk, to keep them supple and avoid cracks. If your nipples become sore during nursing, try alternating the position in which the baby sucks and avoid soaps that irritate them. You can use rubber or plastic nipples over your own; the baby sucks on them, giving your nipples a chance to heal and toughen. After feeding, make sure your nipples are dry; use a hair dryer, which may be helpful in keeping your nipples from cracking. If you experience swelling, redness, or a painful lump, you may have a plugged milk duct. Hot compresses, massaging the area, and more frequent nursing will usually relieve the problem. If you have fever or aches and pains, consult your physician because you may have a breast infection.

Women who choose not to nurse can use icepacks on the breasts, wear a tight bra, and avoid breast stimulation, such as taking a hot shower and letting the water flow directly on the breasts. Reports that breast-feeding reduces the risk of getting breast cancer are true only for women under 20.

BONDING

Bonding is the process of forming a deep attachment with the newborn, and it is equally important to both parents. Although immediate nursing may be your first bonding experience, holding, cuddling, and talking to the infant during the first half-hour of life are all important connections. Since the fetus can hear outside sounds during late pregnancy, it is not surprising that a newborn seems to recognize his or her mother's voice and will also know her partner's voice if he or she has heard it regularly when in utero. Studies have found that fathers and other partners who are involved in the birth and bond early with the infant usually spend more time with the baby later on. Having the baby stay in your room so that both you and your partner can hold and care for him or her is another way of encouraging bonding.

DEPRESSION

Postpartum depression occurs in perhaps 30 percent of new mothers and can sometimes be severe. The causes include the abrupt and precipitous drop in the level of estrogen and progesterone that occurs after delivery, combined with the inevitable fatigue involved in taking care of an infant who wakes up every few hours. You may feel "let down" after the excitement of the birth, and this, too, can raise the level of emotional tension. A fretful baby may make you believe you are not doing a good job. Isolation can also be a serious problem if you have the full responsibility of caring for your newborn. If you are taking an extended pregnancy leave, you may also miss the stimulation of your job.

It helps to talk about your feelings with other parents, grandparents, or neighbors who have raised families, and to make sure you have a support system to help you. This certainly should include your partner, mother, sister, brother, or other close relatives or friends. Usually, postpartum depression doesn't last for long. Getting extra rest is one way of coping; if you sleep when the baby does, you'll be rested. It pays to hire domestic help if you can afford it to take over some housekeeping chores. A baby-sitter is also a good investment so that you can get away for a few hours. This is a suitable time to leave a bottle of breast milk with the sitter, as it gets the newborn used to synthetic nipples, a necessary preparation if you are returning to work and will be skipping feedings.

Documented cases of severe postpartum depression occur in fewer than 1 percent of mothers. Those who are severely depressed need professional treatment, either psychotherapy, medication, or both. As yet, we have no way of identifying who will experience this problem, though women who have had a prior postpartum depression are at risk.

HAIR LOSS

Some women experience hair loss or hair thinning after childbirth. Don't be concerned if this happens, because the hair grows back. Although only about 10 percent of the hair stops growing after delivery in most women, total hair growth ceases in some, perhaps because of the abrupt withdrawal of hormones at the end of pregnancy. If all your hair has stopped growing, there will be a period of noticeable hair loss as the hair is naturally shed. When the hair starts to grow again, the new hair will replace the old, and usually there is full growth. Other factors also cause baldness in women, but only rarely does pregnancy-related baldness persist. (See Chapter 12.)

RECOVERY

Postpartum bleeding, called lochia, continues for four to eight weeks after delivery. It is red for the first four or five days, then it turns brownish. You should use pads for bleeding, not tampons, which may encourage infection. Be aware that the drop in hormones may cause sweating and hot flashes.

You can relieve discomfort from an episiotomy or a stitched tear during the first 24 hours by placing an icepack on the area; pain will usually disappear in a week. Warm showers and sitting in a shallow tub of warm water (a sitz bath) can help stimulate blood flow and healing. Don't sit directly on the perineum but sideways, using your leg or a cushion to avoid direct contact. You can also take pain relievers, preferably acetaminophen, as aspirin can increase bleeding. It takes about four weeks for the underlying tissues to heal.

You may be constipated; if so, increase the bulk in your diet by eating plenty of grains, fresh and dried fruit, and fresh vegetables, and drink six to eight glasses of fluid daily. If hemorrhoids develop, or if they become worse, use over-the-counter cream or suppositories to ease the pain. You will probably urinate more often as your body rids itself of excess fluid. If you experience vaginal burning, it is most likely due to inflammation of the bladder walls and urethra; drinking extra fluid helps to lessen the concentration of urine and to ease the discomfort.

Women who don't nurse resume their menstrual periods within eight to 12 weeks after delivery. For nursing mothers, this time varies; you may have a period within two months or not for eight. The body takes its own time to resume its normal hormone production, and the uterine lining can become quite thick, producing unusually heavy bleeding when you eventually do have a period. If you require more than one pad an hour for longer than six hours, call your doctor.

Exercise can speed recovery. You can start vaginal tightening exercises (Kegel's) right away: Squeeze the muscles around the urethra and anus as if holding back both urine and stool; tighten the muscles and then relax, repeating this 20 times three or four times daily. (See Chapter 5.)

To improve muscle tone in your legs and feet, lie in bed, press the backs of your knees down, and then relax and flex and stretch your ankles. To improve abdominal muscles, lie on your back on a firm surface and lift your head, not your shoulders, then relax. You'll feel the tug on your abdominal muscles. Do this 10 times each session, three times a day.

You can start to have sex again after the cervix has closed and the vagina and perineum have healed. This usually takes about four weeks, and most doctors recommend waiting until after the postpartum checkup at six weeks. *Do not depend on nursing for birth control; it is not a reliable method.* Use condoms with contraceptive foam. If you use a diaphragm, you must have it refitted before you resume using it, because delivery may have altered the size of your vaginal canal. Do not use birth control pills until you stop nursing; the hormones they contain enter the breast milk, and their long-term effects on the baby are still unknown. New mothers who are not nursing should also avoid the Pill in the months after childbirth. There is some evidence of an increased likelihood of blood clots following birth, and oral contraceptives can increase this possibility.

Talking with friends and relatives about their own experiences during the first few weeks with a newborn will help to prepare you a bit for the hectic, sometimes exhausting, and seemingly never-ending period when the baby's needs will seem to tax all the energy that you (and your partner) have to expend. But the pleasures of nurturing are substantial, and you should do your best to savor them in those early days.

10

Infertility

Florence Haseltine, M.D.

There has been a substantial increase in infertility among people of childbearing age in the United States in recent years. Although there have always been couples who wanted children but were unable to conceive them or otherwise sustain a pregnancy, changing conditions in our society have made the problem of infertility both more frequent and more visible than in the past. Two trends have combined to cause this: The first is the large number of young women who have entered the work force and delayed childbearing until their mid-30s; the second is the epidemic eruption of sexually transmitted diseases (STDs) and the infections they cause.

These altered social conditions have met head-on with certain biological realities. A definite decrease of fertility accompanies aging, with a steady decline in conception for both sexes starting in the mid-20s and continuing to age 40; after 40, women experience a sharp drop in their ability to conceive. Infections of the male and female reproductive tracts can leave both sperm pathways and fallopian tubes scarred and/or blocked. We now estimate that approximately 3 to 4 million couples in this country want to conceive children but are unable to do so.

If a growing awareness of the infertility problem was one of the major women's health issues of the 1980s, the infertility issue of the 1990s focuses on solutions. Thanks to the availability of new therapies, more and more couples are taking steps to reverse their inability to have children.

The technique you use when having intercourse has no impact on conception; it doesn't matter what position you are in when making love, or how long your partner's penis remains within your vagina after he ejaculates. What does matter when you are trying to conceive is having intercourse frequently, at least every other day, because sperm live for only 48 to 72 hours. Frequent intercourse ensures that you will have a steady supply of sperm in your reproductive tract, ready to unite with an egg whenever you produce one.

Any abnormality in the process of conception can cause infertility. (See Chapter 9.) If the woman fails to ovulate, or the man does not produce enough sperm; if the woman's cervix or uterine lining is inhospitable; if either party has a hormonal problem; if a physical abnormality is present; or if the fallopian tubes are closed, conception will not occur.

Traditionally, doctors have determined that primary infertility is present when couples have not become pregnant after two years of unprotected intercourse. In what is referred to as secondary infertility, couples may either conceive and then lose the pregnancy or they may have had one child and find themselves unable to start another pregnancy after one year of trying. Many couples seek medical help sooner than the one- and two-year periods by which we have traditionally defined infertility. Certainly those who are over 35 may wish to begin a medical workup earlier, particularly where either one has had a family history of gynecological problems or infertility or when anxiety levels are extremely high because of worry over not becoming pregnant.

When a man and woman consult a physician because of suspected infertility, the doctor will begin a systematic investigation of both partners to determine where the problem lies and to suggest possible therapeutic strategies for correcting it. Each couple will then work out with the doctor a treatment plan that is designed to lead to a pregnancy, taking into account their individual needs and preferences. Infertility, of course, is not simply a medical problem. It involves issues of self-esteem, family background, and cultural conditioning, which make each couple, regardless of the cause of their infertility, unique.

One essential ingredient for successful diagnosis and treatment is establishing open communication between you and your partner and the physician. If you are faced with the problem of infertility, both you and your partner must acquire a comprehensive understanding about what is being recommended and why the doctor believes it is necessary. Be sure to discuss the situation openly with the physician until both of you are satisfied with the answers.

While the reasons for infertility can lie with either the man or the woman, infertility can also be a couple problem; in many cases, what might seem like only minor disturbances in several areas can add up to an inability to conceive.

CAUSES

In addition to physiological abnormalities, such as pathways blocked by disease or infection, an inability to produce sperm and egg, or physical malformations, psychological and emotional factors can play an important role in infertility. Sometimes stress can be severe enough to decrease sperm and egg production. Infrequent intercourse, or not having sex at the time in the month when you are most likely to conceive, also plays a role. If you have a regular menstrual cycle, ovulation usually occurs 14 days after the beginning of your menstrual period. Obviously, repeated intercourse around this time will improve your chances to conceive. If your cycle is irregular, you can determine when you ovulate by using a basal body temperature chart. (See Chapter 7.) Although folk wisdom has it that couples who adopt a child often immediately become pregnant, studies have shown that the pregnancy rates of such couples are no higher than those of other couples who have been infertile.

TUBAL DISEASE

Evaluation of the fallopian tubes is a crucial part of an infertility workup. For conception to occur, at least one tube must not only be open but must also be functioning properly.

Fallopian tubes consist of an inner layer of delicate tissue, the mucosa, surrounded by muscle and peritoneum. The lining mucosa is corrugated and ends in fronds of tissue called fimbria, which lie next to the ovary and are able to move over its surface in a way that allows the egg to be fertilized and subsequently transported through the tube back to the uterus. To function properly, the fimbria must be intact and lacy, with an appearance somewhat like a sea anemone. Any disease that destroys the fimbria or the lining of the tube, even though it does not completely close the tube, can devastate its normal function and prevent pregnancy. Adhesions outside the tube, which keep the end of the tube from moving freely or which cover the ovary, can also interfere with conception, even though the interior of the tube is normal. Proper tubal evaluation, therefore, requires techniques that can look inside, outside, and at the fimbrial end of the fallopian tubes.

HYSTEROSALPINGOGRAM

One of the first infertility tests doctors usually perform is a hysterosalpingogram (HSG). *Hystero* refers to uterus and *salpingo* to tube; thus HSG is a test that reveals the state of the uterus and the fallopian tubes. For this study, the physician injects a radiopaque dye that goes through the cervix, uterus, and fallopian tubes into the abdominal cavity to establish that the tubes are open. The test takes place in the radiology department, where a technician takes a series of X rays as the dye pushes through the cervix. If the tubes are open, the test is relatively painless; if the tubes are blocked, there can be significant pain. With HSG, the physician can diagnose the presence of tubal blockage, determine whether it occurs near the uterus or at the fimbrial end of the tube, and assess whether or not the contour of the uterine cavity is normal.

DIAGNOSTIC LAPAROSCOPY

Although HSG provides information on the interior status of the tube, it does not evaluate its exterior surface, or whether adhesions are present. This information is obtained through a diagnostic laparoscopy, a surgical procedure most often done in an outpatient surgery center with the patient under general anesthesia; it does not usually require an overnight stay. The doctor makes small incisions in the umbilicus and in the pubic hairline and inserts a fiber-optic laparoscope in the upper incision and a small metal probe in the lower incision in order to manipulate the pelvic organs. With this technique, the physician can see the surface of the uterus, tubes, and ovaries; can actually pick up and move the ovaries and tubes to examine all portions of the pelvis; and can determine whether adhesions are present and, if so, their extent. Thus, the diagnosis of tubal disease requires both a hysterosalpingogram to examine the interior of the tube and a diagnostic laparoscopy to look at the exterior surfaces.

Several common organisms, such as chlamydia, N. gonorrhea, and E. coli, are transmitted by sexual contact and cause pelvic inflammatory disease (PID) in women, which often results in adhesions and interior tubal disease. (See Chapter 11.) These pelvic infections, which generate fever and pain, require appropriate antibiotic therapy. Sometimes, however, the infection has no outward symptoms and may cause damage and adhesions before it is detected. Abdominal problems such as appendicitis or endometriosis can also produce adhesions on the exterior of the tubes.

Surgery is the therapy of choice for adhesions or tubal blockage, but selecting the appropriate type of surgical procedure depends on the location and the extent of the problem. Gynecologists can often treat small, filmy adhesions and tubal blockage at the fimbria at the time of diagnostic laparoscopy, using a laser or hot cautery through a laparoscope to remove them. A laser is an intense light beam, capable of immense heat and power, that can remove tissue; cautery uses an electric current to accomplish the same result. These newer laparoscopic surgical techniques allow doctors to vaporize or cut adhesions and to open the tube.

LAPAROTOMY

If the surgery required is more extensive, or if the tube is blocked near the uterus, the doctor must perform the major abdominal surgery called a laparotomy to correct the condition. Today, surgeons use a low transverse, or "bikini," incision near the pubic hairline for most such abdominal procedures. This surgery requires a four- to five-day hospital stay and a four- to six-week recovery period. (See Chapter 14.)

NEW EXPERIMENTAL TECHNIQUE

Reports of a new technique to open blocked fallopian tubes have recently been published. In a study of 77 women in outpatient settings, doctors using local or general anesthesia have passed a catheter with a tiny balloon attached to it through the cervical canal and the uterus and into the tubes. When the catheter tip hits a blockage, the doctor inflates the balloon, opening the blockage. This is the same technique as angioplasty, which cardiologists use to remove clots from blocked blood vessels. Doctors succeeded in opening one or both of the tubes in 64 of the women in the study; 22 of them (34 percent) became pregnant, 17 delivered normal infants, and 5 had miscarriages.

SUCCESS RATES

The chance of a successful pregnancy after either laparoscopy or laparotomy depends on the extent and location of the problem and on how well the tubes heal. Most infertility surgeons use steroids, antibiotics, and other medications in an attempt to prevent adhesions from reforming after surgery. Accurate statistics on the effectiveness of these procedures are not fully available, but a general perspective has emerged. For example, after the simple cutting away of adhesions, pregnancy rates of 60 to 80 percent generally occur, provided the tubes are open and the fimbria are normal. When the end of the tube is closed, whether or not a woman becomes pregnant depends on the amount of intact fimbria remaining inside when the surgeon operates to open the tube. In general, this procedure, called a salpingostomy or fimbriaplasty, produces a relatively lower pregnancy rate, somewhere between 25 and 50 percent of all cases.

The success rate for surgically repairing tubal blockage close to the uterus also varies. In this technique, called microsurgery, the surgeon removes the closed-off portion and reconstructs the tube, looking through a microscope to see this tiny structure clearly. When the blockage is the result of previously having had tubal ligation for birth control, the operation to reopen the tubes results in pregnancy 50 to 60 percent of the time; however, when the blockage has been caused by prior infection, the rate of conception is significantly lower.

OVULATORY DYSFUNCTION

For conception to occur, a human egg must mature properly in the ovarian follicle during the first half of a woman's cycle. Then it must enter the enlarged portion of the tube containing the fronds, or fimbria, where sperm arriving through the fallopian tubes can fertilize it. Conception is impossible without proper ovulation; in fact, 10 to 25 percent of all female infertility seems to occur because of ovulatory dysfunction.

BASAL BODY TEMPERATURE CHARTS

Gynecologists diagnose ovulatory dysfunction by using basal body temperature charts. (See Chapter 7.) In a normal cycle, a woman's body temperature remains below 98°F until ovulation; then, as the level of progesterone increases in the second half of the cycle, her temperature rises an average of 0.6° above 98°F. There is a daily cyclical variation in body temperature, which is almost always lower in the morning and goes up with activity. If you are using this method to detect ovulation, you must take your temperature with an oral thermometer upon awakening in order to compile an accurate record. If your basal body temperature increases at mid-cycle, it is most likely that you are ovulating. Another way of testing for ovulation measures your blood (serum) progesterone level between the twentieth and twenty-third day of your cycle, which is in the middle of the luteal phase, when the hormone progesterone is at its highest level. Or you can use the new ovulation predictor kits; these indicate exactly when the luteinizing hormone (LH) rises during the mid-cycle by changing the color of a urine sample to dark blue, indicating the most likely time for insemination.

INADEQUATE OVULATION

Although all three of these methods register the presence or absence of ovulation, they do not assess the quality of the corpus luteum and the hormones it produces. To do so, gynecologists need an endometrial biopsy. This is an outpatient procedure during which the gynecologist takes a sample from the lining of the uterus, using a small curette, and then sends it to a pathologist for examination under a microscope to determine if you have ovulated and are producing adequate hormones to sustain a fertilized egg. The physician must know the date of your next menstrual period to determine whether you are ovulating optimally, so that the lining of the uterus is ready to accept implantation of the fertilized egg. Although this procedure is somewhat uncomfortable, it provides critically important information because inadequate ovulation, called a short luteal phase, can be corrected by treatment. Two drugs, clomiphene citrate and vaginal progesterone suppositories, prolong and extend the luteal phase of the cycle and improve the quality of ovulation.

THE ABSENCE OF OVULATION

The medical term that describes women who do not ovulate and have irregular periods is *anovulatory*. Therapy to correct the absence of ovulation starts with administering a synthetic progestin (Provera) to see if the drug produces bleeding. If it does, it means you have moderately normal levels of ovarian estrogen and will benefit from 50 to 200 milligrams of clomiphene citrate taken during the first part of your cycle. Although the drug induces ovulation in about 80 percent of anovulatory women, only 50 percent of them conceive.

Doctors can even induce ovulation in women whose pituitary gland is not functioning at all, who produce no estrogen, and who do not bleed after receiving Provera. They prescribe human menopausal gonadotropins (hMG or Pergonal), which simply replace the pituitary hormones that the body fails to make, stimulating the development of the ovaries and producing a pregnancy rate of 70 to 80 percent. In addition, the doctor will prescribe human chorionic gonadotropin (hCG) to be taken at the appropriate time in mid-cycle, which helps the ovaries release mature eggs.

HORMONAL DISTURBANCES

Inadequate ovulation often goes hand in hand with other hormonal disturbances, such as polycystic ovary syndrome, in which the ovaries fail to function optimally. This condition makes the ovaries secrete higher levels of male hormones (androgens) than normal, resulting in poor ovulation and, occasionally, increased facial hair growth and acne. Here, clomiphene citrate induces better ovulation, although it does not correct the excess hair growth.

Women with elevated levels of the pituitary hormone prolactin may also have inadequate or absent ovulation. If prolactin is high, estrogen is low, although no one knows why. The most frequent symptom of elevated prolactin levels is a clear milky discharge from the breasts, a condition known as galactorrhea. To confirm the diagnosis, doctors order a test to determine the serum prolactin level. If the level is elevated, treatment with a drug called bromocriptine (Parlodel) reduces the level of prolactin, stops the breast discharge, and stimulates ovulation.

CERVICAL-BASED INFERTILITY

The cervix, the lowest portion of the uterus that protrudes into the vagina, is more than just a hollow tube through which sperm pass. Stimulated by estrogen, glands deep within the cervix produce mucus, which plays an important role in the sperm's ability to reach the uterus. These cervical glands also store sperm, allowing them to migrate into the uterus and out through the tubes continuously over several days.

In the preovulatory period of your cycle, cervical mucus becomes thin, watery, and vitually free of cells because of high estrogen levels. Specialists call the ability of the mucus to form itself into long strands "spinnbarkeit"; just before ovulation, spinnbarkeit increases to eight to 10 centimeters—between three and four inches. Estrogen also influences dried cervical mucus to form crystalline structures or fern patterns, another sign of good preovulatory mucus. Both spinnbarkeit and ferning confirm the high levels of estrogen and good-quality mucus that are most hospitable to sperm, allowing them to move easily and rapidly into the uterus.

The degree of acidity of cervical mucus is also important. Normally, the secretions of the vagina are too acidic for sperm to survive, and they need the less acidic environment of the cervical mucus. In rare cases, a woman's cervical mucus is too acidic for sperm survival. This is often treated with bicarbonate douches, although there is no scientific evidence that such douches actually increase the pregnancy rate.

POSTCOITAL TEST (PCT)

Doctors can evaluate cervical mucus, as well as sperm, by the postcoital or Huhner test, which is based on taking mucus from your vagina and cervix within a few hours of intercourse before you ovulate. Normal results mean you have good-quality cervical mucus with spinnbarkeit of six to eight centimeters (two to three inches), fern pattern on drying, and more than 20 forwardly active sperm per each high-power field. Normal results are reassuring, because they imply that your partner has good semen quality and adequate ejaculation and that you have receptive cervical mucus. If the results of this test are abnormal, this does not mean that a couple cannot conceive. Sperm have been recovered from the abdominal cavity at laparoscopy following poor postcoital test results. The most common reason for a poor outcome in a PCT is inappropriate timing. If a test is done too early in the cycle, when not enough estrogen is present, or after ovulation, when progesterone makes the mucus thick and impenetrable, then the postcoital test results will be poor, showing few and/or motionless sperm.

OTHER CERVICAL PROBLEMS

Another reason for poor or scanty mucus is prior cervical surgery, such as conization, which removes a cone of cervical tissue with either a knife, cautery, or laser; cryotherapy, the use of extreme cold to eliminate diseased tissue; and cautery. These procedures may obliterate enough of the cervical glands so that they fail to make sufficient mucus.

Cervical factors account for approximately 10 percent of all cases of infertility. If, despite optimal preovulatory timing, the cervical mucus is scanty or thick, the doctor can prescribe estrogen to improve it; often the number of moving (motile) sperm increases as well. Gynecologists should suspect cervical infertility when the PCT shows few motile sperm despite good mucus and a normal semen analysis. If cultures for chlamydia and ureaplasma, agents somewhere between a virus and a bacteria, reveal infections, then antibiotic therapy to both partners can clear up the infections and improve the results of the postcoital test.

ENDOMETRIOSIS

Endometriosis is a disease in which endometrial tissue from the lining of the uterus implants on the lining of the abdomen (peritoneum), where it continues to grow, regress, and grow again, cycling the same way it does in the uterus itself. It affects as many as 25 percent of women of reproductive age. Doctors believe that it is caused by the leaking of menstrual blood and debris out of the end of the fallopian tubes and into the abdominal cavity. Endometriosis sometimes causes severe pain with menstrual periods (dysmenorrhea), as well as pain with intercourse (dyspareunia). The extent of endometriosis does not always correlate with either symptoms or infertility. Many women with very mild endometrial disease suffer severe pain and infertility, while others with much more serious degrees of the disease have little or no pain. Endometriosis can also cause severe pelvic adhesions that restrict the ability of the tubes to transport sperm and egg normally. In fact, as many as 30 to 40 percent of women with endometriosis are found to be infertile at the time they consult a physician.

The symptoms of endometriosis include a history of painful periods and intercourse; a retroverted, or tipped-back, uterus; and painful nodules on the posterior vaginal wall. A laparoscopy is required to make a definitive diagnosis. Gynecologists use anesthesia for this procedure, inserting a fiber-optic scope through the umbilicus and examining the pelvis, which permits them to diagnose both adhesions and active endometriosis. (See Chapter 14.)

THERAPY

Many forms of therapy are available for the treatment of endometriosis. One is the birth control pill, which continuously suppresses ovarian activity; another employs synthetic progestins. Physicians have also relied on a new drug, danazol (Danacrine), to stop ovarian function and alleviate pain in women with moderate to severe endometriosis; although the drug may also improve pregnancy rates, it has not been effective in doing so for women with mild endometriosis. Recently, doctors have tried a new class of drugs, luteinizing-hormone-releasing factor (LRF) analogs (Lupron or Synarel), to treat endometriosis. These drugs, given monthly by injection or daily either by injection or nasal spray, suppress central nervous system and ovarian function completely, essentially creating an artificial menopause. Some improvement in pregnancy rates has been achieved with LRF analogs, but the drugs are still too new for there to be proof of their efficacy.

Danazol or LRF analogs are both appropriate therapies for those women who suffer intense pain from mild to moderate endometriosis and who want to conceive. However, for women who have severe adhesions or enlarged ovaries with endometriomas (endometriosis within the ovaries), surgery is the treatment of choice. When surgeons remove adhesions and endometriomas from the ovaries of women with moderate endometriosis, these women then have a 50 percent chance of becoming pregnant. In women with severe endometriosis, both surgical and medical therapy relieves pain, but surgery produces a successful pregnancy rate of only 30 percent or less.

Doctors can also offer women surgical procedures that may improve their reproductive health or relieve their pain. One such procedure is uterine suspension, in which the surgeon takes the round ligaments, pulls them up against the abdominal wall, and sews them in place; another technique, utero-sacral plication, essentially does the same thing using a different ligament. Both procedures aim to bring the uterus and ovaries out of the pelvis and away from the adhesions but do not guarantee pain relief. Still another method removes some of the presacral nerves that run along the sacrum, the triangular bone at the bottom of the spinal column, which can lessen intense pain.

Women with severe endometriosis, who already have undergone one surgical attempt at reconstruction, do not usually benefit from a second procedure. These patients can try in vitro fertilization, but the chance of pregnancy is only 10 percent. If both medical and surgical therapy fail to control the pain and provide a pregnancy, sometimes the only way to relieve the pain is hysterectomy and the removal of the ovaries, which stops the production of the estrogen that drives and worsens endometriosis. In cases of severe endometriosis with unremitting pain, a total abdominal hysterectomy, which removes the fallopian tubes as well as the ovaries, may be the only path to pain relief. (See Chapter 14.)

DIETHYLSTILBESTROL AND INFERTILITY

Starting in 1940, obstetricians began prescribing diethylstilbestrol (DES), a synthetic form of estrogen, because they believed, incorrectly, that it prevented miscarriage, and they continued to prescribe it until well into the 70s. In 1971, when researchers discovered that the daughters of mothers who had taken DES had an increased risk of vaginal and cervical cancer, doctors stopped using this drug, which was later removed from the market. In addition to suffering impaired fertility from these cancers, DES daughters also may have suffered structural abnormalities in their reproductive organs that prevent conception. These alterations may occur in the shape of the cervix, the vaginal walls, or the uterus. DES daughters may also be at greater risk for ectopic pregnancies, miscarriage, and premature deliveries. The sons of women who used DES have a higher rate of testicular problems, low sperm counts, and abnormally shaped sperm cells, but no large-scale study has shown an overall increase in infertility in these men.

If you were conceived between 1950 and 1975, are still of childbearing age, and your mother had bleeding problems or previous miscarriages for which she received oral medication, check with her or her medical records, if they are available, to find out what medication she took and if you were exposed to DES. If you suspect exposure, you should seek medical care, because preventive and corrective options do exist. DES Action USA, a national organization based at the Long Island Jewish Medical Center in New Hyde Park, NY 11040 (516-775-3450), can supply you with more information.

MALE FACTOR INFERTILITY

Although the public generally perceives infertility as a female problem, in fact, in 40 percent of couples, the difficulty lies with the male.

SEMEN ANALYSIS

Physicians start every fertility workup with a semen analysis to diagnose the possible presence of male-factor infertility. Semen analysis evaluates not only the number of sperm but also how much and how quickly they move, called motility and velocity respectively. The man abstains from sexual activity and ejaculation for two days and then provides the semen sample by masturbating into a sterile cup. A normal semen analysis should show a count (at the very minimum) of 20 million sperm or more per cubic centimeter (cc) of seminal fluid, with a minimum of 40 percent motility, and 60 percent or more of the sperm having normal forms. Optimal counts are over 70 million per cubic centimeter. If the results of the initial semen analysis are abnormal, it is worth repeating the test, since many other factors—such as fever or viral illness, marijuana, or stress—can have a negative impact on semen. If the results of both analyses are abnormal, then the man needs a complete urologic evaluation.

POSTCOITAL TEST

A second method for evaluating sperm is the postcoital test (PCT). As noted earlier, the best time for this test is just before the woman's mid-cycle, when her estrogen levels are highest and her cervical mucus most hospitable to sperm. After intercourse, the woman comes to the doctor's office, where a sample of her cervical mucus is removed. Good pre-ovulatory mucus should be thin and watery, and a hanging drop should stretch to seven or eight centimeters (about three inches) in length. The physician examines the mucus under the high-power field of a microscope and counts the number of forwardly motile sperm. Although 20 or more sperm per high-power field is an excellent result, infertility does not appear to be a problem unless there are fewer than five forwardly active sperm. Male-factor infertility is unlikely when both the semen analysis and the postcoital test are normal.

ANTISPERM ANTIBODY STUDIES

If the results of the PCT are abnormal, an immunological problem may be present, and studies for antisperm antibodies are the next diagnostic step. These studies use immunobeads, tiny latex spheres with antibodies on them that bind to sperm if the sperm themselves carry antibodies. This procedure allows the physician to see tiny white beads on the sperm and to identify various types of antibodies, such as IgG or IgM, two of the four or five classes of antibodies. IgG and IgM behave differently, some attaching to the head and others to the tail of the sperm. Head-directed antibodies appear to interfere with fertilization, while tail-directed antibodies may reduce motility. If the male is producing antisperm antibodies, thus incapacitating his own sperm, the doctor may prescribe steroids, which suppress antibody formation. Steroid therapy works only if it is the man who is producing the antibodies. If the antibodies come from the woman and coat his sperm in the cervix, then a therapy that may be helpful is artificial intrauterine insemination with the male's washed and migrated sperm.

THE HAMSTER PENETRATION TEST

The zona-free hamster oocyte sperm penetration test is another method that assesses sperm quality by examining their ability to fertilize an egg—in this case, the egg of a hamster. Infertility specialists use this test when there is a question of whether or not fertilization has occurred, but the results are sometimes difficult to interpret. For example, some samples of human sperm have not fertilized hamster eggs but have fertilized human eggs, and the reverse has been true as well. Thus, although the hamster penetration test may be helpful in some specialized situations, it is not useful as a primary screening test.

THERAPY

The therapies for male infertility are still at a rudimentary stage. If the results of a man's postcoital test or semen analysis are abnormal, the next step is usually artificial insemination of his sperm, collected after masturbation. The insemination can be done by simply injecting the seminal fluid into the vagina and coating the cervix with it. Conception will not take place if the problem is inadequate sperm, but this procedure can succeed if, for example, the woman's uterus is in an abnormal position so that the sperm have not been reaching her cervix during intercourse or if the man has trouble ejaculating during intercourse. In the past few years, doctors have developed an improved method, injecting washed and concentrated sperm high into the uterus to facilitate conception. In this procedure, after the man masturbates and achieves ejaculation, his seminal fluid is placed in a centrifuge, a machine that spins the sperm rapidly, washing away the fluid and allowing the sperm to swim or migrate into a small volume of tissue culture medium. Thus, only the motile, active sperm reach the uterus for potential conception. Infertility experts believe that using a washed, migrated sperm sample is a potentially more effective method of insemination because it not only concentrates the sperm but also places the sperm high in the uterus, bypassing any barriers that the cervical mucus might present. It is also more comfortable for the woman, because the seminal fluid prostaglandins, which may cause uterine contractions and pain, have been washed away.

Much of the success of intrauterine insemination depends, of course, on timing. Because sperm live for a maximum of 72 hours in the female genital tract, while the egg lasts for 12 to 24 hours, insemination must occur within two days of ovulation. Doctors can estimate the best timing for insemination through one of the several methods described earlier in this chapter.

If a couple has not conceived after four to six cycles of well-timed inseminations using sperm from the male during the ovulatory period, three therapeutic options remain. The first is artificial insemination with the use of donor sperm, an alternative that has been quite successful in cases where the male is infertile. The procedure is exactly the same as for insemination by the male partner except that the sperm comes from donors who have been screened for genetic problems and infectious diseases, such as syphilis and AIDS. Infertility clinics collect donor sperm samples and freeze them, holding them for six months to be certain that no undetected serious medical problem surfaces. Currently, if the donor proves to be negative for AIDS six months after the initial test, the clinic releases the semen sample and thaws it for insemination. Although insemination with fresh sperm produces a higher conception rate, frozen sperm is used to protect the female recipient from sexually transmitted diseases. If donor insemination doesn't work, the couple can try in vitro fertilization (IVF), described later in this chapter.

INFERTILITY OF UNKNOWN ORIGIN

Approximately 90 percent of all couples who consult a physician because of infertility find some abnormality that is preventing them from conceiving. That leaves 10 percent who, even after the most thorough examination and testing, are still unable to conceive even though they have no discernible abnormality. This is not a hopeless situation, however, because studies have shown that some of these couples eventually do conceive a child, sometimes after three or four years of trying. The problem may be that whatever the abnormality is, it is so subtle that more time is required for conception to take place. While the longer the duration of this type of infertility, the less likely it is that conception will take place, several therapies are nevertheless available.

Women who have adequate ovulation, sufficient luteal progesterone levels, and a normal ovulatory endometrial biopsy but still fail to become pregnant, do conceive at an increased rate when they take medications to induce ovulation. Ten to 15 percent of those women with a history of infertility who ovulate normally become pregnant when treated with clomiphene citrate or the combination of human menopausal gonadotropins (hMG) and human chorionic gonadotropin (hCG). Although no scientific rationale explains this fact, it may be that elusive abnormalities in hypothalamic or pituitary function interfere with ovulation, making pregnancy impossible even though gross ovulation still occurs.

Another possible therapy when all discernible problems have been ruled out is inseminating the uterus with washed migrated sperm. The rationale here is the probability that there is some unknown factor in the cervical mucus that prevents conception. However, so far there is no definite proof that this approach results in increased pregnancy rates.

New reproductive technologies, such as in vitro fertilization (IVF) and gamete intrafallopian transfer (GIFT), also have been used to treat couples with infertility of unknown origin. Both these techniques have produced pregnancies in between 5 and 15 percent of couples with long-standing infertility of unknown cause.

An infertility workup is an extremely stressful, emotionally draining, and financially costly procedure. When no obvious reason for infertility emerges, the stress becomes even greater because the physician can neither identify the problem nor offer a rational

therapy to correct it. Although ovulation induction and new reproductive technology have both increased pregnancy rates in such
couples, doctors should offer them with caution, because their
success rates are so low.

PREGNANCY LOSS

Another type of infertility, equally as devastating as the infertility
problems that interfere with conception, is that in which couples
are able to conceive but the woman cannot carry a pregnancy to
viability. Follow-up studies of the results of conventionally available pregnancy tests show that approximately 15 to 20 percent of
all pregnancies diagnosed after a missed menstrual period end in
spontaneous miscarriage during the initial 20 weeks of gestation.
In most cases, this is a onetime event, nature's way of ending
abnormal pregnancies, and it does not reoccur in future pregnancies. However, a substantial number of women miscarry sequential
pregnancies, a phenomenon referred to as habitual abortion. Tech-
nically, the definition requires three consecutive pregnancy losses
before 20 weeks, with the fetus weighing under 500 grams. Most
couples consult a physician after the second miscarriage to find out
what the problem is.

Although recurrent miscarriage is an enormous emotional strain
for a couple, there is nevertheless a good chance of their eventually
having a normal pregnancy. In situations where a hormonal problem is diagnosed as the cause, 90 percent of patients treated ap-
propriately will ultimately carry a fetus to term. In those with an
anatomic uterine problem, 60 to 75 percent will deliver an infant
after a nine-month pregnancy, and even in patients with a genetic
problem, approximately one-third will have a viable child. Of all
couples evaluated, 40 percent will have no demonstrable reason
for recurrent pregnancy loss. Even in this group of patients, there
is hope. Studies show that nearly 70 percent of these couples with
no known reason for miscarrying will eventually have a term birth
without any therapy.

ANATOMIC ABNORMALITIES

Approximately 10 to 15 percent of women who experience habitual abortion have a uterine abnormality. One malformation is a visible septum, a division caused by a piece of tissue hanging down in the middle of the uterus. Doctors believe a visible septum causes pregnancy loss because the embryo implants on it and dies from an inadequate blood supply. Another problem is a bicornuate uterus, in which two little flaps of tissue stick together, causing the fetus to lie in a transverse position across the cervix or to be in the breech position, with the buttocks presenting instead of the head. This condition usually results in an abnormal fetal position or a premature labor rather than an early miscarriage. Although half of all women with these anatomic deviations do not abort, a woman with two or more first-trimester miscarriages needs an evaluation with a hysterosalpingogram (HSG) to determine whether or not an anatomic abnormality is present. This is an important diagnostic procedure, since surgical removal of the septum results in a viable pregnancy at term for 75 percent of those women who have this problem.

There are two methods of removing a septum; in the first, the doctor uses a hysteroscope, going through the cervix and into the uterus to cut the septum. The second approach is an abdominal operation called a metroplasty. This is major surgery in which the surgeon opens the uterus, wedges out the septum, and sews the two halves of the uterus together to create a single interior cavity.

ENDOCRINE ABNORMALITIES

Habitual abortion can also be caused by dysfunction of the endocrine system. An endocrine evaluation looks at thyroid function, because an underactive thyroid (hypothyroidism) can produce habitual abortion, and replacement therapy can restore the thyroid gland to its normal activity and correct the problem. If the difficulty is found to be a short luteal phase with inadequate progesterone production, the doctor can diagnose this with an endometrial biopsy performed two to three days before menstruation. Treatment with either progesterone vaginal suppositories or with ovulation-inducing drugs, such as clomiphene citrate or human menopausal gonadotropins, can remedy this disorder.

GENETIC DEFECTS

Although 50 to 60 percent of first-trimester miscarriages involve genetic defects, these are usually onetime fetal events and have no bearing on the next pregnancy. However, some patients who suffer habitual abortion have genetic defects that they pass on to the fetus repeatedly. A test, called a karyotype, evaluates the chromosomes of both parents, since either can carry the defect. The most common abnormality is a balanced translocation, in which pieces that break off different chromosomes change places without any piece being lost. This causes miscarriage in 25 percent of pregnancies. No therapy is yet available for this genetic abnormality in the mother, but if the father carries the balanced translocation, the couple can elect donor insemination.

OTHER CAUSES

Other, less common causes of habitual abortion include pelvic infections, which may precipitate recurrent miscarriage. If cervical or uterine cultures are positive, treatment with antibiotics, such as Vibramycin or erythromycin, can result in an increased term pregnancy rate. A more recent suggestion, still under study by researchers, is that an immunologic abnormality causes habitual abortion.

ECTOPIC PREGNANCY

A significant number of couples experience another form of pregnancy loss, ectopic or tubal pregnancy, in which the embryo develops outside the uterus, most commonly in the fallopian tube. Although such pregnancies were described as early as A.D. 963, it was not until 1883 that a mother survived surgery for an ectopic pregnancy. Modern surgical treatment saved more patients as surgeons learned to remove the ectopic pregnancy and the tube. This procedure, salpingectomy, was common until 10 to 15 years ago, when new and sensitive tests for pregnancy and sophisticated ultrasound equipment permitted the very early diagnosis of ectopic pregnancy, which brought with it the possibility of saving not only the woman's life but also her fallopian tube. Ectopic pregnancy needs to be approached with great care, however, because it can still result in a lethal situation if the fetus grows to the point of rupturing the tube, with resulting hemorrhage into the abdomen.

Ectopic pregnancy in the United States is increasing. The rate doubled between 1970 and 1978, probably a result of the rise in pelvic inflammatory disease (PID). Studies have shown that women with PID have a high incidence of tubal blockage and pelvic adhesions after an infectious episode. Not only does this render them potentially infertile, but, because damage to the internal surface of the tube seems to be a primary cause of tubal pregnancy, it exposes them to a higher risk of it.

As noted earlier, the usual signs and symptoms of a tubal pregnancy are a positive pregnancy test, abdominal pain, and vaginal bleeding. The availability of early pregnancy testing and new ultrasound techniques allows the physician to diagnose an ectopic pregnancy as early as five or six weeks after the last menstrual period. An additional diagnostic tool is the level of what is called pregnancy titer, the beta hCG level in the woman's blood serum. This is the pregnancy hormone the placenta produces, and it should double every two days. If it does not, or if ultrasound imaging fails to reveal a fetal sac in the uterus at the appropriate time, the pregnancy is probably ectopic. Obstetricians can diagnose an ectopic pregnancy even earlier by using vaginal ultrasonography to visualize the fetal sac.

The treatment for ectopic pregnancy is surgery. Using early diagnostic techniques, before the ectopic pregnancy destroys the fallopian tube, surgeons operate through a laparoscope to remove the pregnancy and reconstruct the tube. Studies have shown that women who have had an ectopic pregnancy removed and at the same time had the tube surgically reconstructed have roughly the same 50 percent chance of conceiving a normal uterine pregnancy as do women who have had the entire tube removed. The advantage of saving the tube is that, in case a second ectopic pregnancy destroys the other fallopian tube, the woman still has one tube and is, therefore, potentially fertile.

Although a second tubal pregnancy is unlikely, it does happen in 12 percent of women who have a prior history of ectopic pregnancy, tubal surgery, or pelvic infection. Since these women have a reasonable chance of conceiving a normal intrauterine pregnancy, they need a second tubal reconstruction.

Although most therapies for ectopic pregnancy require an abdominal incision, surgeons can remove some of these abnormal pregnancies by using the laparoscope but only if the ectopic pregnancy is diagnosed early enough and there is minimal bleeding into the abdomen. The surgeon places a fiber-optic scope through a small incision in the umbilicus while inserting one or two probes through small incisions in the lower abdomen to manipulate the tube. Then, using either cautery or laser, the tiny embryo is extracted. Since conception rates are similar after a laparoscopic or abdominal removal of ectopic pregnancy, using the laparoscope is preferable, since it requires only an overnight stay in the hospital and the woman can return to her normal activities the next day.

NEW REPRODUCTIVE TECHNOLOGIES

Despite a complete medical workup and routine fertility therapy, a couple may still not conceive. Or, the evaluation may show that the woman's tubes are blocked and there are so many pelvic adhesions present that the chances of successful reproductive surgery are poor. Until ten years ago, adoption was the only alternative in both of these situations. However, since Louise Brown, the first in vitro fertilization (IVF) baby, was born in England in 1978, so-called new reproductive technologies have blossomed. In vitro fertilization and gamete intrafallopian transfer (GIFT), as well as the more exotic techniques of donor eggs and embryos, are medicine's newest advances in the attempt to enable an infertile couple to have a child. These techniques, although highly publicized, are immensely expensive and have low success rates; if you are struggling with infertility, you should, therefore, exhaust all of the routine diagnostic tests and treatments before considering them. Both IVF and GIFT range in cost from $5,000 to $7,000 per cycle—that is, for each attempt at pregnancy by these methods. And although more established infertility therapies, such as ovulation induction and some of the surgical procedures, succeed in better than 50 percent of couples, most IVF and GIFT programs quote successful conception rates of only 15 to 25 percent. Moreover, even many of these pregnancies miscarry; you must be careful to inquire about the actual take-home baby rate, since this is the statistic that matters most to you.

In general, the actual rate of successful pregnancies with viable infants range from 5 to 15 percent in these programs, depending on the number of cycles required and the population of patients a progam accepts. If pregnancy doesn't occur with the first cycle, subsequent IVF cycles have the same success rates, so that the overall cumulative possibility of pregnancy increases with the number of cycles used. However, after four or five cycles in the same program, doctors usually suggest the couples discontinue the therapy or try elsewhere.

Additionally, because the likelihood of conception decreases as women get older, a clinic that accepts patients over the age of 40, with problems such as severe male-factor or immunologic infertility, will have a lower success rate than one that admits only women under the age of 35 with tubal disease. Thus, you must be sure to ask not only about an individual program's conception rates and take-home baby rates but also about the composition of the patient population before you decide to try these therapies.

IN VITRO FERTILIZATION (IVF)

This is the most common of the new technological procedures, and it can address many infertility problems, including tubal blockage, male-factor infertility and decreased sperm numbers, endometriosis, cervical or immunologic infertility, and infertility of unknown origin. If poor ovulation alone is the problem, it does not work; here clomiphene citrate or hMG can induce or improve ovulation. IVF also does not prevent recurrent miscarriages.

During an IVF cycle, the doctor uses one or a combination of ovulation induction agents, such as clomiphene citrate, human menopausal gonadotropin (Pergonal), or pure human follicle-stimulating hormone (FSH) to encourage the ovaries to produce many eggs. The physician monitors the medication by taking daily blood estradiol levels and daily ultrasound tests to determine when enough follicles of appropriate size are present to allow ovulation. At that point, you will be given an injection of human chorionic gonadotropin (hCG), which causes the eggs in the follicles to mature in preparation for ovulation, approximately 36 hours later. Eighteen to 20 hours after the eggs have matured, and just before they are released from the follicle, the doctor uses aspiration to recover and collect the eggs. Although physicians originally relied on the laparoscope for aspirations, they now employ the newer techniques of transvaginal ultrasonography, inserting a special ultrasound probe into the vagina and visualizing the follicles on each ovary on a screen. The physician uses a long needle to puncture the vaginal wall and enter the ovarian follicle, aspirating the contents of the follicle, including the egg. This new form of vaginal ultrasonographic aspiration, which takes place in an outpatient clinic, does not require general anesthesia, making it both less expensive and considerably less risky and more comfortable for patients.

After aspiration, the doctor examines the contents of the follicle for eggs, removes them, and places them in small plastic Petri dishes. Then sperm is added, and the contents of the dish are incubated at body temperature until fertilization occurs. Approximately 48 hours after aspiration, the doctor examines the new embryos, which have divided to form four to eight cells. A maximum of three of these embryos are then implanted into the uterus with a long plastic catheter that the doctor inserts through the cervix. Although more than three embryos may have been formed from the harvested eggs, the doctor places only three to avoid multiple pregnancy. The remaining embryos are frozen in liquid nitrogen, which allows couples to use them in subsequent normal ovulatory cycles, increasing the chance of conception from any given IVF cycle and helping to control the cost.

After inserting the embryos, the doctor gives you some type of luteal support as an aid to helping an embryo implant and grow in the uterus. Either progesterone suppositories or sequential hCG injections are used for this purpose.

If you conceive with IVF, your gynecologist must follow your pregnancy carefully, because the method carries a 20 to 25 percent chance of miscarriage. It also raises the risk of ectopic or tubal pregnancy. A third risk is the possibility of a twin or triplet gestation, when three embryos become reimplanted, and if this happens it should be diagnosed early in the pregnancy. However, even with the insertion of three embryos, usually no more than one (or rarely two) will mature successfully.

GAMETE INTRAFALLOPIAN TRANSFER (GIFT)

The theory behind GIFT is that conception may occur more readily if it takes place naturally in the fallopian tube. The GIFT procedure is similar to the one followed for IVF. After stimulating your ovaries with ovulation induction medication to develop many eggs, the doctor recovers the eggs via laparoscopy, visualizing the ovaries through the laparoscope, and then passing a long needle through the abdomen and aspirating the follicles. The physician identifies the eggs, removes them, and places them in a long plastic catheter while you are asleep on the operating table. Your partner's sperm is then added to the same catheter, and both sperm and eggs are injected into the fimbriated end of the tube next to the ovary.

GIFT is not for women with blocked or damaged tubes, because the possibility of a tubal pregnancy outweighs the potential benefits. It is a reasonable procedure for women with normal tubes and normal tubal function who have not been able to conceive because of mild endometriosis, male-factor infertility, or infertility of unknown origin. Success with GIFT appears to be more frequent than for IVF, with pregnancy rates of 20 to 30 percent, although there is also a significant miscarriage rate. This latter is not surprising, since many GIFT patients suffer from infertility of unknown origin.

In the GIFT procedure, your own tubes transport the eggs and sperm into the uterus where, if successful, the embryo implants. As in IVF, the doctor usually injects only three or four eggs into the tubes to prevent multiple pregnancies. The remaining eggs with sperm are incubated in a Petri dish, and the embryos are frozen for implantation during subsequent cycles.

OTHER METHODS

IVF and GIFT are the two most common procedures used in the new reproductive technologies. However, there are many variations on this theme. They include direct injection of sperm into the peritoneal cavity at the time of ovulation; zygote intrafallopian transfer (ZIFT), which involves collecting the eggs by using ultrasound and then reimplanting the embryo into the tube two days later with a laparoscope; and incubating developing embryos in capsules in the woman's own vagina rather than outside her body.

The common denominator in all these procedures is the attempt to provide the most natural and, therefore, successful environment for the egg, the sperm, and the developing embryo, thus allowing an optimal chance for pregnancy.

Although IVF and GIFT benefit patients who still ovulate but have other difficulties, such as poor male-factor or cervical problems, there are a significant number of women who experience premature menopause in their early 20s or who have their ovaries removed surgically. These women do not produce eggs and as a result cannot become pregnant. In such a situation, doctors can prescribe oral estrogen and progesterone for several cycles until the woman's uterus resembles that of a woman having a normal cycle. The doctor then implants a donated embryo, which has been conceived from harvested eggs incubated with her partner's sperm, paralleling the IVF and GIFT procedures. The donors can be relatives or friends, or can be anonymous; thanks to our ability to freeze embryos, the procedures of donation and implantation do not have to occur simultaneously. In this way, women who cannot produce their own eggs, or who have a genetic abnormality they do not want to pass on to a child, can attempt a pregnancy.

A recent California study found that older, postmenopausal women can also become pregnant using donated eggs from younger women, which were then fertilized in the laboratory by their partners' sperm. Both the older women and the egg donors received hormones, the donors so that they would produce many eggs, the older women to simulate a menstrual cycle that was synchronized with that of the donor. The women also received hormones for the first 100 days of their pregnancies to mimic the luteal support their ovaries would have provided had they not experienced menopause.

In this study, four out of seven women between the ages of 40 and 44 gave birth to healthy babies, one of them to twins. There was one stillborn infant and one miscarriage, and one woman failed to conceive because her husband's sperm was defective.

When the results of the study were published in late 1990, the media focused on the success of the efforts to extend childbearing beyond menopause, ignoring the practical problems of older couples caring for the lively teenagers these infants eventually will become. Researchers cited the study's real significance as showing that women have a more difficult time conceiving in their 40s because their eggs, and not their uteri, are declining. These results may encourage premenopausal women with infertility problems to try using donor eggs from younger women to improve their chances of conceiving.

STRESS AND THE NECESSITY FOR COUNSELING

After a thorough infertility workup and routine therapy, followed by IVF or GIFT if so required and/or desired, approximately 50 to 70 percent of all couples will eventually conceive. Interestingly, a 1985 article in the *New England Journal of Medicine* reported that couples who take no supplementary steps to conceive have the same 50 to 70 percent conception rates as those who receive treatment at a fertility clinic. This leaves 30 to 50 percent who, despite all treatment and many years of trying, are unable to have children.

If you and your partner have an infertility problem, be aware that the rapid development of the new reproductive technologies has allowed physicians to help many people conceive who could not have hoped for pregnancy ten years ago. Nevertheless, engaging in these therapies creates both emotional and financial stress. In addition, these new technologies and their consequences have far exceeded the current coping abilities of our society's legal, social, and ethical framework. Thus, many of the programs that offer these technologies offer accompanying counseling and support during the procedures.

OTHER SOLUTIONS

Early in an infertility workup, you should understand the emotional and financial costs and the chances of success as well as what other alternatives are available so that, if you are not among those who conceive, you have thought about other possible solutions. For the man who has no spem, there is donor insemination. For a woman who has not been able to conceive despite all treatment, seeking a surrogate mother is a possibility—although it is fraught with potential legal, ethical, and emotional consequences. Most couples who do not conceive on their own usually consider adoption, and those who do adopt find this a very satisfactory and fulfilling option. You should think about adopting early in your infertility therapy, since healthy newborns are at a premium and it may take years for you to find an adoptable child. In addition, many adoption agencies in this country reject couples over the age of 40 on the basis of their age alone. People who cannot find babies in the United States should inquire into programs based in foreign countries.

GAY AND SINGLE PARENTS

Most gay women who consult infertility specialists do so because they wish to be artificially inseminated in order to have a baby. The vast majority are in stable, monogamous relationships, but some are single. Single women who are not gay also see infertility specialists for artificial insemination.

Many, but not all, infertility specialists send all gay and single women seeking insemination for a complete psychological/psychiatric workup before proceeding with the insemination. They do this to be certain that the woman is stable, that she understands the serious responsibility single parenthood entails, and that she has a support system in place—either a long-term partner, family members, or devoted friends in her community—to help her raise the child. Sometimes the deep-seated and long-frustrated desire to have a baby obscures the very real difficulties that single parents encounter, and a psychological workup helps to bring these issues into focus.

Beyond this, infertility specialists treat their gay and single patients the same way they treat their heterosexual patients.

PREVENTING INFERTILITY

You can protect your fertility in a number of ways. If you are a teenager or in your 20s, use condoms during intercourse to protect yourself from sexual infections. Avoid having many sexual partners, and don't have intercourse with anyone who has symptoms of a sexually transmitted disease (STD). (See Chapter 11.) These precautions apply to women of any age. If you and/or your partner develop an infection, see a doctor immediately for a full course of antibiotic therapy. You should also be sure you are immune to

German measles (rubella) and that your partner has had or has been immunized against mumps, as both of these childhood diseases in adults can cause infertility. If you have been using an IUD, switch to another form of birth control. Seek medical care promptly if you develop genital warts or any unusual bleeding, discharge, or pain. If you need medical or surgical care, discuss with the doctor its possible impact on your fertility, and be sure your questions are answered to your satisfaction. If your partner has any unusual discharge or bleeding from his penis, or experiences urinary burning, pain, or warts, he should see a urologist immediately. Finally, be sure to weigh your desire to pursue a career or other options before you have a child against the impact of advancing age on your fertility.

11

Infections of
the Reproductive Tract

Mary Jane Gray, M.D.

Human beings have always suffered from sexually transmitted diseases (STDs), but these conditions have become epidemic in the United States during the 1980s, particularly for those between the ages of 15 and 34. This does not mean that if you are older or younger than this you are free of risk; everyone who is sexually active, whether frequently or seldom, can be exposed to contagion. But you are in greater danger if you have more than one sexual partner, either concurrently or in rapidly changing sequential relationships.

In the days when we used the term *venereal disease* (VD), the popular stereotype of the VD victim was largely male, the diseases were gonorrhea and syphilis, and the image of the victim was generally unsavory. If women were portrayed as having VD at all, they were usually prostitutes. Today, the range of possible infections is much broader, and they strike (as they always did) across all social and income groups. The trouble they can cause presents a major health hazard to women.

STDs vary in their degree of seriousness. Some are only annoying; others can cause major infections and sterility. Some never go away completely, returning periodically, even with treatment;

some increase the risk of developing cancer; and some cause death. Therefore, the best defense against any infection of the reproductive tract is prevention.

PREVENTIVE MEASURES

The guiding principles of prevention against STDs include choosing a sexual partner with care and selectivity, establishing good communication with your sexual partner, assessing your partner's sexual history prudently, and using condoms. These principles, and the advice that follows, apply to all STDs. Here are some of the specific steps you can take to protect yourself:

1. Try to establish a long-term, steady relationship with one sexual partner who is willing to have an exclusive relationship with you. The more people you have sex with, and the more people *they* have or have had sex with, the greater your exposure. Before you become intimate with someone, talk about the risks and try to find out whether your intended partner has, or has had, an STD and, if so, how it was treated, when it happened, and whether he is cured. This is difficult at the beginning of a relationship, when you are sometimes unrealistically trusting and optimistic, but it is necessary, particularly since your partner is probably just as concerned as you are, or should be. In fact, you can start such a conversation by giving him your own sexual history.

Some authorities recommend examining a new—or long-term—partner's penis for sores, discharge, odor, or other signs of possible infection before having sexual intercourse, believing that this precaution is necessary in today's climate. If you see obvious penile abnormalities, of course you should avoid intercourse, but we must point out that penile examination, even adroitly engaged in as part of foreplay, cannot provide you with total protection. For example, a man can have the HIV virus or syphilis and have a perfectly normal-looking penis.

2. Even if you use birth control pills, if you know you are infertile, or if you have been sterilized, use condoms with a spermicide before you begin intercourse, because, used together, they can reduce your risk of contracting an STD by 50 percent. Men who refuse to wear condoms are ignoring the basic realities of healthy contemporary sexual activity and need to be brought up-

to-date about them, regardless of local peer practices based on the conventions or misinformation of an earlier time. When insisting on using condoms, you can point out to your partner the obvious protective advantages they give both of you.

3. If either you or your partner has any symptoms at all of infection, or if you have any reason to suspect that either of you has been exposed to infection by a previous sexual contact, *do not engage in any form of sexual intimacy, from kissing to intercourse.* This is difficult indeed, but it may save you months and years of illness, worry, and pain. Remember that STDs not only cause sickness, they can make you infertile as well, and some of them can kill you.

4. If you learn that you have an STD, seek out any previous sexual partner and notify him. Doing so may prevent his transmitting it and preserve his health and fertility.

IRRITATIONS AND INFECTIONS

The relationship between irritations, infections, and STDs is often confusing. Irritation or increased sensitivity of the vulvar skin (the external female sexual area) and the mucous membranes of the vagina can be caused by soaps, dyes, perfumes, spermicides, or other substances to which one is allergic; or by friction, radiation, or various infectious agents.

On the other hand, microorganisms such as bacteria, viruses, fungi, and parasites cause infections, which can then spread from one place to another. The most common route of infection in the female reproductive tract is through sexual intercourse, which is why these infections are referred to as sexually transmitted diseases. Some STDs—AIDS and hepatitis B, for example—do not affect the genital organs primarily; they just gain access to a woman's body through the walls of the vagina or rectum.

The vulva has many nerve endings responsive to sexual stimulation, and therefore it is highly vulnerable to pain. Many agents that cause irritation, itching, swelling, and increased discharge in the vulvar area also involve the vagina. Some of these infections lodge in the glands of the cervix. Infected urine can be very irritating to surrounding tissues. If you have pain in the vulvar region and suspect infection, you should see your doctor, because all of these areas should be examined. This is not a condition that can be diagnosed and treated by telephone, and it should be evaluated as quickly as possible.

DISCHARGE

Some discharge from the vagina, consisting of fluid containing cast-off vaginal cells, is normal. The quantity varies from woman to woman; it may be enough to moisten underwear, or it may require a panty liner. Because of the changes that occur in the cervical mucus at the time of ovulation, the quantity of thick discharge from the vaginal opening is usually increased at the midpoint of the menstrual cycle. A young girl may be surprised by the increase in secretions that takes place at puberty; in fact, she may erroneously believe that the lubrication accompanying sexual arousal is abnormal. The internal alterations that occur during pregnancy also include an increase in vaginal discharge.

When, then, is a discharge abnormal? A discharge that is yellow, that is streaked with blood, that has an unpleasant odor, or that causes itching or irritation of the skin is usually a sign of infection. Allergies, radiation treatment, and tumors can also produce abnormal discharge. Soaps, fabric softeners, perfumes, douches, and some spermicides are the most common reasons for allergic reactions, although some women are actually allergic to their partner's semen. In the latter case, the couple should use condoms, which will protect the woman from her partner's semen, unless, of course, they are trying to conceive.

INFECTIONS

Before puberty and after menopause, the vaginal lining is very thin and particularly susceptible to infection by all manner of organisms, a vulnerability that is described as atrophic vaginitis. Radiation treatments also render the vagina thin and vulnerable. If an infection is present, after determining its cause the doctor will prescribe suitable antibiotic treatment to help clear it up and may advise using estrogen cream, which will act to increase the thickness of the vagina.

"YEAST," MONILIA, OR CANDIDA

A fungus, or "yeast," organism called candida albicans or monilia is the most common cause of vaginal infection. This condition is not spread primarily by sexual intercourse but comes from an organism that occurs throughout the environment. Often it lives in the vagina without causing problems, but when vaginal conditions change it may grow rapidly. Moisture from wet swimming suits and synthetic-fiber underwear facilitates its growth, as does the increased sugar and glycogen that accompanies pregnancy and diabetes. Oral contraceptive pills seem to increase the incidence of yeast infection in susceptible women; what makes some women vulnerable and others resistant is still unclear. Perhaps the most frequent predisposing event is the use of antibiotics that kill the normal vaginal bacteria, allowing the fungus to grow unchecked. If treatment with an antibiotic is necessary, such an infection is sometimes a necessary risk.

Symptoms

The usual symptoms associated with a yeast infection are severe itching in the vaginal area, irritation, and soreness of the mucous membranes, along with a thick, white discharge. Skin reaction to a yeast infection includes redness, a raised rash, and small cracks in the sensitive mucous membrane. The itching and redness sometimes spread to the upper thighs. The intensity of the symptoms occurs because of an allergic response of the tissue to the fungus. In fact, this response is so common that doctors use a skin test employing this fungus to demonstrate the existence of a normal immune system. Thus, itching may be very severe from only a minimal infection. Conversely, many women harbor this organism without symptoms.

Diagnosis

Doctors diagnose a vaginal fungal infection by placing a drop of vaginal secretion in an alkaline solution, such as potassium hydroxide solution (KOH), that will dissolve all cells except those of the fungus, which they can then identify under a microscope. This method takes only a few minutes. If there is any difficulty in establishing the diagnosis, the clinician can obtain a culture that a lab can identify in two days, a procedure that is necessary only if too few organisms are present to be seen under the microscope.

Treatment

Physicians treat yeast infections by prescribing various antifungal and antibiotic agents in the form of vaginal suppositories and creams. They include miconazole (Monistat 7), clotrimazole (Gyne-Lotrimin, Mycelex), butoconazole (Femstat), and perconazole (Terazol). Monistat 7 and Gyne-Lotrimin are now over-the-counter (OTC) drugs. If you are certain you have a yeast infection, you can use an OTC; however, this is a difficult diagnosis and you will waste time and money, and will continue to have unpleasant symptoms, if you guess wrong and wait to seek medical care. Your doctor will usually prescribe a 100-milligram daily dose of one of these medications for seven days, or 200 milligrams a day for three days. A single 500-milligram dose of clotrimazole usually suffices. Medications combining yeast-killer and cortisone (Mycolog) will reduce itching and increase comfort. You should not use any of these drugs during the first trimester of pregnancy and when breast-feeding, as their safety has not been confirmed.

Although all these agents are between 80 and 85 percent effective, they do not eliminate the underlying conditions that promote the infection, and, because these often persist, such infections tend to recur. Certain oral agents are also prescribed for the treatment of fungal infections, but they are much more expensive than the medications available in suppository or cream form and no more effective. Other remedies include gentian violet suppositories, with which you must wear a sanitary pad, as any discharge will turn your clothing purple; boric acid powder, dissolved in a douche or inserted in the vagina in gelatin capsules; and potassium sorbate, the yeast-killer vintners use in wine. Home remedies, such as yogurt douches, are messy and not particularly effective.

Although symptoms usually disappear within two days after treatment, recurrences are unfortunately frequent. If you have a repeat infection, it is important to establish that the problem is being caused by the yeast infection and not something else or something in addition to it. You should consider a longer course of treatment and a monthly dose of further medication for one or two days to prevent reinfection. Your partner should also be treated. If he is not, and still harbors the infection, there is a danger you will become reinfected; in fact, the yeast infection can ping-pong back and forth between you unless you are both cured. It is important to make your partner understand that it is in his best interest, as well as yours, to seek and accept treatment.

In the future, you should use an antifungal medication whenever you take antibiotics. It is particularly important during this time to maintain basic genital cleanliness and good general health. Since eliminating the ubiquitous yeast organism completely is virtually impossible, the aim of treatment is to control its growth so that a few yeast organisms can exist compatibly with normal vaginal bacteria.

Although yeast infections are not usually transmitted sexually, male partners of women with yeast infections may develop itching and a rash on the penis and scrotum. Some men experience inflammation of the urethra (urethritis). Symptoms subside spontaneously in most males when the woman is treated, but men can speed up the process by using a little of the prescribed vaginal cream on the affected area. Healing will also occur more quickly if you avoid intercourse during treatment.

BACTERIAL VAGINOSIS (NONSPECIFIC VAGINITIS)

The other common vaginal infection that may occur without intercourse has recently undergone a change in name from nonspecific vaginitis to bacterial vaginosis. The current term reflects the fact that the cause is more one of an imbalance of vaginal bacteria than an infection with a single organism. The bacteria most associated with the general infection is Gardnerella vaginale (formerly called Hemophilus vaginalis and Cornybacterium vaginale). All this name-changing should not disguise that few firm facts have been established about this condition. Studies show that, in addition to the Gardnerella organism, intestinal bacteria must also be present to constitute this kind of infection, yet we know little as to why some women suffer it repeatedly and others not at all.

Method of Infection

Several studies have shown that the Gardnerella organism can be sexually transmitted, although recently this has been disputed.

Since women who have never had intercourse, as well as women who are sexually inactive, acquire this organism, other routes of infection are clearly also to blame, although these have not been identified.

Symptoms

Bacterial vaginosis can be present without causing symptoms. When symptoms do occur, they include a discharge with an unpleasant, fishy odor. The discharge is usually thin in consistency, gray-white in color, and irritating to the vaginal lining and the vulva. Irritation around the urinary opening may cause burning with urination, and intercourse may be painful.

Diagnosis

The fishy odor that characterizes this infection is intensified, if present, by adding a drop of alkali to a bit of vaginal secretion, which is the basis for diagnosis. Microscopic examination reveals "clue cells," vaginal cells that appear as polka dots because the bacteria cover the surface of the cell. The pH of the vaginal secretions is less acid than normal, and wriggly bacteria also frequently appear. Some laboratories can grow the Gardnerella organism, but such cultures delay the diagnosis, increase the expense, and add little information.

Treatment

The Centers for Disease Control (CDC) does not recommend treating partners for bacterial vaginosis, but in those women whose infections recur after intercourse, treatment of partners is only sensible and often proves helpful. The treatment of choice is 0.5 grams of metronidazole (Flagyl) twice a day for seven to 10 days. Physicians must warn both partners not to drink alcohol while taking this drug because of possible severe nausea. Other side effects may occur, including diarrhea, an allergic reaction, dry mouth, metallic taste, and a decreased white blood cell count. Further concerns have been raised about this drug because of animal research showing it causes cancer in mice and rats, but it does not appear to be carcinogenic in humans. Still, clinicians do not prescribe it during pregnancy and breast-feeding but try to control symptoms with vaginal creams, which are less effective. Ampicillin, amoxicillin, or a sulfa/trimethoprim combination may be used in women who do not tolerate metronidazole. Recent reports suggest that clindamycin vaginal cream may also be effective. The infection seems to recur in some women despite adequate treatment. Although this condition has usually been considered unpleasant but relatively harmless, some evidence links bacterial vaginosis to post–cesarean section infections. We have no real evidence yet that bacterial vaginosis leads to uterine infection, but it has been found in the fallopian tubes.

TOXIC SHOCK SYNDROME (TSS)

The infectious staphylococcus strains produce a toxin or poison that is absorbed into the bloodstream, where it causes a generalized illness characterized by a rash resembling sunburn, fever, aching, and diarrhea. In severe cases, which are rare, women can experience dangerously low blood pressure and kidney, heart, liver, and blood-clotting difficulties. About 2 to 3 percent of TSS patients die of complications resulting from the infection. If the vagina becomes infected with certain strains of staphylococcus, tampons left in place for more than four hours during the menstrual period provide an excellent place for the organism to grow. Cases of TSS have also been reported with the use of vaginal contraceptive sponges and diaphragms, but it has not been established that these contraceptive devices cause an increased risk.

Diagnosis

Doctors should always consider the diagnosis of TSS whenever an acute illness occurs during the menstrual period. Diagnosis is based on the symptoms described above. A vaginal culture to identify staphylococcus aureus organisms may confirm the diagnosis.

Treatment

Doctors can reverse the illness by removing the tampon, if present; giving intravenous fluids; and, perhaps, prescribing antibiotics effective against staphylococcus aureus. The medical decision whether or not to use antibiotics is extremely difficult because, by the time you have TSS, it is too late for antibiotics to clear up the existing infection. The reason clinicians use antibiotic therapy at all is that it may prevent recurrences.

Prevention

Since the removal of superabsorbent tampons from the market, which were implicated in causing TSS, women are using less absorbent tampons that they must change more frequently. As a result, physicians do not see as much TSS as they did in the past. Tampons are a great boon to women, but they must be used only when needed and changed at least every four hours.

If you use sanitary pads instead of tampons, the risk of TSS is almost eliminated, although women who use tampons still have little chance of getting TSS with the kind of frequent change recommended. If you use tampons, try using a pad at night to give the vagina a time period with nothing in it that can harbor bacteria. Always wash your hands before inserting a tampon, to avoid introducing bacteria from your fingers into the vagina. (If you have any leftover superabsorbent tampons, throw them away.) Don't leave your diaphragm or contraceptive sponge in your vagina longer than the recommended six hours, and don't use either of them during your menstrual period or for three months after giving birth. If you have had one episode of TSS it is probably wise to stop using tampons, diaphragms, and sponges altogether.

CYSTITIS

Cystitis is an infection of the urinary bladder. It is much more common in women than in men because the female urethra connecting the bladder to the urinary opening is much shorter than it is in males; thus, bacteria have only one or two inches to travel to reach the bladder. Although cystitis is not a sexually transmitted disease, it is usually provoked by intercourse traumatizing the urethra, because sexual thrusting can push bacteria up into the bladder. Frequently, first attempts at intercourse precipitate this problem; hence the term *honeymoon cystitis*.

Many different bacteria can be responsible for cystitis, but the majority of infections are caused by intestinal organisms, chiefly

E. coli. The use of a contraceptive diaphragm, which exerts pressure on the urethra and partially obstructs it by allowing retention of urine even after voiding, increases the likelihood of a bladder infection.

Symptoms

Cystitis causes frequent voiding of small quantities of urine accompanied by pain and burning during and after urination. Blood in the urine is also common and indicates nothing more than an irritated lining of the bladder. The urine may be cloudy or have an unusual odor. The symptoms may be the same if the infection is in the kidneys (pyelonephritis), but the potential for long-term problems in kidney infection is much greater. Pyelonephritis may also produce pain in the back or flank as well as chills and fever; if you have these symptoms, you should have a complete evaluation of your urinary system to determine whether you have a kidney infection.

Diagnosis

Your doctor can sometimes diagnose cystitis from your medical history, but the best and most accurate way is from a urine sample, which can be examined under the microscope, and from a culture, which can determine which antibiotic will be most effective for treatment. Rapid but less accurate tests have also been developed, in which the clinician dips a strip of tape into the urine and observes it for color changes. Other infections also cause irritation around the urinary opening, and this sometimes makes it difficult to distinguish cystitis.

Treatment

Recent studies have shown that single-dose therapy of simple acute urinary tract infections in women is as effective and less expensive than the traditional seven to 10 days of antibiotics and has fewer side effects. The antibiotic of choice to treat cystitis is trimethoprim/sulfamethoxazole, although ampicillin and tetracycline are also useful. Macrodantin is another good antibiotic, since it reaches its highest concentration in the urine; however, its side effects, including dizziness, faintness, and nausea, are more severe than those from other medications. Diabetics, pregnant women, and those with other special problems have more relapses and should not use the short treatment, nor is it sufficient to control kidney infections. Some doctors use three-day therapy as an effective compromise between the short course and the standard treatment.

Prevention

The following strategies may help to prevent cystitis, and they are especially important if you have experienced repeated episodes:

- Drink lots of fluid, particularly water, milk, and fruit juice, especially before intercourse.
- Void promptly after having intercourse.
- Void at regular intervals during the day, because urine left in the bladder can provide a site for infection.
- Don't use a diaphragm, because it causes retention of urine; women who use them have more cystitis.
- Minimize your risk of contracting STDs.
- If you don't produce enough fluid naturally during intercourse, use lubrication liberally; any water-based product, such as K-Y Jelly or contraceptive foam, will suffice.
- Observe basic feminine hygiene: always wipe from front to back after a bowel movement to avoid spreading bacteria from the rectum to the urethra, and shower or bathe daily.

If these measures don't prevent infection, you may have to take prophylactic antibiotics either just before or after intercourse or on a more regular basis.

SEXUALLY TRANSMITTED DISEASES (STDS)

TRICHOMONAS

A trich infection, as it's called colloquially, is a sexually transmitted vaginitis caused by a one-celled organism that travels rapidly with the help of tiny moving appendages. The infection is not as common as it once was because a specific cure has been available for 25 years. The organism can be demonstrated by analyzing a culture from the male reproductive tract, but this is rarely done because trich usually produces no symptoms in the male, who can harbor the infectious agent for years. Occasionally, however, men experience discharge, burning with urination, or irritation.

Symptoms

A profuse yellow-green discharge, together with severe itching and irritation of the mucous membranes, indicates an infection with the trichomonas parasite. Sometimes you will also urinate frequently; pain and/or odor are rarely present. Symptoms may continue until treated or they may gradually resolve on their own. Some women may also carry the organism for years without symptoms.

Diagnosis

If the health-care provider places a drop of the vaginal discharge in a dilute salt solution and examines it under the microscope, the moving organisms can be seen. Sometimes the pathologist makes the diagnosis from a Pap smear. In case of doubt, the organism can be grown in a special solution.

Treatment

Clinicians use 2 grams of metronidazole (Flagyl) given within a 24-hour period to both the woman and her partner, and this treatment is almost always effective. Again, both partners must be warned not to drink alcohol while taking this drug because of the possibility of severe nausea; other possible side effects include diarrhea, an allergic reaction, dryness of mouth, metallic taste, and a decreased white blood cell count. If symptoms recur, it usually means either that the partner did not use the medication or that the couple was not treated simultaneously, which causes the infection to ping-pong back and forth between them—or a third partner is involved. In the rare instances when patients exhibit a resistance to metronidazole, doctors can usually bring the infection under control by increasing the dose, but this will intensify the same possible side effects, which may appear even more frequently.

CHLAMYDIA

Identified as an important cause of infection in the female reproductive tract only 15 years ago, chlamydia is one of the most common STDs and is probably the most frequent cause of PID. Currently, 5 to 15 percent of sexually active women harbor the chlamydia infection. The bacteria that causes chlamydia lives inside cells, especially those of the cervical canal and those lining the fallopian tubes. This organism causes at least 50 percent of nonspecific urethritis (NSU), infection of the urethra in males. Both persistent and dangerous, chlamydia can result in sterility.

Symptoms

The most common symptom of chlamydia infection in women is a heavy yellow discharge that may be somewhat irritating to the vagina and vulvar membranes. The cervix may be tender during intercourse or during a pelvic examination. If the infection has spread up into the tubes, mild or severe pelvic pain may be present. Both males and females may complain of burning when they urinate. A negative urine culture in a woman who has symptoms of a urinary tract infection should suggest chlamydia, because the organism cannot be grown with the usual urine culture. The infection, however, may be totally without symptoms in either sex, and lead over time to sterility. Chlamydia is also a threat to a baby born through an infected vagina, because the infant may acquire the infection. However, the diagnosis of chlamydia in pregnant women is not an indication for a cesarean section.

Diagnosis

A reddened cervix with a discharge of pus is a clue to start treatment. Doctors can confirm the diagnosis with a culture, but the organism is difficult to grow and the culture is expensive. Certain tests can also indicate the presence of antibodies to the organism in the blood, a sign of a past or present chlamydia infection. Other tests detect such antibodies in cervical mucus.

The diagnosis of mild PID resulting from chlamydia is one of the most difficult to make, because the symptoms are subtle. Despite infection, test results may be negative. Sometimes physicians must use a laparoscope to look at the tubes to see whether infection is present. (See Chapters 10, 14.) Because of the severe consequences of the infection, and because symptoms may be absent, every woman who is having heterosexual intercourse should be tested for chlamydia and gonorrhea annually and sooner after acquiring a new partner. These two STDs often occur simultaneously.

Treatment

Tetracycline or its derivative doxyclycline, used two to four times daily for 10 days, cures more than 95 percent of chlamydia infections. Tetracycline must not be used during suspected or confirmed pregnancy because it affects the teeth and bones of the developing fetus. Erythromycin is an acceptable alternative. Obviously, the male partner must be treated at the same time, and the couple should use condoms until the infection is gone. A test that determines cure should be performed after about three weeks. Persistent disease in a woman usually means that her partner did not take his medication, or that another partner is involved. Anyone who has had sexual contact with a man or woman with chlamydia should always be treated, regardless of the results of the diagnostic tests, because such tests are not infallible.

If the infection has progressed into the tubes, a woman must enter the hospital, and intravenous antibiotics may be necessary. Once the tubes have been invaded by chlamydia, other organisms may move in and cause a life-threatening infection of all the pelvic organs.

MYCOPLASMA

The mycoplasma organisms, Mycoplasma hominis and Ureaplasma urealyticum, are small infectious agents between the size of bacteria and viruses. They cause about 50 percent of the non-specific urethritis (NSU) in men. In women, they are responsible for postsurgical infections and cervicitis, an inflammation of the cervix; they may also cause PID. Their role in STDs, however, is not clear, in part because the organisms are difficult to grow in the laboratory and therefore to study. Doctors often make the diagnosis of mycoplasma by excluding other agents—a shaky basis at best. Highly specialized cultures are available for diagnosing this infection, but clinicians rarely use them because their accuracy is questionable. Tetracycline or erythromycin are both effective in treating mycoplasma.

GONORRHEA

Gonorrhea, also called the clap and abbreviated to GC, has been identified as a sexually transmitted infection for centuries. The responsible organism is a bacterium that lives within cells of the cervix, the urethra, and the fallopian tubes in the female; in males, it survives in the urethra and in the elongated cordlike structure along the posterior border of the testis, which contains the ducts that store sperm (the epididymis). Gonorrhea is highly contagious with only one act of intercourse. Symptoms appear in three to five days. Despite the fact that physicians have been able to diagnose and cure gonorrhea with antibiotics since the 1940s, the infection is so common, and the organism so skilled at developing antibiotic resistance, that the infection is on the increase and remains widespread, with about 2 million cases occurring annually in the United States.

Symptoms

The classic symptoms of gonorrhea are a puslike discharge or "drip" from the penis, accompanied by burning upon urination in the male and a yellowish discharge and/or urinary burning in the female. This infection may spread, typically during menstruation, into the fallopian tubes, causing pelvic pain, fever, gastrointestinal symptoms, general peritonitis, and even death.

Although doctors once believed that the infection always produced symptoms in the male and rarely in the female, they now know that many males are infected without knowing it; thus the "drip" is not always present.

Diagnosis

Gonorrhea may be suspected on the basis of a discharge of pus, but it must be confirmed by microscopic examination of the discharge on a specially stained slide or by culture. Although the organism requires a special culture medium to grow, many clinics and private health-care providers perform this test routinely; results are available in 48 hours. Recent advances in antibody detection may provide cheaper and easier tests in the future.

Treatment

Because the gonococcus is an elusive and adaptable bacterium with the ability to change its metabolism and acquire resistance to antibiotics, the Centers for Disease Control (CDC) has recently changed its recommendation for the treatment of gonorrhea to a single shot of Ceftriaxone, a new antibiotic with no reported record of patient resistance as yet. The advantage of this therapy is that one shot cures all. Doctors can still use the earlier prescribed treatment—penicillin, ampicillin, or spectinomycin—but those who receive these drugs must be monitored closely with cultures that test for antibiotic resistance. They must also take probenecid with penicillin-type antibiotics, to slow kidney excretion and retain a high level of these medications in the bloodstream.

Everyone with whom the infected person has had sexual contact must also be treated. In addition, because at least 25 percent of those who are infected with gonorrhea will also have a chlamydia infection, all gonorrhea patients should also receive tetracycline/doxycycline, regardless of culture results.

PELVIC INFLAMMATORY DISEASE

Pelvic inflammatory disease (PID) is a general term describing infection anywhere in the pelvis—for example, in the lining and/or muscle layers of the uterus, the fallopian tubes, or the ovaries. PID is a major health problem in the United States, affecting a million women annually. It is estimated that infections from chlamydia and gonorrhea are responsible for more than half of all PID.

Symptoms

The symptoms of PID caused by chlamydia and gonorrhea differ. Chlamydia symptoms are usually more gradual and subtle, with women experiencing mild abdominal pain or backache or pain they notice only during intercourse. A woman's vaginal discharge may increase only slightly or may not change at all. Chlamydia may cause as much—or more—permanent damage to the fallopian tubes as gonorrhea.

The symptoms of PID caused by gonorrhea are usually more striking; women often experience severe pelvic pain and high fever, between 101° and 104°, as well as chills, vaginal discharge, and, sometimes, vaginal bleeding.

Diagnosis

The differences in symptoms should make the diagnosis of gonococcal PID easier than for PID caused by chlamydia. However, because the characteristics of gonococcal PID mimic those of appendicitis and ectopic pregnancy, differentiating among them can be difficult. Since treatment varies markedly—appendicitis and ectopic pregnancy require surgery, while gonococcal PID needs a course of antibiotics—the doctor may have to perform a laparoscopic examination to look at the pelvic organs. (See Chapter 14.)

The clinician must also conduct a pelvic exam, because tenderness in the uterus, tubes, or ovaries is a sign of pelvic infection. Taking a culture may help determine which bacteria are responsible for the problem; if it does, deciding on appropriate antibiotic therapy is easier. However, culture results are not always clear-cut, since many bacteria normally live in the vagina. Your physician will certainly test for chlamydia and gonorrhea to find out which of them is the culprit, or if both are present. Another diagnostic tool here is a blood count; if your white cell count is high, it means your system is fighting an infection. If an abscess containing pus and bacteria is suspected, the doctor may suggest a sonogram to assess its size and location and decide whether or not to drain it surgically.

Treatment

Of the 1 million women who suffer from PID annually, almost a third end up in the hospital. If the infection is widespread and severe, or if oral antibiotics are not working, hospitalization is required so that intravenous antibiotics can be administered. While many specialists recommend hospitalization for all PID patients, specific indications for hospitalization include an uncertain diagnosis; a suspected pelvic abscess; an adolescent patient, because as a group adolescents find it difficult to comply with doctors' orders and also suffer particularly severe long-term consequences; and inability to obtain clinical follow-up 72 hours after starting antibiotic therapy.

The drugs used must be effective not only against gonorrhea but also against the other organisms that move into the infected area, which can include streptococci and mycoplasmas, among others. Anti-PID drugs include cefoxitin plus doxycycline or clindamycin with gentamicin. Some doctors use tetracycline or erythromycin. Without treatment, pus may spread throughout the pelvis—sometimes traveling up under the liver—causing severe illness, infertility, and possible death. Even when symptoms are borderline, the clinician may decide on treatment to prevent more serious problems from developing. If you are pregnant, or if your doctor suspects an ectopic pregnancy or appendicitis, you must be hospitalized. Part of any treatment is getting plenty of rest to help your immune system fight the infection.

Prognosis

Twenty percent of women become sterile because of blocked tubes after one episode of PID, and that incidence jumps to just over 50 percent after three episodes. Usually, a woman does not learn she has a tubal problem until she attempts to become pregnant, because the tests one takes to find out whether or not the tubes are open are not without complications. When women with blocked fallopian tubes who have no history of diagnosed PID are checked for antibodies showing evidence of a previous chlamydia infection, 80 percent show signs of such infection, while only 20 percent of women with normal tubes turn out to have had chlamydia.

SEXUALLY TRANSMITTED RASHES, ULCERS, AND OTHER SORES OF THE VULVA

The vulva is made of skin and mucous membrane, and thus it is susceptible to all the irritiations and allergies that affect other parts of the body. Allergic reactions usually take the form of redness and itchiness.

Shaving the pubic hair in the bikini area can cause pimples on the vulva and mons. Infection is common if the hairs grow back crooked in the hair follicles, as they sometimes do. The openings of the glands on the vulva and around the vagina may be blocked so that secretions pile up and become infected. The Bartholin's glands drain on either side of the vagina, producing some lubrication. If one of these is obstructed, a Bartholin's abscess may occur, requiring antibiotics and, often, surgical drainage. Sometimes this can be done in the doctor's office with local anesthesia. After the infection subsides, a collection of clear fluid may remain as a Bartholin's cyst. Unless this causes problems during intercourse, you need not have it treated. (See Chapter 14.)

DOUCHING

The odors associated with sexual activity are normal and may be washed away, but they should not be disguised with perfumes. Doctors sometimes prescribe washing the vagina, or douching, to introduce medication to treat infections. It is relatively safe to use douches occasionally after a menstrual period or after intercourse, but they are never necessary. Bathing or showering regularly will maintain sufficient cleanliness. If douches are used frequently, they may upset the normal balance of acids in the vagina and may even force fluid up the tubes, damaging these delicate structures.

HERPES

Herpes is a sexually transmitted viral infection. The typical small blisters appear in the genital area three to 14 days after intercourse with someone who has the disease. The blisters rapidly lose their tops and become very painful, especially when irritated by urine. Ulcers, areas where the top layer of skin has been lost, most often follow the tiny blisters. The initial infection lasts for about 10 to 12

days. The lesions gradually clear, and the virus particles travel up
the nerve fibers to hibernate in nerve cells near the spinal cord.
Whenever one's immunity to infection is low, the virus migrates
back down the nerve fiber to the site of the previous infection,
precipitating a similar but shorter outbreak.

Herpes types I and II are closely related, but it is the type I virus
that causes the common fever blisters. The most common cause of
genital herpes is the type II virus. Both viruses can grow either in
the mouth or in the genital area, although the type II virus usually
causes more general symptoms, such as fever, aching, and swollen
lymph nodes. Infection with type I virus seems to make subsequent
infection with type II less severe. It is estimated that 20 million
people may have this ubiquitous virus, and about 200,000 new
infections occur annually.

Symptoms

After the appearance of the tiny blisters (some women can identify a vague tingling in the area before the blisters appear), painful
small ulcerated sores develop in the genital area, which are typical
of herpes. Voiding may be so excruciating that a woman cannot
pass urine except in a tub of warm water. If there are infected areas
in the vagina or on the cervix, a very profuse vaginal discharge
may be present. The vulva may swell, and there may be fever as
well as tender and enlarged lymph nodes in the abdomen. Severity
varies among women; some have only one or a few sores, some
have many, and some remain asymptomatic.

Diagnosis

The ulcers of herpes are usually so typical that the experienced
health-care provider can diagnose the infection simply by seeing
them. Cultures are the clear proof of infections but are most likely
to be positive only during the first two to three days after the ulcers
appear. Antibodies in the blood indicate contact with the virus,
but they do not indicate when the contact may have occurred. It
is unusual to obtain a positive culture for the virus between out-
breaks, although this happens on occasion.

Because the virus can be passed from a woman to her infant
during labor and delivery, obstetricians take cultures during the

last weeks of pregnancy from the vaginas of women with a history of herpes infection. If the culture is positive, the doctor may recommend a cesarean section to avoid the possibility of infecting the infant. Although herpes was once a clear indication for surgical birth, the criteria are slowly changing. If you have herpes and are pregnant, you should carefully discuss the options with your doctor in deciding on the safest type of birth.

Treatment

There is no cure for herpes. Symptoms can be mitigated and attacks shortened by the use of oral acyclovir, an antiviral agent that is relatively nontoxic; acyclovir cream is not as effective as the pills. Treatment with one capsule five times per day for seven to 10 days is usually effective for either the initial attack or for recurrences. The earlier the treatment begins, the more effective it is. Since the drug is not a cure, there is no reason to treat partners with no symptoms.

Some people never have a second attack of herpes; others will have a recurrence every two weeks for years. If recurrences are a major problem, acyclovir capsules taken three times a day will usually reduce the frequency and severity of infections. The drug has now been used in this way for up to three years without severe side effects. The drawback is that acyclovir is expensive; preventive care costs $50 to $100 per month. Recurrences are likely to appear at times of physical stress—after riding a bicycle, for example—with emotional stress, or when a woman has another illness (thus the term *fever blister* to describe herpes). Some women have a recurrence each month just before their period. The control of herpes is based on the ability of the individual immune system to keep the infection in check.

Prevention

The virus is most prevalent and infectious during an outbreak of the open ulcers. Therefore, men and women should avoid intercourse and oral sex during this time. The virus has also been cultured in vaginal secretions when no lesions can be found. Consequently, many doctors recommend that all individuals who have ever had herpes, and their partners, use condoms for life, unless a couple is trying to conceive a child. Although studies show that the herpes virus renders animals vulnerable to cancer, and although women with herpes have a higher than average risk of precancerous conditions and cervical cancer, herpes is still less likely to cause such problems than is the wart virus.

WARTS

Warts (condylomata acuminata) are areas on the skin or mucous membranes that may be flat or raised; pink, white, or pigmented in color; large or small; single or multiple. The human papilloma virus (HPV) causes warts. Almost 60 strains of the wart virus have been identified, but only a few are commonly found in the genital area, where the infection is spread by sexual intercourse. Until recently, warts were regarded as only a vaguely unpleasant condition, because no one wants to have "warty" genitals. But doctors have started taking the presence of warts much more seriously for two reasons: first, because up to 60 percent of those who have ever been sexually active may harbor the virus; and second, because the virus has recently been linked to precancerous and cancerous changes in the cervix, vulva, and penis.

Vaginal warts may also spread the virus to the vocal cords of infants during delivery, but since they are not a serious threat to the infant, this is not an indication for cesarean section.

Symptoms

The mere presence of the raised rough areas on the vulva is alarming to many women. Warts can also appear in the vagina and on the cervix. Men can experience warts on the penis and scrotum, and they are frequently found around the anus and on the rectal mucous membrane in both sexes. They can even appear in the mouth, although this is rare.

Diagnosis

An experienced health-care provider accustomed to making this diagnosis can almost always do so on the basis of appearance. A clinician can recognize warts more easily after painting the skin with 3–5 percent acetic acid. Occasionally, however, normal, slightly rough areas of the vulva may be mistaken for warts. If the diagnosis is uncertain, the doctor can take a tissue sample of the area to send to the lab for further study, a procedure called a biopsy. (See Chapter 14.)

The presence of the wart virus is related to specific tissue changes and the later development of precancerous dysplasia. Researchers have known this from many years of animal studies; the connection in humans has gradually been getting stronger as investigators gain a better understanding of Pap smears. For example, thanks to improved methods for typing the virus, researchers have found that Types 16 and 18 are associated with cancer more often than other varieties, but these investigations have also shown that all strains are occasionally associated with dysplastic and malignant conditions. (See Chapter 13.) As long as there is no sure way to cure the HPV infection, typing the virus at great expense in every woman with warts is probably not warranted; besides, routine Pap smears pick up changes suggestive of wart viruses 15 percent of the time. When this happens, the doctor will use a colposcope, a diagnostic instrument resembling binoculars that is mounted on a tripod or a movable mechanical arm, to see details of the cervix magnified 10 times. (See Chapter 14.)

All abnormal Pap smears indicate the need for careful clinical follow-up with more Pap smears at frequent intervals and colposcopy and biopsy as indicated. How often you should have a Pap smear depends on how poor the results of the last one was, and on your doctor's opinion. Because up to 85 percent of women with warts may have some degree of cervical abnormality, doctors must follow these patients carefully and treat them as needed to control the condition.

Treatment

As with other viral infections, there is no cure for warts. The virus survives not only in the wart, but biopsies have shown that it also lives in apparently normal surrounding skin. Since the virus is only local and does not travel through the bloodstream to other parts of the body, warts may often be destroyed at the initial site with persistent treatment. All of the methods doctors use—treating with trichloroacetic acid, bichloroacetic acid, podophyllin, liquid nitrogen, cryotherapy, electrocautery, laser, and 5-fluorouracil (5-

FU) cream—are designed to kill the infectious agent locally. All cause pain and soreness in the affected region until healing takes place. Patients usually need frequent retreatment, which is costly and time-consuming, but untreated warts tend to grow and spread. Ultimately, as in herpes, the control of warts depends on the ability of your body's immune system to keep the virus in check. Treatment tips the balance in favor of the body.

Overtreatment of the vulva, as may occur when a doctor uses a laser to remove the whole superficial skin layer, has proven almost as bad as no treatment, because, after a long period of pain and healing, women often experience a recurrence of the warts. An anticancer drug, 5-FU cream, is helpful in treating vaginal warts but may produce a severe inflammation of the vagina (vaginitis). Interferons—a group of biologically active proteins that enhance the immune system—have been somewhat efficacious when injected into warts that are resistant to other forms of therapy, but this approach is still experimental. It is expensive, has unknown side effects, and shows no clear advantage over other methods of treatment.

When the male sex partners of women with warts are screened with colposcopy and biopsy, 67 percent have the HPV. In spite of this high figure, insufficient numbers of medical professionals and medical institutions are concerned enough about this condition in men to make appropriate therapy available. Ideally, all visible lesions should be treated with the same drugs used in women, but until more treatment facilities and better means of treatment are available, relying on condoms to prevent spread may be the best course. However, if the warts extend beyond the penis onto the scrotum, a condom will not suffice, and protected intercourse will not prevent infection.

MOLLUSCUM CONTAGIOSUM

A third common STD transmitted by a virus is molluscum, characterized by small bumps on the vulva and skin of the thighs. The infection shows up in children without sexual contact, and it may occur on any part of the body. Because this condition does not appear to cause any serious problems and is not as common as herpes and warts, it is not as well known. Although not in itself a significant infection, it may indicate that the person has other STDs and, therefore, should be examined by a physician.

Symptoms

Generally, no symptoms are present except for the multiple round white bumps with solid centers that seem to be indented on the vulva and the skin of the thighs.

Diagnosis

Microscopic examination of the contents of the lesions shows inclusion particles indicative of the molluscum virus.

Treatment

Doctors often freeze the white areas, a technique called cryotherapy, and then scrape out the contents to speed healing. Occasionally, the practitioner will use caustic substances like those employed to treat warts; these are sometimes successful in eradicating the lesions. Since treatment takes a long time and the infection tends to clear in about six months without it, therapy is not urgent.

SYPHILIS

Syphilis, or lues, is a serious, and sometimes fatal, STD that usually starts with a sore or chancre in the genital region and spreads to become a general infection. First described in the sixteenth century, it is caused by a very small, rapidly moving bacteria called a spirochete, Treponema pallidum. The incubation period is about three weeks.

Until the advent of penicillin 40 years ago, syphilis was a very common disease with a high mortality. This "wonder" drug provides a true cure with one shot, so that the number of cases fell dramatically and health officials began predicting that this scourge would be wiped out. A few thousand new cases continued to be reported each year until the 1980s, when the incidence began to climb again. Although there were only about 13 cases per 100,000 people in 1985, by 1989 this figure had jumped to almost 20 per 100,000 of population.

Because of this recent, substantial increase in the number of syphilis cases, and the devastating effects this condition has on the fetus, obstetricians are reinstituting routine testing of pregnant women in various parts of the country. The greatest incidences of syphilis in 1989 occurred in the Southeast, New York, Pennsylvania, and Connecticut. Request this test if you are pregnant and are not totally sure that your partner is free of syphilis.

Symptoms

The only symptom of early or primary syphilis is the presence of a raised, smooth, painless sore about half an inch in diameter on the vulva or penis. This chancre may also occur out of sight on the cervix, so that the primary infection may pass unnoticed in women. The initial, painless sore disappears in two to five weeks. The next, or secondary, phase sees the general spread of the organism; symptoms include a skin rash, often involving the palms of the hands and the soles of the feet, fever, aching, skin ulcers, and patchy loss of hair. If untreated, in the third or tertiary phase of the disease, which occurs years later, syphilis involves the heart valves, the brain, and the spinal cord, often causing death. Syphilis can cross the placenta to infect the fetus, producing babies born with congenital syphilis. These infants have various birth defects and may be very ill. The incidence of congenital syphilis, like that of all syphilis, is currently increasing. In New York City alone, 13,000 new cases were reported in 1989, a 20-fold increase over the incidence of congenital syphilis in the 1970s.

Diagnosis

If a physician examines an infected person when the primary sore or chancre is present, the secretions will contain spirochetes, which can be viewed in motion with the use of a special "dark field" preparation under a microscope. Usually only dermatologists and STD specialists can perform this diagnostic test because of the expertise it requires. Six weeks after the infection begins, the results of blood antibody tests become positive. If the first test is negative, and if you or your physician suspects syphilis, the test should be repeated in six weeks.

Treatment

Penicillin remains the treatment of choice; if late syphilis of the central nervous system is diagnosed, even those who are sensitive to penicillin must be desensitized and treated. Experts must direct this desensitization, which is a difficult process that carries a considerable risk. Some physicians use 500 milligrams of tetracycline four times a day instead of penicillin, and follow these patients to be certain of cure. Doctors can treat less advanced cases with doxycycline. Partners must always be treated simultaneously.

OTHER STDs CAUSING VULVAR SORES

Three other STDs, which are rarely seen in the United States, may cause swellings and sores on the vulva: granuloma inguinale, lymphogranuloma venereum, and chancroid, or "soft chancre." All three may be diagnosed through biopsies or cultures, and they usually respond to antibiotics.

OTHER VULVAR LESIONS

Sores that do not begin to heal within a week or two, that are irregular in outline, or that bleed should be examined by a healthcare professional because they may indicate the possibility of cancer. A biopsy using local anesthesia may be required to establish the diagnosis. (See Chapter 13.)

PUBIC LICE

Pubic lice (pediculosis pubis, or crabs) infest the pubic hair and cause severe itching. Although they are usually transmitted by sexual proximity, actual intercourse is not required; they can also be passed on by infected bed linen or clothing.

Symptoms

The usual complaints are severe itching in the pubic area, with redness and irritation secondary to scratching.

Diagnosis

The diagnosis is made by seeing the tiny creatures move or finding the egg cases fastened to pubic hairs.

Treatment

Scratching should be avoided because it can increase local irritation and can possibly spread the lice to hair elsewhere on the body. A number of preparations, including lindane (Kwell), made up as shampoos, kill pubic lice. Partners should be treated at the same time, and all clothing, towels, and bed clothing should be washed in hot water. Repeat treatment may be needed one week later after all the eggs have hatched. The shampoo is a powerful substance that is very irritating and should not be used more often than necessary. Be sure to follow the warnings on the label, or to discuss its use with your doctor.

STDS WITHOUT PELVIC SYMPTOMS

Two important sexually transmitted diseases, AIDS (HIV infection) and hepatitis B, may be acquired by intercourse but do not start with a primary infection of the genitalia. This is also true of certain less common infections, and it is not surprising, because the vulva and vagina and the tip of the penis, like the respiratory tract and the mouth, are composed of moist mucous membranes through which viruses may pass without drying out. In contrast, viruses rarely, if ever, penetrate intact skin.

HIV INFECTION (AIDS)

Infection caused by the human immunodeficiency virus (HIV) is of relatively recent origin, with the first cases in the United States reported in 1981. The virus is transmitted via vaginal mucosa during vaginal intercourse, via rectal mucosa during anal intercourse, less readily by oral-genital sex, by direct injection with infected blood and blood products (although rarely now that these are routinely screened for HIV antibodies), by contaminated needles from infected IV drug users, and, occasionally, by direct contact with infected blood under unusual conditions. The virus can also cross the placenta to the fetus, and the chance that the fetus may be infected by a mother with HIV is 30 to 50 percent. It is probable that the HIV virus is spread by breast-feeding. In those parts of the world where there is a reasonable alternative, HIV-positive mothers should not nurse their babies. There is no evidence that saliva, food or drink, mosquitoes, or casual contact with infected persons can transmit the virus (see Table 11.1).

The reason the HIV virus is deadly is that it invades T cells, those white blood cells that normally fight infection, and not only renders them unable to do so but also turns them into AIDS virus production centers, which multiply rapidly and then attack other T cells. The difference between HIV and other viral infections is stark: It is not so much that the antibiotics we have today cannot cure it but that, by destroying the body's immune system, which usually controls infections, the HIV organism finally grows unchecked, as do a myriad of other organisms, until the infected person dies. The immune system is also of primary importance in regulating malignant cell growth and preventing cancer.

Once the HIV virus establishes itself in the cells of an infected individual, many years may pass before the victim develops the unusual infections and tumors that herald the breakdown of the immune system and give rise to the final stage of HIV infection, labeled acquired immunodeficiency syndrome, or AIDS. After a person reaches this stage, death usually occurs within months or within a very few years.

Symptoms

HIV infection usually has no early symptoms. Some people develop a vague ache and low-grade fever, similar to the symptoms of other viral infections, about two to five weeks after exposure. Following this brief phase is a period, often lasting many years, when the infected individual has no symptoms. In the next period of the infection, sometimes called AIDS-related complex or ARC, the person has swollen lymph nodes, fever, weight loss, and fatigue. This stage may last for up to four years.

A succession of unusual and unusually severe infections, and the development of tumors of types that were previously rare, mark full-blown AIDS. There is continued weight loss, weakness, fa-

**How Women
Contract AIDS**

**Heterosexual Contact:
How Women Get Infected**

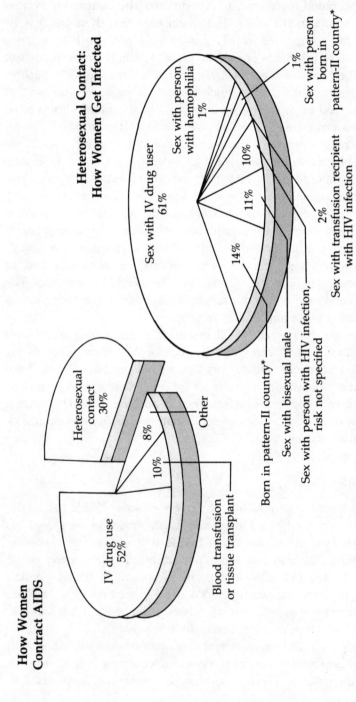

Heterosexual
contact
30%

IV drug use
52%

Other

8%

10%

Blood transfusion
or tissue transplant

Sex with IV drug user
61%

Sex with person
with hemophilia
1%

Sex with person
born in
pattern-II country*
1%

10%

11%

14%

2%

Sex with transfusion recipient
with HIV infection

Born in pattern-II country*

Sex with bisexual male

Sex with person with HIV infection,
risk not specified

*e.g., Haiti and countries in Central Africa where heterosexual transmission is believed to
play a major role in the spread of AIDS.

tigue, and often neurological symptoms, including confusion and other manifestations of brain involvement. Death at this stage is inevitable.

As many as 50 percent of the babies born to mothers with HIV show evidence of the infection soon after birth. Almost half of these babies die within a few months. Therefore, all pregnant women with risk factors for HIV infection should be tested, and the consequences of a positive result should be discussed with a physician. Pregnant women who test positive for HIV should consider the option of terminating the pregnancy.

Diagnosis

Diagnosis of an HIV infection is possible as early as three months after exposure to the virus, but the development of detectable antibodies may take up to a year. The test for antibodies is an Enzyme-Linked Immunosorbant Assay, or ELISA. If this test is positive, a more exact procedure, the Western Blot test, can confirm it. Because of the serious consequences of HIV infection, explanations and counseling usually precede all tests. If the tests are positive, you should be sure to seek expanded counseling. The confidentiality of test results is particularly important, because the widespread prejudice against those with AIDS in our society may make housing, job security, and the availability of health insurance very difficult for HIV-positive individuals. Testing should be done only where confidentiality is complete.

Treatment

There is currently no cure for AIDS. However, research has shown that zidovudine (AZT) prolongs survival and may be effective in extending the symptom-free period that precedes AIDS. Doctors give AIDS patients antibiotics to protect against certain rare infections, such as pneumocystis carinii, which occur frequently in AIDS patients. Investigators are testing many other drugs and vaccines providing hope for progress against this rapidly spreading infection.

Prevention

At the present time, abstinence provides the only sure protection against HIV infection. Serial monogamy is not a guarantee against your contracting the virus, as often it cannot take into account a partner's previous—or clandestine—sexual history or current practices. However, if your partner has not had other sexual contacts for at least two years, and tests negative, you can be relatively certain that he has escaped infection. Three years is an even safer measurement although there have been rare reports of the HIV virus remaining latent for as long as 12 years. Careful partner screening and the use of latex condoms give relatively good protection. It is important that everyone knows what constitutes "safe sex" and what is risky or dangerous. (Be sure to study the detailed recommendations contained in Table 11.2.) Since any body fluid (blood, urine, semen, saliva, feces) can contain the virus, if you work in the health field you should observe additional common-sense precautions, such as wearing gloves and eye protection, using masks for mouth-to-mouth resuscitation, and exercising particular care when disposing of needles and other medical equipment. The Public Health Service has compiled a list of recommendations for health-care workers, available from your local health department or by writing to the U.S. Public Health Service, Centers for Disease Control, 1600 Clifton Road, NE, Atlanta, GA 30333.

VIRAL HEPATITIS

Hepatitis B is an extremely common disease worldwide. In the United States, about 200,000 new cases occur annually, and one-fourth of them have serious symptoms. Hepatitis B, or serum hepatitis, as it was formerly called, is a viral infection primarily affecting the liver. Blood and contaminated hypodermic needles can transmit the virus, but it is more frequently acquired through sexual intercourse. It can also be transmitted to family members, although exactly how is unknown; the virus may exist in tears, sweat, and saliva, as well as in semen and vaginal secretions. Infants can get hepatitis if their mothers are infected. Viral hepatitis is more contagious than AIDS, and it can be fatal, although 90 percent of previously healthy individuals recover without such serious consequences as liver failure. Some victims suffer from persistent infection, which can damage the liver and put them at greater risk of getting liver cancer. Health-care workers who may come in contact with infected blood or contaminated needles and medical equipment should be vaccinated against the condition.

Food prepared and served by infected food handlers, or close contact in institutions and day-care centers, can transmit other strains of hepatitis, such as hepatitis A, a mild and transient illness.

Symptoms

Low-grade fever, muscle aches, fatigue, headache, nausea, vomiting, diarrhea, and abdominal pain, together with a yellow hue to the skin and eyes known as jaundice, are the typical symptoms of all types of hepatitis, although only half of infected patients experience jaundice. Symptoms normally appear two to three months after exposure, but they can emerge anytime between 30 days and slightly more than a year.

Diagnosis

Doctors suspect hepatitis on the basis of the symptoms noted and confirm it with blood antibody tests and tests of liver function. Abdominal tenderness high on the right side can indicate an enlarged liver.

Treatment

There is no cure for viral hepatitis once it occurs, but recent research has found that treatment with interferon alfa-2B may provide lasting benefit. A study of 169 patients divided into four treatment groups found a decline of both the hepatitis B virus and its antigen in a greater number of those who received interferon alone or in combination with prednisone, a steroid medication, than among patients who received either a lower dose of interferon or none at all.

Supportive treatment, including plenty of rest and a nutritious diet, may also be helpful. Since the liver breaks down estrogen, you should stop taking birth control pills or estrogen replacement therapy for menopausal symptoms if there is evidence of liver

Table 11.2 Sexual Practices

Safe Sex Practices

1. massage, hugging, body-to-body rubbing
2. dry social kissing
3. masturbation (touching your own genitals)
4. acting out sexual fantasies (which do not include any unsafe practices)
5. using vibrators or other sex toys (but not sharing them)

Low-Risk Sex Practices

1. wet (French) kissing (to be avoided if either partner has any sores in the mouth)
2. mutual masturbation (touching each other's genitals) (use latex gloves if there are any cuts on the hands)
3. vaginal intercourse using a condom (anal intercourse with a condom is riskier)
4. oral sex (mouth to penis) using a condom
5. oral sex (mouth to vagina) using a thin piece of rubber between the mouth and vagina (higher risk during menstruation)
6. skin contact with semen or urine, if there are no breaks in the skin

Unsafe Sex Practices

1. vaginal or anal (riskier) intercourse without a condom
2. unprotected penetration of the vagina or anus with a finger or hand
3. unprotected oral sex
4. semen (or urine or feces) in the mouth
5. mouth-to-anus contact
6. blood contact of any kind
7. sharing sex toys (or needles for drug use)

The Only People Who Do Not Need to Practice Safe Sex Are

1. people who are not sexually active with a partner
2. couples who are both virgins when they begin their relationship, have no other sexual partners afterward, and have not shared a needle or received a blood transfusion since before 1980
3. couples who have been in a monogamous relationship (no other partners for either) since before 1980, neither of whom has shared a needle or received a blood transfusion during that time

*These lists are adapted from Betty Clare Moffatt et al., *AIDS: A Self-Care Manual* (Santa Monica, Calif.: IBS Press, 1987), p. 125.

damage. You should also avoid alcohol until you know your liver is functioning normally. The liver usually recovers in two to three months, although about 10 percent of hepatitis victims have some degree of permanent liver damage.

Prevention

One way to prevent hepatitis B—as well as the other infections that are sexually transmitted—is to exercise care in your sexual contacts and avoid multiple partners. Use condoms. An immune globulin injection after exposure can provide you with temporary protection by giving you antibodies to both types of hepatitis, but you must get this injection within two weeks for the A strain, and within eight days for the B variety. This should prevent between 75 and 80 percent of cases. You can be immunized against hepatitis B by following a three-shot immunization schedule, the first two shots of the vaccine given one month apart and the third six months later. This is expensive, usually costing about $150, but it is much cheaper than getting sick. Immunity should last five years or more. You should be tested annually for antibodies starting five years after your initial three shots. If you lose your immunity (i.e., have a negative antibody titer), you should receive a single booster shot. Besides doctors, nurses, emergency personnel, and other health-care workers who may be exposed to this disease regularly, you should consider immunization if:

- You have a family member or sexual partner with hepatitis B.
- You have more than one sexual partner, or your partner does.
- You or your partner is an intravenous drug user.
- You plan to travel to Southeast Asia, parts of Africa, and the Pacific Islands, where the disease is rampant.

12

Abnormalities and Diseases

Mary Jane Gray, M.D.

From her first period to her last, most of the problems that send a woman to a doctor relate to her reproductive tract. This remarkable system, responsible for so much joy and so necessary for the survival of the human race, is a highly intricate one, and its sheer complexity makes it vulnerable to functional errors: having too few menstrual periods or too many, bleeding too little or too much, being infertile or too fertile, and developing infections and tumors. Because all of these conditions are matters of concern, it's best to be familiar with the features of the most common of these problems and with methods of diagnosis and treatment that can help make sense of some of them.

ABNORMAL BLEEDING

Blood from the uterus during a normal menstrual period should be unclotted and dark in color. If the blood is bright red, if large clots are present, if a flow occurs at an unexpected time of the cycle, the uterine lining may be bleeding abnormally. This general category of abnormal bleeding encompasses a wide range of patterns.

SCANT BLEEDING

Scant periods that occur at the expected time are rarely abnormal. It is quite common, for example, for your periods to be very light while you are taking the oral contraceptive pill. There is, however, an important exception. If you become pregnant, you may experience heavy spotting at the time the embryo implants in the uterine wall. Since implantation usually occurs two weeks after fertilization, at the same time that you expect your period, you may find it hard to distinguish between implantation bleeding and a regular period, particularly if the pregnancy was not planned. When in doubt, it is best to have a pregnancy test.

HEAVY BLEEDING

Some women have very heavy periods throughout their reproductive years. If you have consistently heavy periods, it's important to have your blood count tested regularly because heavy bleeding often depletes the body's iron stores, and you may need to eat more iron-rich foods or use iron supplements. Indeed, most women have slightly low hemoglobin levels and low values for the red cell portion of the blood (hematocrits) from menarche to menopause, reflecting the intermittent blood loss from menstruation during these years.

Experiencing a change in the amount of bleeding you have with your period is usually significant as well. If the change occurs gradually, be sure to schedule an appointment with your doctor to look for causes. On the other hand, if you experience sudden heavy bleeding that requires a change of pad or tampon every half hour for more than six hours, or bleeding that you cannot control by the usual means of protection, see your physician immediately. If such hemorrhage continues, you can become anemic and weak, go into shock, and even require blood transfusions. The early symptoms of hemorrhagic shock are dizziness, fatigue, restlessness, anxiety, weakness, and clammy skin. This type of bleeding must be investigated and controlled at once.

Sometimes the doctor will prescribe high doses of hormones to control heavy bleeding, at least temporarily. Performing a dilatation and curettage (D&C) will provide tissue for diagnosis and cure the bleeding as well, but this is rarely necessary in young women.

Sometimes doctors perform a hysterectomy to control excessive bleeding (see Chapter 14). A possible nonsurgical alternative to hysterectomy is a new procedure called endometrial ablation, in which the doctor uses a hysteroscope to inflate the uterus, then cauterize the endometrium with an electric wire or laser. This destroys the endometrium and eliminates menstruation; it is therefore suitable only for women who do not want more children and do not wish to menstruate any longer. In fact, some women are requesting this procedure as a form of birth control, since without a healthy endometrium the uterus cannot support a pregnancy. But the endometrium grows back in some women, making endometrial ablation an unreliable method of birth control; there have been pregnancies reported after the procedure in a small number of women. Also, endometrial ablation does not always end menstrual bleeding; a recent study in the British medical journal *Lancet* found that 50 percent of patients who had had the procedure experienced reduced menstrual flow, 30 percent had no flow, and 20 percent were unchanged. (See Chapter 14.)

Incomplete Abortion

One of the common causes of heavy bleeding is threatened or incomplete abortion. The further a pregnancy has progressed, the more bleeding there will be if you miscarry. Doctors usually control this type of bleeding by suctioning or curetting the uterus to remove any remaining tissue so that the uterus can cramp down effectively. (See Chapter 14.) Sometimes such drugs as Pitocin and Ergotrate are prescribed to help the uterus contract.

Lack of Progesterone

Heavy periods often reflect a lack of progesterone, the hormone produced by the follicle after ovulation and by the placenta during pregnancy. At both the beginning and the end of the menstruating years, early adolescence and just before menopause, there are frequent cycles in which a woman does not ovulate. These cycles produce what are referred to as anovulatory or estrogen-only periods, which are usually heavier and longer than normal ovulatory periods and have more irregular intervals between them. Doctors consider the bleeding that takes place during these anovulatory periods dysfunctional. Since drugs that induce ovulation are very expensive and produce many side effects, physicians rarely use them unless a woman is trying to become pregnant. Instead, doctors administer a synthetic progesterone such as medroxyprogesterone for heavy bleeding, or alternatively, they seek to control the problem by prescribing oral contraceptive pills, which substitute the Pill's estrogen and progestins for the body's own erratic hormones.

Uterine Fibroids

Uterine fibroids (leiomyomata uteri) are benign smooth muscle tumors that enlarge and distort the uterus (see Figure 12.1). These tumors occur freqently, often produce no symptoms, and require no treatment. The most common problem associated with them, however, is heavy bleeding during menstrual periods, probably because fibroids increase the surface area of the uterine lining—the endometrium—and because fibroids contain abnormally large blood vessels located just under the endometrium. Sometimes the bleeding can be controlled temporarily with progestins or a D&C, but in the long run, if bleeding is a continuing problem, a woman may need a myomectomy (removal of fibroids) or hysterectomy (removal of the uterus). Although having the surgeon remove only the fibroids while leaving the uterus sounds like a relatively less extreme solution to this problem, in reality a myomectomy is a difficult operation that leaves a woman with the potential for further trouble. (See Chapter 14.)

Recently doctors have become interested in using antigonadotropin substances, such as leuprolide and buserelin, to treat fibroids. These medications act by inhibiting the body's gonadotropins and thus reducing the amount of estrogen that feeds and encourages the growth of these benign tumors. However, reducing the amount of estrogen also precipitates menopausal symptoms that continue for as long as a woman takes these medications. The fibroids will start to grow again as soon as the medications are discontinued. One advantage of using antigonadotropins for a few months is that they are likely to make any surgery that might

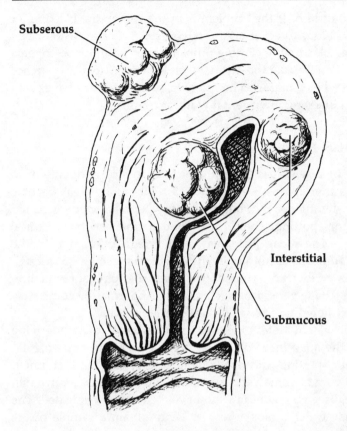

Subserous

Interstitial

Submucous

Fig. 12.1   Fibroids

subsequently be necessary to remove the fibroids or the uterus much easier, with less blood loss.

Metrorrhagia

Metrorrhagia is irregular bleeding that occurs between periods or that goes on so continuously, or so randomly, that it is difficult for a woman to define when and if she is actually menstruating. One frequent cause of metrorrhagia is the presence of polyps on the cervix or the endometrium. Polyps are small benign growths extending into the cavity of the uterus or into the cervical canal.

Intrauterine devices and infections of the uterus can also cause spotting, but the presence of any irregular bleeding means that the physician must consider the possibility of cancer of the cervix or the endometrium. If the problem is in the cervix, the bleeding or spotting is likely to occur after intercourse. A woman who has an underlying bleeding or clotting problem, such a thrombocytopenia purpura, von Willebrand disease, or leukemia, may experience uncontrolled bleeding with her periods, just as she may have problems with bleeding after dental work or trauma.

Menopausal Bleeding

At menopause, it is normal for periods to stop suddenly or to become farther apart. (See Chapter 15.) The periods may become lighter or slightly heavier, but very heavy periods, or any irregular bleeding or spotting, should alert you to the need for medical evaluation. The most likely reason for irregular bleeding is the erratic production of hormones that occurs as women go through menopause. However, your doctor must rule out cancer or precancerous changes as a possible cause. Abnormal bleeding may also reflect hereditary blood diseases or leukemia.

Doctors cannot determine the seriousness of the underlying cause by the quantity of bleeding. If you experience any irregular bleeding or spotting, except that which occurs for the first time if you are a young woman and are taking the oral contraceptive pill, you should see your clinician and have the cause investigated. The doctor may order a biopsy or a D&C to obtain a sample of the endometrium. If these tests and the pelvic examination are normal, additional blood tests and tests of clotting may be ordered.

VAGINAL DISCHARGE

With the onset of puberty, estrogen influences the vaginal wall to become thicker, and the blood supply to the area increases. The vagina sheds dead cells and accompanying fluid, which increases the clear discharge appearing at the vaginal opening. Other causes of normal discharge are sexual stimulation and pregnancy. The observant woman will note that the discharge increases in thickness at mid-cycle when she ovulates; it is usually odorless and clear to white in color, about the consistency of egg whites.

Discharges that are reddish (bloody), brown (old blood), or yellow or green (infection) usually suggest a problem. A strong odor, itching, or irritation of the surrounding skin are also signs of infection. If any of these problems are present, a health-care professional should examine some of the discharge under a microscope and take a sample for culture so that the responsible organism can be identified and treated.

Sexually transmitted diseases (STDs) cause many vaginal discharges. (See Chapter 11.) Certainly a discharge that appears for the first time two to five days after intercourse with a new sexual partner should make you suspicious that a sexually transmitted organism is involved. Nevertheless, the most common causes of vaginal infections are fungus or yeast, and these infections occur just as often in those who have never had intercourse as in those who have. A tampon left in the vagina for several days or weeks by mistake may also cause a discharge with an unpleasant odor. You can sometimes locate the offending article by putting a finger in the vagina, but usually you will need professional help to remove it if the string is missing. Once the tampon is out, the discharge clears up promptly.

A change in discharge may reflect the presence of a benign or malignant tumor of the vagina, cervix, endometrium, or fallopian tube. If no cause for the change can be promptly determined, the doctor will do a Pap smear. Occasionally, the change has been caused by an allergy to chemicals in vaginal creams or foam and will disappear when you change to another form of contraception. A woman can also be allergic to something in her partner's semen, although this is rare. Using a condom prevents this reaction, though this is not a practical solution if the couple is trying to become pregnant.

OVARIAN CYSTS

Most ovarian cysts, especially in young women, are merely a variation of normal. Every month when you ovulate your body forms a small cyst called a follicle, which releases the egg. Often, instead of rupturing at the time of ovulation, the follicle keeps on growing, producing a cyst, which can be seen by ultrasound techniques or felt at the time of a pelvic examination. Most of these cysts are painless, but those that grow to one and one-half to three inches (four to six centimeters) in diameter may become painful, and you may feel this pain on whichever side of your lower abdomen houses the cyst. Whether painful or painless, most ovarian cysts go away uneventfully. Occasionally, however, the cyst will rupture, causing sometimes severe pain as blood hits the peritoneum. Even less frequently, the cyst and the ovary from which it originates will twist and cut off the blood supply to the ovary. This condition is extremely painful and requires surgery to save the ovary.

If you develop simple cysts, be sure to visit your doctor repeatedly so they can be followed to be certain that they are indeed transient. If they don't disappear within two or three months, if they increase in size, or if they do not feel like the usual simple cyst, the doctor may use an ultrasound examination to determine whether a different kind of ovarian tumor may be present. Ultimately, it may be necessary to insert a laparoscope in order to see the area and determine whether or not surgery is advisable. (See Chapter 14.) Anything suggesting that the ovarian enlargement may be a malignancy requires surgery. (See Chapter 13.)

ENDOMETRIOSIS

Endometriosis, a condition affecting 20 to 25 percent of women, occurs when tissue from the endometrium, the lining of the uterus, travels from its normal location. For a long time gynecologists have theorized that, at the time of menstruation, some of the endometrial tissue finds its way through the fallopian tubes and out into the abdominal cavity, where it implants, grows, and recedes just as it does in the uterus. This theory has received support as researchers have shown that this reverse menstruation occurs in 90 percent of normal women. But investigators do not know why relatively few women have growth of this tissue significant enough for it to become clinical endometriosis. Some think a variation in the immune mechanism is involved. Most endometriosis occurs on the peritoneum covering the uterine ligaments and bladder and on the fallopian tubes and ovaries. Some burrows deep into uterine muscle, a condition known as adenomyosis. Rarely will endometrial tissue travel to the umbilicus, and very rarely to lung tissue. Fortunately, this endometrial tissue is not malignant and almost never becomes so.

The typical pain of endometriosis occurs just before a period starts and lessens after menstruation begins. Doctors believe that the release of estrogen and progesterone occurring with each menstrual cycle produces growth and swelling of the endometrial tissue and causes pain. It is clear that endometriosis does not grow in the absence of estrogen, because it gradually goes away after menopause.

The amount of endometriosis a woman has does not always correlate with the amount of pain she experiences from the condition, and not all pain follows a typical pattern. If ovaries are involved, for example, the pain can be persistent throughout the cycle. Endometriosis in the wall of the rectum can cause pain with bowel movements, and pain on deep penetration with intercourse is frequent. But many women with endometriosis have no pain at all.

Another serious problem associated with endometriosis is infertility. (See Chapter 10.) Again, only rough correlation exists between the presence of endometriosis and the rate of infertility. Doctors once believed that endometrial implants interfered with the mechanics of conception, but recent evidence indicates that an immune-system effect on fertility may be involved.

A doctor suspects endometriosis when a woman complains of pain as she relates her medical history. If examination shows nodules behind the uterus or on the uterine ligaments and ovaries, or that the uterus is fixed tightly against the rectum, the diagnosis becomes more likely. Most often, in milder cases, the pelvic exam is entirely normal. The only way a certain diagnosis can be made, however, is by seeing the endometrial implants at surgery, usually with laparoscopy. (See Chapter 14.)

THE TREATMENT OF ENDOMETRIOSIS

Surgery

Gynecologists have traditionally treated severe cases primarily by surgically removing as much endometriosis as possible while attempting to preserve a woman's childbearing capacity. If you are incapacitated by your symptoms and if the possibility of future pregnancy is either not desired or otherwise not feasible, the gynecologist will usually advise a total hysterectomy, during which both ovaries and as much disease as possible are removed. This treat-

ment results in a surgically produced menopause and inactivates
the remaining endometriosis. You can take estrogen-replacement
therapy (ERT) a few months after surgery, but this sometimes
reactivates the disease process. Recently, doctors have found that
laparoscopy combined with laser treatment of the endometriosis
is an effective treatment for relatively small amounts of the disease.
(See Chapter 14.)

Pregnancy

One medical theory, not very well documented, is that pregnancy has a beneficial impact on endometriosis. In the past, some
doctors advised patients to have a baby as soon as possible after
the condition was diagnosed. Because these women already suffered from decreased fertility as a result of their disease, and most
were unable to become pregnant, this advice for the most part
produced only frustration and further suffering. Since pregnancy
involves major changes in life-style, and since no adequate proof
exists that it is beneficial to those who suffer from endometriosis,
be wary of this recommendation, and be sure to seek a second
opinion from a physician who is not a colleague of the doctor who
suggested it.

Medication

In the past as synthetic hormones became available, doctors attempted to create pseudo-pregnancies as treatment for endometriosis, first by using large doses of DES and then by prescribing
increasing doses of synthetic progestins. These schedules reduced
pain in many women, but the side effects of the treatment—including swelling, weight gain, nausea, and irregular bleeding—significantly limited the length of time women could tolerate these large
doses of hormones. Clinicians found that a much better course
was to prescribe the oral contraceptive pill, which reduced pain
and, in cases of early endometriosis, slowed progression of the
disease.

The first drug that was found to reverse endometriosis effectively
was danazol, a synthetic steroid derived from testosterone. The
drug affects the immune system, which may play an important

role in its efficacy. Originally approved by the FDA in 1976 for use in treating endometriosis, danazol inhibits the action of the gonadotropins and produces a low estrogen state in a woman's body. It is effective in treating mild to moderate disease, but it produces a pseudo-menopause with the hot flashes, cessation of periods, moodiness, depression, and bone loss that resemble the characteristics of true menopause. In addition, because it is closely related to testosterone, danazol causes hair loss, oily skin, and acne. Moreover, while pain decreases during the time the medication is taken, symptoms gradually return once it is discontinued. The pregnancy rate increases for a time after its use. Doctors often use danazol to treat the endometrial implants that remain after surgery has removed the bulk of the disease.

A new class of drugs called gonadotropin-releasing hormone antagonists, or LRH analogs, blocks the action of the gonadotropin-releasing hormones and is also proving useful in treating endometriosis. Nafarelin and buserelin are two that have been studied extensively, and the FDA has approved nafarelin for the treatment of endometriosis while allowing doctors to use the other preparations to treat cancer of the prostate. Although they do not produce the same testosterone-like side effects as danazol, these compounds induce a premature menopause accompanied by hot flashes, decreased libido, vaginal dryness, mood changes, and headache. They also decrease bone density, and researchers are attempting to modify the loss of bone mass by giving progestins at the same time. Unfortunately, this seems to reduce the drugs' effectiveness against endometriosis. And again, the disease tends to recur when treatment stops. Researchers hope that the large, long-term studies under way will eventually establish the place of these drugs in the treatment of endometriosis.

Researchers in Europe and elsewhere are testing other synthetic steroids with the hope that they can find some pattern of treatment that stops or slows the progression of endometriosis without producing side effects so severe that they are almost as bad as the disease. At the present time, doctors use a combination of surgery and drugs that is often able to improve a woman's fertility enough so that she can become pregnant. Fortunately, once conception has taken place, endometriosis does not affect either pregnancy itself or delivery.

FIBROIDS

The benign muscle tumors called fibroids cause more heavy bleeding than pain, but the degeneration that sometimes occurs during pregnancy, when fibroids outgrow their blood supply, can be severe. Despite the discomfort they may cause, surgery is rarely advised for this problem during pregnancy.

More than 25 percent of women over 35 have fibroids, and they are the most common cause of hysterectomy. Fibroids rarely become malignant, but they may cause bleeding and pain. Although they start in the uterus, they can also grow into the abdominal cavity, and, if they become large enough, they can press on the bladder or bowel, generating secondary problems, such as frequent urination, changes in bowel patterns, and an expanding abdomen. If they outgrow their blood supply and start to die, causing the fibroid to bleed into its own inner portion, they can cause tremendous pain.

PAINFUL INTERCOURSE (DYSPAREUNIA)

Whether you have experienced pain from your very first intercourse or whether it started with an infection or after intercourse with a new partner, the problem should be evaluated by a healthcare professional, because relief is usually available. (See Chapter 5.)

CHRONIC PELVIC PAIN

Doctors use the term *chronic* when pelvic pain has continued without significant improvement for at least six months. When clinicians make a determined effort to find the cause of chronic pelvic pain, a specific condition such as endometriosis can be found in 50 to 75 percent of women. This still leaves a significant group with pain of unknown origin.

Many women who have had severe pelvic pain and have not found relief can now attend pain clinics that have been established over the past few years at some of the country's large medical centers. There, various specialists are available to help women in the management of pain. A variety of techniques, from local anesthesia to acupuncture, can decrease symptoms. Keep in mind that chronic severe pain cannot be managed with narcotics, not only because such strong substances work for just a limited time, but also because they pose the danger of creating narcotic dependency. Medicine has a great need for more effective pain medications that are not addicting. Meanwhile, women who suffer chronic pain need to develop a network of family and friends who have been educated about the seriousness of the problem so they can offer assistance in managing this often debilitating condition.

MIGRAINE HEADACHES

Migraines occur more frequently in women than in men. Many women have migraine-type headaches that occur just before, or during, their menstrual periods. These are related to the drop in estrogen that happens at this time, and such headaches can sometimes be controlled by hormonal manipulation. If you are troubled by this type of headache, consult your physician about possible relief.

Women who develop migraine headaches for the first time after starting to take oral contraceptives, and continue to have them every month when they menstruate, are not good candidates for the Pill and should stop taking it. On the other hand, women who have occasional migraine headaches after beginning the Pill are considered to have a relative contraindication. If you are experiencing occasional migraines that are related to oral contraceptive use, you should discuss this with your physician, because there is an increased risk of stroke in some women. Be sure to have your doctor explain the risks and benefits in your individual case. Fortunately, for most women, migraine headaches tend to disappear after menopause.

EXCESSIVE HAIR GROWTH

Excessive hair growth, hirsutism, describes an increased growth of hair in areas where it is not usually found, such as between the breasts, along the midline of the abdomen, on the back, and in the area beneath the nose and upper lip. In hirsutism, the hair on the arms and legs often becomes more profuse, and it tends to become coarser. The complaint is relative; Western women have more hair than Asian women, and brunettes have hair that is more visible than that of blonds. The female hair follicles are very sensitive to the small quantity of male hormones (androgens) that the female body produces—for example, to the testosterone produced by the ovaries and the dihydroepiandrosterone manufactured by the adrenal glands. Diminutive increases in these androgens, so small that menstrual periods may be normal and the woman fertile, are enough in some women to stimulate the hair follicles to make coarse hair.

It is normal for women to experience greater hair growth during puberty, pregnancy, and after menopause, when estrogen levels fall more rapidly than androgens. In addition, some families produce a greater amount of body hair among their members than others. Recently, researchers have found that women who have excessive hair produce an increased amount of an enzyme in the skin that can change testosterone to a more potent androgen, which then stimulates the hair follicles to grow more hair. Certain abnormal conditions may also cause increased hair growth, including polycystic ovarian disease (many cysts on the ovaries), adrenal hyperplasia (overactive adrenal glands), and androgen-producing tumors.

Any woman who experiences a rapid change in the quantity of her hair should consult her physician, who will look for the cause by examining hormone levels. If the results of these are abnormal, a further search is important, using ultrasound, laparoscopy, and other diagnostic tools. If the hormone assays are normal, hair growth can be reduced in a number of ways. Because the ovaries make most of the androgens in the female, suppressing ovarian function with the oral contraceptive pill is often helpful. Alternatively, the diuretic spironolactone blocks the action of testosterone on the hair follicles and is effective in treating hirsutism. Often both are needed. If the androgen is coming mostly from the adrenals, corticosteroids can suppress it. Relatively few side effects are associated with this drug, but because of the slow growth of hairs, therapy must continue for six to nine months before any improvement occurs. If any of these medications are discontinued, the problem returns. Treatment only prevents new hair growth and does not make the hair already there disappear. Electrolysis proves helpful in modifying the appearance of many hirsute women.

If the androgen levels are found to be several times that of normal levels, a process known as virilization may have taken place. In addition to hirsutism, the other symptoms include acne, baldness, deepening of the voice, loss of periods, increased muscle, and growth of the clitoris. If you have any of these changes, or manifest the early stages of any of them, your doctor should promptly start a search for the source of the androgen.

HAIR LOSS

Although there is a hereditary factor in baldness in women as well as in men, unfortunately, in most cases, the cause is undetectable. If you experience thinning of the hair or baldness, see a doctor. After eliminating the possibility that drugs or radiation therapy are causing the problem, your doctor should obtain tests of your thyroid function and other hormone levels. The treatment for hair loss has been unsatisfactory, although a relatively new drug, minoxidil, approved by the FDA in 1988, produced moderate to dense hair growth on the crown of the head in 39 percent of men studied in clinical trials after 12 months of use; 61 percent of the men had little or no growth. The study showed that minoxidil had no effect on frontal baldness. The drug has not been studied in women.

PROLAPSE

Prolapse, or falling, of the uterus, bladder, and rectum are common problems. Because the trauma of childbirth tears and weakens the structures that support these organs, prolapse usually occurs only in women who have had vaginal deliveries. Often the symptoms do not begin until after menopause, when decreasing estrogen levels further weaken the supporting structures. Mild prolapse of the uterus causes pelvic pressure or a dragging sensation; more severe prolapse, in which the cervix of the uterus and the vaginal walls hang out through the vaginal opening, may make walking difficult (see Figure 12.2). Bladder prolapse (cystocele) often results

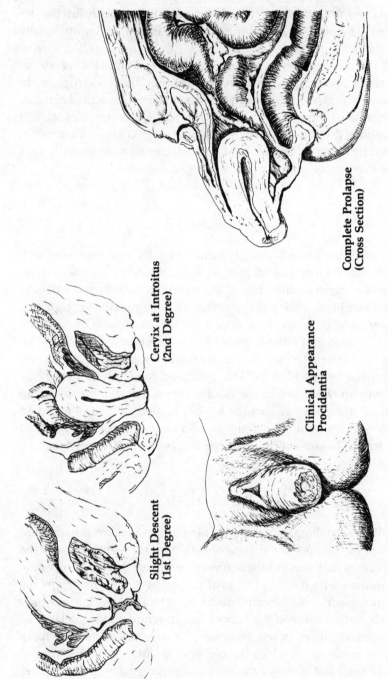

Complete Prolapse
(Cross Section)

Cervix at Introitus
(2nd Degree)

Slight Descent
(1st Degree)

Clinical Appearance
Procidentia

Fig. 12.2 Prolapse of the Uterus

in loss of urine with coughing, sneezing, laughing or strenuous activity, and rectal prolapse (rectocele) may make bowel movements difficult.

If you have a prolapse with bothersome symptoms, a pessary— a rubber device fitted around the cervix that adds support to the uterus—can be inserted. Because wearing a pessary sometimes results in infections, you should determine, in consultation with your doctor, whether you are a good candidate for it. It is important to take the pessary out weekly and wash it carefully so as to avoid infection. Signs of infection are a discharge and/or an unpleasant odor; if you experience either or both of these, you should see your doctor.

In severe cases of prolapse, many doctors recommend a vaginal hysterectomy and repair of the supporting layers of the bladder and rectum. You should seek a second medical opinion before consenting to this surgery, particularly if you still wish to have children. In fact, women who want to retain their fertility are one group for whom a pessary can be a satisfactory solution to the problem of prolapse, at least until they have had the desired child, or decided against future childbirth. Hysterectomy for prolapse is one situation in which a surgeon removes a "normal" uterus because a better repair can often be achieved once the uterus is gone. You may have to have a catheter inserted for a few days after the surgery, but other major complications are not common. (See Chapter 14.) While this is major surgery, and should not be accepted without a careful review of all your options, the real danger here is waiting too long, until illness or age makes surgery unwise. The other group of women for whom a pessary is suitable are those who are considered poor surgical candidates.

PROBLEMS OF THE KIDNEY AND BLADDER

The urinary tract consists of the kidneys, ureters, bladder, and urethra. The kidney filters waste products from the blood into the urine; the ureters are the tubes that connect the kidneys to the bladder; the bladder is a hollow muscular storage organ for collecting urine; and the urethra is the tube that leads from the bladder to the urinary opening above the vagina. The kidneys are the site of many impairments related to the cardiovascular system, and also of general metabolic diseases such as diabetes. The chief problems associated with the urinary tract are infection and incontinence.

URINARY TRACT INFECTIONS

Infections of the Bladder

Bladder infections, also called cystitis, are more common in women than in men because women have a much shorter urethra than men do. This permits bacteria originating in the rectum and deposited on the perineum to travel up into the bladder. The thrusting and other general activity of intercourse can further aggravate this process. The symptoms of infection include increased frequency of urination, burning with urination, blood in the urine, and nocturia, the need to void at night. The irritation of the bladder in chronic cystitis may contribute to incontinence, the involuntary loss of urine.

If you experience these symptoms, see your doctor promptly because if an infection is present you need immediate treatment with antibiotics. Failure to control cystitis can allow the infecting organisms to spread up the ureters into the kidneys. Here the infection, now called pyelonephritis, is much more serious, causing high fever, pain, and general malaise. Unless it is quickly brought under control with effective antibiotics, it can cause permanent damage to the kidneys. You can help to prevent cystitis by observing a number of practices that will contribute generally to your good health. (See Chapter 11.)

Urethritis

Urethritis, infection of the urethra, is also relatively common. The same organisms that generate gonorrhea and chlamydia cause urethritis, as do other bacteria. Symptoms include burning during and after urination and some frequency of urination.

In treating urethritis, doctors order cultures to identify the specific organism involved so the proper antibiotic can be prescribed. Some women have a sac extending off the urethra called a diverticulum, which may be present from birth; this may harbor bacteria and predispose to infection. If a diverticulum is causing problems, it can be removed with a surgical procedure done through the vaginal wall.

URINARY INCONTINENCE

Urinary incontinence, the involuntary loss of urine, is a very common disorder in women. Surveys have determined that as many as 16 percent of young women, and at least half of older women, suffer occasionally from this symptom, but only recently has the medical community begun to turn its attention to the problem.

The most encouraging sign that urinary incontinence is beginning to receive the attention of the medical community is that the National Institutes of Health (NIH) held a conference on the subject in 1989. The conference conclusions encouraged patients to discuss their incontinence openly with their medical caregivers and recommended that doctors evaluate and treat all patients with symptoms of urinary incontinence, giving them sufficient information about the various available therapies so they can make informed choices. The conference also supported the development of strategies for nursing-home patients that will circumvent the lack of staffing at night, which can lead to incontinence if there are not enough employees to bring patients bedpans or help those who need assistance when going to the bathroom. Most important, the NIH panel concluded that a great improvement must take place in the availability of public toilets.

We believe the current shortage of public toilets poses a particular problem for women. Women always have to wait on line at rest room facilities because architects never take into account the fact that it takes women longer to attend to their excretory needs than men; therefore, public buildings need twice as many toilets for women as for men.

All these developments indicate that, as women become aware of the increased availability of help for incontinence from all causes, the social climate surrounding this sometimes serious problem will change to allow them to discuss incontinence with their health-care providers. Medical practitioners, too, need to have their consciousness raised about the necessity to pay serious attention to the problem. Proper care that can control or reverse incontinence should make it less likely that older women will be pushed into nursing homes simply because they are incontinent.

Three conditions combine to make urinary incontinence a significant problem for women. First is the injuries that occur to the layer of tissue supporting the bladder with almost every vaginal delivery; next is the fact that, after menopause, a loss of tissue tone takes place as well as a decrease in blood supply because of dropping estrogen levels; third is that the relatively short female urethra allows urine to escape more easily.

There are three basic types of incontinence:

- incontinence caused by fistulas, or holes, in the bladder, ureters, or urethra
- stress incontinence, which involves loss of urine with coughing, sneezing, or laughing
- bladder instability or urgency incontinence, where the bladder goes into spasm, which is followed by immediate involuntary voiding

In addition, many neurological diseases, such as polio, diabetes, stroke, coma, or paralysis on one side of the body (hemiplegia), can cause incontinence as patients suffer nerve damage and lose voluntary control of the urinary system.

Fistulas are relatively uncommon in this country, and when they do occur it is usually the result of injury during surgery. If the surgeon recognizes and repairs the damage at once, residual problems can be avoided. If the damage goes unrecognized, and the woman needs a later procedure, the surgery is more difficult, and the result may be less satisfactory. This kind of operation should be performed only by a highly experienced gynecologist.

Most women who experience stress incontinence usually do so when the bladder is very full. Any increase in abdominal pressure pushes out a little urine. After childbirth, the structures that support the neck of the bladder may not do so sufficiently, and as a result, even slight increases in abdominal pressure are transmitted in a straight line through the bladder and urethra to the urinary opening. Women with stress incontinence often remain relatively continent until after menopause, when the tissues supporting these structures become very thin and sag even more.

Diagnosis

Doctors suspect stress incontinence when a woman reports urine leakage as part of her medical history. If you have such a history, the clinician may ask you to demonstrate the leakage by asking you to strain down or cough with a full bladder. The physician will then check a subsequent urine specimen for evidence of an infection that may be contributing to the symptoms. If there is any doubt about the diagnosis, the doctor can order a cystometrogram, which studies the pressure relationships of the bladder to incontinence. Many doctors believe that all women who are considering vaginal repair surgery to correct serious incontinence should have this test, which can be performed without admission to the hospital, is relatively painless, and ensures that a medical practitioner will recommend surgery only when it has a good possibility of correcting the problem.

Diagnosing bladder instability or urgency incontinence from the medical history is more difficult, and the kind of surgery that works for stress incontinence does not help this condition. Consequently, diagnostic pressure studies are needed to aid in the diagnosis, a tool that is only now becoming available and produces results that many urologists and gynecologists cannot yet interpret accurately.

Treatment

Treatment should be sought only if the symptoms are substantially interfering with a woman's daily life. It includes exercises, estrogen supplementation, biofeedback, behavior modification, drugs, and surgery, if necessary.

Exercise

Kegel exercises are the most useful treatment for incontinence because they strengthen the muscles of the pelvic floor. You can identify these muscles by stopping voiding in midstream, and you can then practice contracting and releasing them 20 times, three or four times a day. A new exercise employs graduated weights shaped like tampons that you can insert into the vagina and hold in place by using these pelvic muscles. By the time you can hold the heaviest weight in place for 10 or 15 minutes in the morning and evening, you will have strengthened your muscles significantly. About 60 percent of women will acquire at least some relief from their stress incontinence by exercise. (See Chapter 5.)

Estrogen

You can often attain marked improvement in tissue tone and the reduction of the symptoms of incontinence by using estrogen. Many physicians prescribe the use of vaginal estrogen cream because this places the estrogen where you need it. There is some validity to this approach, although you should remember that estrogen is absorbed through the vaginal wall, gets into the bloodstream, and affects other parts of the body. The overall dose prescribed, however, is likely to be lower than that used for oral estrogens, so any unwanted side effects should be minimal.

Surgery

For those women who have serious defects in the structures that support the bladder, and whose symptoms fail to respond to exercise and estrogen, vaginal repair surgery is successful in about 85 percent of the cases. (See Chapter 14.) Most of the failures can be cured by a second, somewhat different operation to suspend the neck of the bladder. If you need surgery, you should not put it off until old age greatly increases the symptoms—the surgical risks will be greater then. This surgery is relatively superficial, because the doctor does not have to open the abdominal cavity, and even some very elderly women tolerate the surgery well.

Other Methods

Treating bladder instability or urgency incontinence is more difficult than treating stress incontinence, but 60 percent of patients can benefit from therapy. Behavior modification that employs practicing bladder control and other methods of controlled voiding may help some women. Biofeedback, which makes women aware of their bladder symptoms by teaching them to recognize bladder sensations, helps others. Doctors also have used anticholinergic drugs, muscle relaxants, and prostaglandin inhibitors such as Naprosyn with some success. Surgeons have been able to relieve debilitating symptoms in some women by cutting the nerves to the bladder, although this procedure is rarely necessary.

DEPRESSION

Most people, both physicians and laypeople, believe that depression is more common among women than men, and that much of it is connected to the hormonal alterations in women's reproductive biology. A recent task force report to the American Psychological Association (APA) found that women are twice as likely as men to suffer from major depression. About 7 million American women are afflicted with depression, and the condition leads to 30,000 suicides annually. But this APA-sponsored research identified cultural rather than biological causes for depression, citing unhappy marriage, reproductive stress, and sexual and physical abuse as stronger factors in accounting for the gender difference. Other researchers hesitate to endorse the cultural hypothesis, pointing out that, while biology may not be the entire answer, women do develop severe mood changes accompanying alterations in their reproductive status, and these indicate a real physiological base to depression. Undoubtedly, both culture and biology play a role in this serious problem for women.

Although the APA task force noted that depression in women was directly related to the way they experience being female in U.S. culture, it did not cite any single factor and observed that menstruation, pregnancy, abortion, and menopause were only modestly associated with severe emotional distress. The researchers did cite infertility as a major risk factor for depression, reporting that 40 percent of the women in one study reported their inability to conceive as "the most unsettling experience of their lives." Other risk factors included marriage, with unhappily married women three times more likely to be depressed than married men or single women; poverty, with low-income women at significantly higher risk for depression; and women's socialization to avoidant, passive, and dependent behavior patterns that dispose them to focus on depressed feelings rather than to cultivate "action and mastery" strategies.

In addition, a recent review article in the *American Journal of Psychiatry*, reporting on European studies of depression in women, found that both a diagnosis of cancer and having a mastectomy were causes of depression in women. Women who had mastectomies for breast cancer were much more vulnerable to psychiatric problems than were those who had the less disfiguring lumpectomy and radiation, and many women who had had mastectomies said they wished they had opted for lumpectomy. Among mastectomy patients, however, those who had breast reconstruction experienced less distress, and the sooner they had the procedure, the better they felt.

Whatever the cause, depression is a genuine illness, and one that should not be ignored. The symptoms of depression include changes in eating patterns, loss of appetite or substantial overeating; sleep disturbances, either the inability to sleep or sleeping too much; restlessness and hyperactivity or a severe decrease in the desire for physical activity; decreased sex drive; loss of energy and fatigue; feelings of worthlessness, self-reproach, or excessive guilt; diminished ability to think or concentrate; recurrent thoughts of death or suicide; and attempted suicide. If you are experiencing some of these symptoms, talk to your doctor and seek therapeutic help. Antidepressant medications can sometimes provide relief, and psychotherapy can be effective in relieving and/or curing depression.

Certain events in life tend to precipitate depression, including the death of a spouse or a close family member; marriage, pregnancy, divorce, marital separation, reconciliation with a partner, and sexual difficulties; personal illness or injury or sickness of a family member; and job loss, retirement, business readjustment, or a change in financial status. Since everyone experiences some of these events at various times in life, it is wise to be aware that they may cause depression and to seek professional help if the depression continues for more than a few weeks. Any depression that causes one to contemplate suicide should be taken very seriously. It is imperative to seek medical care immediately.

13

Cancer

Mary Jane Gray, M.D.

Cancer frightens women more than any other disease, partly because we still think of it as fatal and partly because the treatment
can be either disfiguring or have other significantly unpleasant
effects. It is important for all women to understand that cure rates
for many cancers are encouraging, particularly when the disease
is discovered early. Eighty to 90 percent of women with Stage I
and II cervical cancer survive; for the very common endometrial
cancer, 85 percent of women who have total hysterectomy and 75
percent of all women who have the disease conquer it. Ninety
percent of women with vulvar cancer who have a vulvectomy live
for five years and, overall, 75 percent of all women who have this
cancer are cured. *There are 6 million people living with cancer in this
country, and half of them have survived for five years from the time they
were first diagnosed.* If your doctor diagnoses cancer, find out everything you can about your particular disease and locate the specialist
with the highest degree of training in your cancer. Discuss the
possible treatment options and cure rates carefully and choose,
with the best advice of your doctor, the therapy you think will give
you the best chance of survival and that you can best tolerate.

Often, in the period immediately after diagnosis, you will be so busy with medical tests that you may be too exhausted to get the psychological help you need. Don't ignore this aspect. Lean on family, friends, and counselors; search out support groups by asking a social worker at your hospital for information, by calling your local chapter of the American Cancer Society (listed in the phone book), or by contacting the National Coalition of Cancer Survivorship (323 8th Street S.W., Albuquerque, NM 87102 [505-764-9956]); and locate and talk to cancer survivors. Two recent studies have confirmed that support groups benefit cancer patients. One found that people who attended support groups lived one and a half years longer than patients without this experience; another, that patients in a six-week support group reduced their level of stress and enhanced their immune systems by actually increasing the number of cells that attacked tumors. While this improvement held up when they were tested six months later, it will be years before researchers know whether this type of intervention affects long-term survival.

Read everything you can on your particular disease, because the more you know, the better your decisions will be. Find out what to expect from therapy. Make sure, once your therapy is over, that you see your doctor regularly for follow-up, so that any recurrences can be diagnosed and treated quickly. And by all means, keep using the support system you built while you were in treatment to help you deal with the aftermath of the illness.

Cancer is the leading cause of death in women between the ages of 35 and 75. After 75, women, like men, usually die of heart disease. Cancer is not a single disease but many disparate types of uncontrolled growths that behave very differently. The most common cancers in women include skin cancer, lung cancer, colon and rectal cancer, breast cancer (see Chapter 4), and cancer of the reproductive organs. Of these, skin cancer is rarely fatal and, because of its relationship to exposure to excessive sunlight, is almost entirely preventable. Cancer of the lung is currently the most frequent malignancy in women, more widespread even than breast cancer. As a primary tumor—that is, the place where the cancer starts—lung cancer is so closely related to cigarette smoking that it, too, can usually be prevented. *This is a crucial fact for women to understand for two reasons: first, that lung cancer can rarely be cured; and second, that once they begin smoking, women have a more difficult time quitting than men do. Thus the best way to prevent cancer is not to*

smoke, and to stay out of the sun or, when exposed to sunlight, to wear
sufficient protection, either clothing or lotions that block the sun's dam-
aging rays.

WHAT IS CANCER?

Cancer is an uncontrolled growth of cells that originates in normal
tissue and is capable of killing in two ways. Either it enlarges locally,
extending and destroying essential organs, or it metastasizes—that
is, cells with the same growth potential as the original tumor break
away and travel to other parts of the body, especially the liver and
lungs, where they continue to spread in an uncontrolled fashion.
Sometimes fibrous tissue surrounds these abnormal cells, limiting
their growth for long periods of time without killing them. If the
individual's general health becomes impaired, or if the immune
system weakens, the cancer may begin to grow again.

Physicians refer to tumors—any tissue enlargement—as either
malignant or benign (bad or harmless), to indicate whether or not
the growth is cancerous. (Large benign tumors, such as ovarian
cysts or fibroids of the uterus, may occasionally cause death from
pressure or bleeding, but this is relatively rare and usually confined
to people who lack access to medical care or who are so frightened
by the prospect of entering the medical system that they fail to
seek treatment.) Whether or not a malignancy is present is determined by a pathologist—a doctor who studies body tissues. When
a cancer occurs in the skin or mucous membrane (epithelium), it
is referred to as a carcinoma; if it is found in muscle or bone, it is
called a sarcoma.

The uterus, although it lies within the pelvis, connects through
its opening, the cervix, to the vagina. The signs and symptoms of
uterine cancer include abnormal bleeding; the shedding of abnormal cells, picked up through Pap smears; and the gynecologist's
observations of abnormal tissue during a pelvic exam. During a
vaginal exam using a speculum, the doctor may note an unusual
appearance of the cervix indicating cancer, or in feeling the uterus
and evaluating its size, shape, and consistency the doctor might
recognize certain changes or abnormalities that may spell danger.
You should take advantage of the ready accessibility of this portion
of your reproductive tract and be sure to have annual Pap smears

and pelvic exams to permit your doctor to detect problems and potential problems, and start early treatment.

Partly because the fallopian tubes and ovaries are smaller and less accessible than the vagina, the cervix, and the uterus, accurate methods of diagnosing cancers of these organs early have not yet been established, and cure rates are lower than for other cancers. Although many factors—including the state of an individual's general health, her specific immune response, and the innate aggressiveness of different tumors—affect the potential for surviving malignant tumors, one of the most important is early diagnosis.

DIAGNOSTIC DELAYS

With the advantages of accessibility and with effective treatment for the many cancers of the reproductive tract that are diagnosed early, why do so many women still die of malignant tumors originating here? One big reason is that many women avoid routine medical care, including annual mammograms, pelvic exams, and Pap smears, because of the lingering myth in our society that cancer is fatal, and that it will do no good to face the bad news. A great women's cancer specialist of an earlier era, James Corscaden, put it this way: Suppose 100 women have a type of cancer that can be cured in 80 percent of the cases. Those 80 women can be divided into two categories—those who never realize that they have a malignancy, or the "Don't worry the patient" group; and those who know but don't want to discuss it, which means that only their inner circle of family and friends are aware of the diagnosis. Of the 20 who die, most will do so after one or two years of protracted illness. All their friends and acquaintances, family, health-care providers, and those supplying support services will be aware that Mrs. X died of cancer. Thus the public impact of the relatively small percentage of women who die from cancer far exceeds that of those who get well, and the myth that cancer is incurable continues. And if cancer is irreversible, the reasoning goes, why look for it?

Another reason women do not take advantage of medical services that can fight cancer effectively is a general distaste for the pelvic examination. Put simply, many women detest it, and the range of responses goes from "Let's get it over with" to "I *hate* this." As a result, women use all kinds of rationalizations, from "I just had an examination," which can mean two to three years ago, to "I'm having my period; I'd better put it off." (Actually, only very heavy bleeding interferes with a Pap smear.) Much more dangerous is the "I don't want my doctor to see me when I'm bleeding." To avoid falling into this self-defeating trap, do your best to make the appointment for your annual checkup for a time when you are between periods. If you are irregular and you are bleeding heavily on the day of the appointment, reschedule it for a few days later. If you continue bleeding, it may be an indication of hormone imbalance, benign fibroids, muscle tumors of the uterus, or a more serious condition. All of these situations need evaluation. The point is that a woman can bleed enough to become anemic or even die while she waits for the bleeding to stop so she feels it is proper for the doctor to examine her. *If you have any abnormal bleeding, consult your health-care provider at once.*

The medical profession is also responsible for dangerous delays in diagnosis. A pelvic examination should be part of any general physical exam, yet many internists and family practitioners draw back from this "personal" examination of "private" parts. A male physician usually requests the presence of a female nurse or other female chaperon to comfort the patient as well as to protect himself from any possible charges of wrongdoing. Performing a proper pelvic examination means that he needs an examining table with stirrups and special vaginal instruments in his office—equipment that many physicians consider an additional nuisance. In hospital clinics, these problems are magnified. If the patient says she has her period and would rather wait, the practitioner often agrees, and far too often the medical record reads "Pelvic and rectal exams deferred"—indefinitely. You must take the responsibility of making sure a pelvic exam is rescheduled, because many clinics won't do it for you.

A third and major problem is money. Our overburdened and costly medical system largely excludes economically disadvantaged women who do not qualify for Medicaid, have no medical insurance, and cannot afford the time they have to wait during a clinic visit, or cannot pay even modest clinic fees for routine medical care.

The most important step you can take to protect yourself against cancer is to see a competent health-care provider at least annually for a breast exam, a mammogram, a pelvic, and a Pap smear.

TREATMENT

The medical profession uses surgery, radiotherapy, chemotherapy, and immunotherapy to treat cancer. Obstetricians and gynecologists provide routine care of the female reproductive tract during pregnancy and throughout life, operating when necessary; oncologists (cancer specialists) generally treat all cancers; some gynecologists specialize in gynecologic cancer, performing radical surgery when indicated and directing the use of chemotherapeutic agents; radiologists provide radiotherapy and other X ray–related services; and pathologists do the microscopic diagnostic work so important in understanding the disease and choosing among treatment options.

SURGERY

For many relatively early tumors, doctors consider surgery the best approach. The idea of surgery in the treatment of cancer is to remove all of the cancer—every cell—so that it is gone and cannot return. This is, however, not always possible. Removing a malignancy is practical only when the area involved is not necessary for life, when the cancer has not spread to other distant and unknown areas of the body, and when the woman's physical health is such that she can withstand the surgery. Improvements in anesthesia and increased knowledge of postoperative care have extended the limits of age and illness relative to cancer surgery, but side effects can be serious. They may include infection, bleeding, a long recovery period, numbness and swelling in the operative field area, restricted motion if the surgeon removes muscles, and disruption of normal body functions if structures affecting them have been excised. In addition, the risks of being a hospital patient in the United States today must be taken into account. Cost-cutting procedures and the bureaucratization of hospital care mean that the potential for unnecessary and sometimes harmful testing is high, as is the possibility of error in administering medications, all of which should be monitored by you or the family member or friend you appoint as your advocate while you are a hospital patient.

Before using any therapy, doctors should make every effort to determine the extent of disease. With malignant tumors of the female reproductive tract, clinicians do this by using X rays, ultrasound examinations of the organs involved, and direct viewing of adjacent organs. For example, they can see the lining of the bladder with a cystoscope and that of the rectum using colonoscopy or sigmoidoscopy. If this kind of examination reveals that the cancer has already spread to such regions, surgery will be either useless or harmful in its potential to further spread the disease.

When cancer spreads, malignant cells break off and travel throughout the body via the bloodstream; they also go to the lymph nodes through the lymph channels. The rate of cure for many cancers, including breast, cervical, and vulvar cancers, improves significantly if surgeons remove the lymph nodes that drain the tumor-bearing area as well. Doing so, however, increases the magnitude and the possible complications of the surgery significantly.

The discovery that malignant cancer cells get into the bloodstream whenever the cancer is handled or manipulated, and probably at other times as well, was initially dismaying, but doctors now know that this occurs even in patients who are eventually cured of cancer. This shows how effective the body's defense mechanisms can be in eliminating *a few* malignant cells. It is naive to think of surgery as "cutting out all the cancer." Instead, patients should consider surgery as a method of tipping the balance in favor of the body.

RADIATION

Radiation consists of the process of administering small, rapidly moving, high-energy-containing particles. Radiation kills cancer cells that are dividing rapidly more readily than it kills other cells, but it can eliminate all cells with a high enough dose; thus, radiation therapy exploits the difference between cancer cells and normal cells in their susceptibility to high energy by attempting to find a dose of radiation that will destroy the malignant cells without damaging too many normal cells. Some normal cells are always injured during the process, but the tissue that has been irradiated usually recovers over time. Thus a radiation patient will often suffer from the effects of both tissue injury from local radiation and the general systemic consequences of dying tissue. Anemia, fatigue, nausea, aching, and bowel and bladder symptoms all commonly accompany radiation treatment. Nonetheless, radiation can be useful in areas where surgical removal is neither possible nor advisable. Furthermore, some tumors, especially highly malignant, rapidly growing ones, respond very dramatically to radiation; others react only minimally.

Several sources of therapeutic radiation are employed in cancer treatment today, among them X rays and radioactive isotopes. Radium is one of the frequently used isotopes. The higher the energy expended, the more tissue the radiation will penetrate, and the more accurately the rays of energy can focus on specific tumor-containing areas during treatment. The application of physics to medicine is a specialized field practiced by radiotherapists, those physicians who are first trained as radiologists and then spend additional years learning about cancer treatment.

CHEMOTHERAPY

Chemotherapy exploits the same difference in susceptibility to injury between cancer cells and normal cells as radiotherapy does. Many of the substances used in contemporary chemotherapy block the growth process of rapidly dividing cancer cells. Oncologists give most of these agents to patients either orally or by injecting them directly into the bloodstream, where they circulate throughout the body. Because the substances are unable to distinguish between normal cells and cancer cells, they therefore act as general poisons, causing anemia, weakness, nausea, and, sometimes, hair loss, but they can destroy tumor cells that have escaped from the main mass of a tumor.

Most of the information we have about the effectiveness of different chemical agents on various types of cancer comes from two sources. The first is research involving the treatment of animal tumors; the second relies on clinical trials of promising experimental drugs that individuals with little hope of recovery using conventional treatment elect to use after giving their informed consent to such experiments. If initial trials are favorable, oncologists administer these drugs more widely. Employing them effectively, with the fewest possible side effects, requires great skill and knowledge, so it is important for the doctor who administers them to be highly experienced in their use.

IMMUNOTHERAPY

Immunotherapy is a recent approach to treating cancer, and it is not yet well established. It relies on methods that will reinforce the natural immune system, which is, in large part, based in the white blood cells of the body. At present, doctors use immunotherapy after surgery has reduced the size and volume of the tumor, or in conjunction with chemotherapy. For example, clinical trials suggest that colony-stimulating factors, natural substances known as biological response modifiers, can help cancer patients recuperate more rapidly from bone marrow transplants and chemotherapy. The field is in its infancy but shows great promise; in fact, some researchers are comparing the future impact of biological response-modifiers to that of antibiotics. Very few oncologists have experience in this field. Interferons are another example of substances that have been found effective in the treatment of some cancers.

NONTHERAPY

Physicians find it very difficult to determine when treatment is likely to benefit patients and when little can be expected from further therapy, especially in cases where a cancer has not responded to earlier treatment or has stopped responding. Here the clinician's skill, compassion, and experience should support the informed desires of the patient, so that together they can decide whether to "try everything" or concentrate on making the patient as active and comfortable as possible. Sometimes patients conclude that they want their doctor to proceed slowly and carefully with treatment to see if the tumor responds and to determine how well they can tolerate the particular therapy involved.

PREMALIGNANT AND MALIGNANT TUMORS OF THE CERVIX

As we have noted, the cervix, the portion of the uterus that opens into the vagina, may seem to be buried deep within the body; yet with the help of a speculum, an instrument built like two shoehorns to hold the vaginal walls apart, the cervix is quite accessible. (See Chapter 2.) Fifty years ago, George Papanicolaou discovered that not only malignant but also premalignant changes in the superficial layer of the cervix produced the shedding of abnormal cells. He put these abnormal cells on slides and studied them under a microscope, giving rise to the "Pap" smear, a major milestone in the detection and, later, the prevention of cervical cancer. At the same time the Pap smear was being developed in this country, the Europeans invented the colposcope, a magnifying instrument that allows doctors to see and study the surface of the cervix. (See Chapter 14.) These two techniques formed the basis for present-day prevention and detection of cervical cancer.

A more recent advance in understanding this disease has come from our awareness of the link between sexual intercourse, the wart virus, and the development of cervical cancer. A British gynecologist, Stanley Way, noted that a very high rate of cancer of the cervix was present in women married to sailors who were known to have intercourse with prostitutes in ports of call. He also observed that some seafarers had more than one wife who had died of cervical cancer, indicating that these men were probably spreading some causative factor to their wives, who subsequently developed cervical cancer. Way found that the malignancy behaved as if it were an STD, and he postulated that it was induced by something related to sexual intercourse, possibly sperm themselves. In recent years, researchers have shown that some strains of sexually transmitted wart viruses are very frequently accompanied by premalignant and malignant changes in the superficial layer of the cervix. Researchers have also found that women who smoke have an increased rate of cervical cancer, although how this occurs is not clear.

CLASSIFICATIONS

For many years, gynecologists have studied and described the appearance of the cervix viewed through a colposcope. They compared changes in the way the cervical surface looked with the pattern of cells found in biopsies taken from these areas. Doctors found a progression of microscopic alterations, which they first called dysplasia, a term indicating abnormal development. Later they used the more specific categories of mild, moderate, and severe dysplasia. Mild dysplasia often reversed and became normal development, but as the severity of the cellular changes and the degree of cellular multiplication increased through the stages of moderate and severe dysplasia, so did the likelihood that the process would, with the passage of time, progress to cancer. Often, viral particles caused by the wart virus accompany dysplasia, but the exact interaction between these two processes has not been established.

Current terminology for these premalignant changes in the cervix is cervical intraepithelial neoplasia (CIN) I, II, and III. In general, changes in the cervical surface proceed slowly, over months and even years, from mild to severe and on to true invasive cancer, but great variation takes place in the rate of progression and regression. This variation may be based on the type of cancer-producing stimulus, a woman's nutritional status, and how her immune system responds.

There is one further stage between severe dysplasia and true cancer, in which cells with all the characteristics of cancer have not yet begun to invade the deeper tissue of the cervix. This is called carcinoma in situ (noninvasive carcinoma), intraepithelial carcinoma, or Stage 0 cancer of the cervix. If the cervical variations have progressed this far by the time the doctor examines the patient and makes this diagnosis, immediate treatment is imperative to prevent progression to true invasive cancer.

The results of Pap smears usually pick up these abnormal, precancerous changes in the cervix, which is why it is so vital for women to have a Pap smear at least annually. In the past, the results of Pap smears have been reported roughly as Class I—Normal; Class II—Inflammation; Class III—Dysplasia; Class IV—Carcinoma in situ vs. cancer; Class V—Invasive cancer. As the continuity of these superficial changes became more apparent, a committee convened by the National Institutes of Health, consisting of pathologists and gynecologists, studied the issue and recommended abandoning the old "Class" system, advising instead that pathologists simply describe any abnormalities. Since this change is happening slowly, your doctor may still use the old classification system to describe any cervical change.

There has been disagreement within the medical profession about how often women should have Pap smears. The usual recommendation has been for an annual pelvic examination and Pap smear. Some practitioners have believed that *if* a woman has three completely normal Pap smears at yearly intervals, and *if* she did not begin sexual intercourse before age 18, and *if* she has had only one partner and no sexually transmitted infections, a Pap smear every three years may be often enough. However, very few women fit into this group. Because of this, and because the Pap smear is one of the very few cost-effective cancer screens, we recommend that you continue to have annual exams.

TREATMENT

When the results of a Pap smear are abnormal, your doctor will do a biopsy, using the colposcope to find out just what the smear is indicating. (See Chapter 14.) The practitioner places the colposcope at the vaginal opening, where it provides magnification of the surface of the cervix. With instruction and practice, a healthcare provider can learn to identify the patterns in the cervix that are typical of dysplasia, carcinoma in situ, and true cancer, and thus can identify those areas from which biopsies will be most useful.

After you receive the biopsy results, you and the gynecologist can discuss available treatments. With mild dysplasia (CIN I), your clinician may recommend following the condition with frequent Pap smears, once or twice a year, since many abnormalities of this degree will revert to normal on their own. If you have moderate dysplasia (CIN II), or warty changes of the cervix, the treatment of choice is usually cryosurgery, freezing the cervix and killing the abnormal superficial cells. When the diagnosis is severe dysplasia or carcinoma in situ (CIN III), your physician will recommend freezing, using a laser, removing the abnormal tissue with cervical conization surgery, or, if you are older and no longer want children, a hysterectomy. (See Chapter 14.) Patients who are not likely to return regularly for repeat smears, biopsies, and follow-up should have surgery.

CANCER OF THE CERVIX

Cervical cancer starts in the superficial layer of cells and spreads deeper into the cervix, then to the vagina and the tissues beyond. It often travels to those lymph nodes along the major vessels and nerves supplying the legs. More distant spread occurs very late, if at all.

The first step in treating cervical cancer is to determine the extent of the disease. In addition to a biopsy, your doctor will take a careful history, do a complete physical examination, and order routine laboratory tests for diabetes and other potentially complicating medical problems. You will also be sent for X-ray studies of the lungs, kidneys, and bowel; cystoscopy to look inside the bladder; and sigmoidoscopy to look inside the rectum and sigmoid, the lower portion of the large bowel. Your doctor will then define or "stage" the cancer, from I (confined to the cervix), to IV (advanced). These stages do not relate to the classification of premalignant changes but reflect the clinical extent of disease before treatment. Physicians use them to choose the best therapy.

Primary treatment of Stage I and II can be either radical surgery, including removal of the lymph nodes, or radiation therapy, with irradiation of the pelvic lymph nodes. In these early stages, cure rates of 80 to 90 percent are roughly comparable for both surgery and radiotherapy. Each is accompanied by some risk of complications (including infection, bladder problems, and, rarely, death), but each is associated with an excellent chance of cure.

Choosing therapy is not easy. It will depend on your particular situation, what your doctor recommends, and how you evaluate the risk-benefit ratio of the two procedures. Cure rates drop for the later stages of cervical cancer, where surgery is no longer an option and even radiotherapy may not be able to encompass the area of spread. (See Table 13.1 for cure rates for one cancer hospital, the M. D. Anderson.) In general, doctors treat recurrences after surgery with radiotherapy, and recurrences after radiotherapy with surgery. Chemotherapy has not been particularly successful with this tumor.

Table 13.1 Cervical Cancer Cure Rate
(M. D. Anderson Hospital)

Stage	5-year Cure Rate (%)
I	91.5
IIA	83.5
IIB	66.5
IIIA	45.0
IIIB	36.0
IV	14.0

Source: S. L. Romney et al., *Gynecology & Obstetrics: The Health Care of Women* (New York: McGraw-Hill, 1980), p. 1043.

ADENOMATOUS HYPERPLASIA AND CANCER OF THE ENDOMETRIUM

Like the cervix, the lining of the uterus, or endometrium, passes through premalignant stages before becoming true cancer. During the menstrual cycle, high estrogen levels make this endometrial tissue divide rapidly for 10 days each month, while progesterone stops the process. Throughout a woman's life, however, the endometrium will grow rapidly whenever it is exposed to estrogen, and it may escape normal controls. Estrogen exposure can take place if a woman has an "aging" or otherwise malfunctioning ovary, or an ovarian tumor, which produces estrogen but no progesterone, or if she is taking unopposed estrogen (without progesterone) for treatment of problems resulting from menopause or osteoporosis. Whatever the source of the estrogen, the effect may be uncontrolled growth of the endometrium, called hyperplasia. This usually causes irregular bleeding, which the doctor will investigate by performing either an endometrial biopsy or a D&C (dilatation and curettage) of the endometrium to obtain tissue for a diagnosis. (See Chapter 14.)

One of the ways you can protect yourself from endometrial cancer is to keep a careful record of your menstrual periods and any other bleeding, especially during the years just before and during menopause. Currently, the average age of menopause is 50 in the

United States, but it may occur as early as 35 or as late as 60. (See Chapter 15.)

Normal menopausal patterns range widely. The large majority of women, 70 percent, experience increased intervals between periods and scanty bleeding during periods; 12 percent of women find that their periods stop suddenly; while 18 percent have heavy blood flow, longer periods, or irregular bleeding between periods. *It is this latter group that experiences almost all of the endometrial cancer. By far the most ominous pattern is irregular bleeding or spotting. If you experience heavy or irregular bleeding, longer periods, or spotting at menopause, see your gynecologist at once for a complete medical evaluation.*

The use of oral contraceptive pills has reduced the rate of endometrial cancer; in fact, the Pill has been associated with a 50 percent reduction in the rate of endometrial cancer, probably because the combination pills have enough synthetic progesterone to oppose the estrogen effect on the endometrium. The earlier sequential Pills supplied estrogen alone in the first part of the cycle, followed by estrogen and progesterone together for the next 10 days, but they were associated with a slightly increased rate of endometrial cancer. These pills are no longer available. Other conditions associated with an increased risk of endometrial cancer are infertility, whether voluntary or involuntary, diabetes, and obesity, possibly related to the body's storage of estrogens in fat. In other words, anything that increases unopposed estrogen in the body seems to increase endometrial cancer rates, and anything that opposes estrogen with progesterone seems to decrease this risk.

ADENOMATOUS HYPERPLASIA

Mild forms of hyperactivity of the glands lining the uterus (hyperplasia) may revert to normal without treatment, but gynecologists usually prescribe progesterone or synthetic progesterones like medroxyprogesterone to change the endometrium to a less actively growing state. If you have adenomatous hyperplasia, your doctor should schedule follow-up biopsies. Whenever the degree of hyperplasia is such that it is difficult to differentiate from cancer, you should not take estrogen without accompanying progesterone. If you don't plan to have children, a simple hysterectomy may be the treatment of choice. (See Chapter 14.)

CANCER OF THE ENDOMETRIUM

Cancer of the glands lining the uterus is the most common cancer of the female pelvic reproductive tract. It occurs most often in women between 50 and 60, but it may happen anytime between puberty and death; the average age is about 60. Since most cases are detected early, the overall cure rate is about 75 percent, making endometrial cancer one of the most curable cancers in women. Risk factors include obesity, never having had children, late age of menopause, and diabetes. Multiple term pregnancies and using oral contraceptive pills decrease the risk of this cancer.

Diagnosis

Clinicians suspect cancer of the endometrium in any woman who has abnormal vaginal bleeding despite the fact that only one in five women with postmenopausal bleeding turns out to have cancer. Because there are so many other causes of bleeding, including benign growths, such as polyps, and the hormonal stimulation of the endometrium, the first step in diagnosis is to secure tissue to examine under a microscope by obtaining a biopsy or performing a D&C. In the past, physicians did D&Cs in the operating room under general anesthesia to secure sufficient tissue for adequate examination and diagnosis, but increasing hospital costs have pressured clinicians to develop better techniques and instruments for outpatient procedures. The results of such techniques are not always infallible. If the results of tissue examination are negative, but *you continue to bleed abnormally, or if bleeding stops and then recurs, you must see your doctor for further diagnostic work to find the cause.*

If your clinician has diagnosed a cancer in the uterus, as much as possible must be learned about the extent of the disease. Your doctor will order chest and kidney X rays, and may also use new techniques, such as magnetic resonance imaging (MRI) and hysteroscopy, a scope that allows visualization of the inside of the uterus. (See Chapter 14.)

Treatment

If your uterus is normal in size and the tumor relatively superficial, total hysterectomy, including removal of the cervix, tubes, and ovaries, will produce a cure in about 85 percent of women, with very few complications from the surgery. With more extensive disease, preoperative radium treatment or postsurgical radiotherapy give better results than surgery alone. This cancer does not spread to local lymph nodes early, and removing lymph nodes increases complications without improving survival.

If the tumor recurs, your doctor may use radiotherapy to treat it. Many advanced cancers of the endometrium also respond to synthetic progesterone, which has the advantage of being associated with very few side effects. Chemotherapeutic agents, given singly or in combination, are also effective for variable periods of time.

SARCOMA OF THE UTERUS

Sarcomas are malignant tumors of muscle and connective tissue. Although much less common than carcinomas—the incidence of uterine sarcoma is only about two in 100,000 women—they tend to be more malignant and more difficult to treat. These tumors grow rapidly, and they are almost impossible to distinguish from the very common fibroid tumors of the uterus. Thus, many hysterectomies are performed because of suspected sarcomas that turn out to be fibroids. This is one instance when getting a second opinion does not have much value, because a doctor cannot determine the nature of the tumor until it has been removed surgically and examined by a pathologist. If a sarcoma of the uterus is diagnosed, total hysterectomy—removal of the sarcoma with the uterus, cervix, tubes, and ovaries—offers the only hope of cure. Radiotherapy may occasionally be of help; chemotherapy is of little documented use.

CANCER OF THE OVARY

Cancer of the ovary currently accounts for 25 percent of all malignancies of the female reproductive tract, but because it is often difficult to detect early enough to cure, it causes 50 percent of women's deaths from cancer. One in 70 women will develop cancer of the ovary in her lifetime. The incidence is higher in infertile women and in those with a family history of the disease, and it decreases by half in women who have used the oral contraceptive pill for at least one year. Women who have had either breast cancer or endometrial cancer have a higher risk of developing cancer of the ovary. Research suggests that these three cancers may be related to a high-fat diet. (See Chapter 6.) The tumor is more frequent in white than in African American women, and it continues to occur in older women at least up to age 79.

Ovarian cancer is not a single disease. The ovary is a very active organ, ovulating and manufacturing hormones, and its many different cell types produce a variety of disparate benign and malignant tumors that behave diversely and require assorted approaches to therapy. For this reason, the treatment of ovarian tumors requires very specialized knowledge. *If you have this tumor, you should see a gynecologic oncologist, a physician with highly specialized training in treating malignancies of the female reproductive tract.* Because ovarian cancer is so difficult to find prior to surgery, surgeons often come upon it accidentally when treating another problem. In these cases, the surgeon should refer the woman to an oncologist as soon as possible. In what follows, we have generalized the description of cancer of the ovary by considering it as if it were a single disease.

DIAGNOSIS

At the present time, there is no effective method of mass screening for cancer of the ovary. Careful and routine annual pelvic examination remains the most effective method to date. Pap smears rarely help to detect the presence of this tumor. Although pelvic ultrasound can yield more information about enlargements found on pelvic examination, it does not differentiate reliably between benign and malignant tumors. Vaginal ultrasound gives more information, but it is not at present a routine screening method. Several tumor markers in the blood show promise in detecting ovarian cancer; the most useful to date is CA 125. (See Chapter 14.) Unfortunately, this blood test is neither sensitive nor specific enough to be used for mass screening.

There are no early symptoms of ovarian cancer. Symptoms such as bleeding, a sensation of abdominal fullness and discomfort, or the discovery of a lump that can be felt through the abdominal wall occur only after the tumor has grown large and spread over the surface of the bowel. Other cancers, especially those from the breast and the gastrointestinal tract, often spread to the surface of the ovary. When the doctor evaluates the cause of enlarged ovaries, these areas should be considered as well, and examined when indicated.

Whenever cancer of the ovary is suspected, the physician should obtain X rays of the lungs and kidneys and should order blood studies to detect possible tumor markers—not for diagnosis, but because these may later help determine the progress of whatever treatment you and the doctor select. These initial studies show a baseline value, while subsequent ones indicate whether the tumor is growing or shrinking.

The most difficult decision for a physician to make in this area is figuring out whether a particular ovarian tumor is benign or malignant. Since benign cysts, thin-walled collections of fluid, are far more common than cancer in women under 40, and since these tumors regress spontaneously or can be encouraged to regress by hormonal treatment with the oral contraceptive pill, the gynecologist's first step in treating a young woman is to observe the patient carefully and examine her repeatedly until the enlargement disappears. Simple benign ovarian cysts occur very frequently when a small cyst containing an egg fails to rupture or ovulate but instead continues to fill with fluid. Such a cyst may grow to four inches in diameter and may be painful, but it rarely involves any threat to life. It is very important that gynecologists *not* remove an ovary because of such a cyst, as this may subsequently impair a woman's fertility. In older women, doctors must evaluate persistent cysts and ovarian enlargements more vigorously, with ultrasound, laparoscopy, and/or surgery.

In general, any enlargement of an ovary that appears after menopause, any enlargement at any time that is more than four inches in diameter, or any enlargement in the pelvis that cannot be accounted for after observation and careful workup requires surgical exploration. If the tumor has spread, the diagnosis is obviously cancer. If it is local, the doctor may take a frozen section of the tumor, a biopsy that is sent to the lab for an immediate decision while the patient is still under anesthesia, to decide on appropriate further treatment.

The exact diagnosis will determine the extent of the surgery required. If the diagnosis cannot be made rapidly in a young woman, it is better to leave her with her childbearing potential and do a repeat operation as soon as a firm diagnosis has been made, if it is necessary.

TREATMENT

The first line of treatment of cancer of the ovary is surgery. The surgeon almost always removes both fallopian tubes, both ovaries, and the uterus because this cancer sometimes spreads to the opposite ovary and the adjacent structures. The gynecologist will explore the rest of the abdominal cavity for evidence of spread. If the tumor is already widely scattered, she or he removes as much of it as possible in order to increase the effectiveness of subsequent radiation and/or chemotherapy (see Table 13.2).

Currently, in all but the earliest ovarian cancers, studies have shown that chemotherapy, using agents such as cisplatin, cyclophosphamide, or melphalan, significantly improves the chances for survival. Oncologists employ many different programs in this treatment, using lower doses of multiple drugs. This approach yields good results, while reducing the toxic effects of any one agent. Another effective agent is radioactive P32, a radioactive isotope of phosphorus that is injected into the abdominal cavity. The use of these medications requires a great deal of skill and experience, and this therapy must be directed by an oncologist. Some types of ovarian cancer are very responsive to radiotherapy.

Except in cases when only minimal disease is present, once a woman has finished treatment with chemotherapy the gynecologic

Table 13.2 Survival in Terms of Stage of Epithelial Ovarian Cancer

Stage	2-year	5-year
I	80%	70%
II	40%	25%
III	18%	12%
IV	5%	0%

Source: William Creasman and Philip Disaia, eds., *Clinical Gynecologic Oncology*, 3rd ed. (St. Louis: Mosby, 1989), p. 356.

oncologist often performs surgery again to take a "second look," to find out whether further disease remains, to excise any tumor that can be removed, and to assess the patient's condition in order to plan further therapy. This approach cannot help with rapidly progressing widespread disease, but at the present time, a majority of gynecologic oncologists credit the "second look" with saving the lives of a significant number of women. A few, however, are questioning its use and, wishing to spare the woman from further surgery, rely on an alternative approach that can provide follow-up to tumor growth using blood tests to detect CA 125 and other tumor markers. This approach also appears to be useful in monitoring response to therapy.

In general, ovarian cancer remains a frustrating disease. Only about one-third of cases are diagnosed in an early state, and almost half of the early tumors recur. The newer techniques of chemotherapy are beginning to improve results. In addition, the widespread use of the oral contraceptive pill should reduce the incidence of this cancer. Women with a first-degree relative (mother or sister) with ovarian cancer are at greater risk of getting the disease and should consult a gynecologist so that they can be followed very closely. If you are in this group, you should see your gynecologist every six months for a pelvic exam and Pap smear, and you should consider having your ovaries removed when you have completed childbearing. In fact, the reason many gynecologists recommend excising the ovaries when performing a hysterectomy in menopausal women is precisely to prevent this cancer. The only disadvantage, loss of whatever hormones the ovaries still produce, is negligible, since these hormones can be replaced.

CANCER OF THE FALLOPIAN TUBES

Cancer of the fallopian tubes is a very rare malignancy. This is fortunate, because fallopian tube cancer produces few if any symptoms, is diagnosed early only if found by chance at the time of other pelvic surgery, and is almost never cured. Some doctors maintain that it occasionally gives evidence of its existence by causing pain that subsides when the muscles of the tubes contract, pushing out a spurt of clear vaginal discharge. The only feasible therapy for cancer of the fallopian tubes is surgery.

CANCER OF THE VAGINA

Cancer of the vagina is an infrequent tumor. When it does occur, it is difficult to treat and cure because of the vagina's proximity to the bladder and the rectum. Doctors usually find this malignancy by Pap smear, or see or feel it during a routine pelvic exam. The presence of genital warts probably predisposes a woman to cancer of the vagina as well as to cancer of the cervix.

This is one of the cancers that occur with greater frequency among DES daughters than among women who have not been exposed to DES. As we noted earlier, obstetricians prescribed the synthetic estrogen diethylstilbestrol (DES) for many pregnant women during the late 1940s and up through the 1960s because they believed it prevented miscarriage; toward the end of this period, carefully controlled studies showed that the medication was ineffective for this purpose, and doctors gradually stopped using it. In 1970, an astute researcher observed that clear-cell carcinoma of the vagina, which previously had been extremely rare, was 20 times more common in young women whose mothers had taken DES during the first 20 weeks of pregnancy compared to women whose mothers did not take the drug. If your mother used DES, your chance of getting this cancer, even as a member of this high-risk group, is only one in 1,000. Nevertheless, all DES daughters must have at least one examination of the vagina with a colposcope, and annual Pap smears, to find out if you are one of those women who is at risk.

If gynecologists can identify changes in the superficial layer of the vagina while in the noninvasive stage, it may be sufficient to treat the disease with laser or with the cancer therapeutic agent 5-FU. For invasive cancer of the vagina, the gynecologist can either operate to remove affected tissue or treat the condition with radium implants, but many complications are associated with either approach, and the overall cure rate is only about 50 percent.

CANCER OF THE VULVA

Cancer of the vulva is a form of skin cancer, and, as such, the prognosis for cure is usually good. Although this cancer can occur in young women, the average age of women who have it is about

70. The incidence in younger women may be increasing, however, possibly because of the increase in genital warts as a result of the general spread of sexually transmitted diseases. In general, doctors do not diagnose this cancer as early as they should because women fail to examine this part of their body, because they are often reluctant to call lumps in this area to the attention of a physician, and because so many fail to have regular pelvic examinations. If you have any lump on the vulva that does not go away within two to three weeks, bring it to the attention of your physician. Most such lumps will turn out to be benign cysts or benign fatty tumors, but some will need to be biopsied. As we noted earlier, we recommend that every woman over the age of 18 use a mirror for self-examination of the vulva once a month between menstrual periods to detect early changes in this area.

Often biopsies of slightly abnormal areas of the vulvar skin will not reveal cancer but will indicate changes in the superficial layer characteristic of noninvasive cancer, or even earlier abnormalities, such as dystrophies and dysplasias. Gynecologists can treat these early changes with hormone or chemotherapeutic creams, or can remove them during local surgery with a scalpel or laser.

Invasive cancer of the vulva can occur on the vaginal lips, in both the labia majora and minora, on the clitoris, and on the skin around the vaginal and rectal openings. This area drains to the lymph glands of the groin, and for this reason, the treatment that gives the best results—a 90 percent five-year survival rate if caught in the early stages—is removal of the entire vulva and the lymph nodes of the groin. More extensive disease involves the deep nodes along the major vessels connecting the legs with the aorta and the veins that return blood to the heart, and sometimes oncologists recommend removal of these nodes as well. Although the vulva itself does not involve any vital organs, and while complications are usually related to blood loss, infection, and slow healing, this is, nevertheless, major surgery. A simple vulvectomy consists of removing only the skin; a radical vulvectomy eliminates all tissue down to the muscle layer, and usually includes taking the lymph nodes of the groin. The surgeon can frequently save the urinary opening, the rectum, and most of the vagina. After a vulvectomy, women can still have intercourse, and many continue to experience orgasm.

Doctors can sometimes treat very early tumors with minimal

invasion of the underlying connective tissue with good results. Radiotherapy can be a successful treatment even with extensive tumors and growths in elderly patients who are poor surgical risks.

The overall cure rate for cancer of the vulva is about 75 percent, making this a cancer well worth finding and treating.

Annual mammograms, annual pelvic exams, and annual Pap smears go a long way toward early detection of cancer so that it can be promptly treated. All three, as well as proper diet and exercise, are first-rate investments in your health. Resist whatever impulse you may have to skip, delay, or postpone them.

14

Tests, Procedures, and Operations

Florence Haseltine, M.D.

Technology has invaded today's medical practice and flourishes there, giving the health-care community a great array of new tests and procedures that help in diagnosing problems and recommending treatment. These new tests, medications, and the bureaucratization that has accompanied them also have introduced new medical risks, and the more you know about their potential benefits and risks, and the procedures themselves, the easier it will be for you to decide if they should be part of your medical care.

Since you should be the only person who decides whether or not to have elective surgery, you certainly need this kind of knowledge if you are to make an informed judgment, both in deciding about the surgery and, if you have it, in ensuring that your experience will be as anxiety-free as possible. Besides understanding exactly what your surgeon will do, in order to give your truly informed consent you should be sure you know:

- the operation's expected benefits
- the risks involved, both rare and common
- the cost of the surgery and whether your health insurance will cover all or part of the expense

- how much time your recuperation will take, and how you will feel during the recovery period
- whether you will need household help while you are convalescing, particularly if you have children
- how long you should plan to be away from your job if you are employed
- the alternative treatment options and their benefits, risks, convalescent time, and cost
- your surgeon's training, whether she or he is board-certified and a Fellow of the American College of Surgeons or the American College of Obstetricians and Gynecologists (which you can find out by consulting the Directory of Medical Specialists at a large general or medical library), as well as how experienced the surgeon is in performing the operation you are planning to have
- whether the surgery will be performed by the surgeon or by a hospital resident
- whether the hospital at which the surgery will take place is accredited (which you can learn by contacting the Joint Commission on Accreditation of Hospitals, 1 Renaissance Boulevard, Oakbrook Terrace, IL 60181 [708-916-5600])
- who will give the anesthesia, whether the anesthesiologist is a Fellow of the American College of Anesthesiologists, and when you can discuss the pros and cons of local, regional, or general anesthesia
- and what is likely to happen to you if you choose to do nothing

Obviously, acquiring all this information takes time and is appropriate only for elective surgery. If your illness constitutes a real emergency, you will have to make the surgery decision on the basis of your doctor's recommendation and the immediately available facts.

Most doctors report that medical and family histories form a vital part of any diagnosis. This means that not only should you learn as much as you can about any medical condition you have, but that you should also keep a record of all tests and treatments, a diary of your medical care, including records of any medication that caused an allergic reaction. If you have such allergies, even wearing an engraved bracelet or hospital identification is no substitute for your own vigilance.

Because a great deal of unnecessary surgery is done in this country, and because hysterectomy and cesarean section are the most common surgical procedures performed on the female reproductive tract, you should be sure to get a second opinion whenever either of these operations is recommended to you. Most physicians pay very little attention to the quality-of-life issues involved in the surgery they recommend to women in their 40s, for example, and to how it will affect their patients when they reach later life. If you are not totally convinced that you need a hysterectomy, you will find few physicians willing to spend time with you to discuss the long-term effects of this operation and some of its possible side effects. Worse, one reason for this is that the studies on the long-range effects of hysterectomy—in terms of sexual functioning, response to hormonal medication, and pelvic disease—are so inadequate. However, there is another side of the unnecessary surgery coin. The current high level of malpractice suits and today's medical review procedures have also made many doctors hesitant to operate. Paradoxically, unless you are in a life-threatening situation, you may have to repeat your requests for a procedure you want or feel you need.

Doctors find it difficult to explain the risk-to-benefit ratio of an operation, and patients find it even more difficult to balance all the pros and cons and arrive at a decision. As a result, a "wait and see how the patient does" attitude has become increasingly common among physicians. Sometimes this wait-and-see attitude is perfectly appropriate; however, sometimes it just delays necessary treatment.

TESTS

Doctors order tests to help them diagnose illness, and while they generally recommend those that they believe are appropriate for each patient, many doctors and hospitals routinely order tests that are only of marginal relevance to your medical condition, partly because they are motivated by profits and partly to establish a record in the case of future legal action. A few tests are part of any regular physical examination—pulse, blood pressure, temperature, and respiration (called vital signs); urinalysis; and blood count. Beyond these, no tests are routine, and each should have a reason for being given.

VITAL SIGNS

Pulse

The pulse measures pressure as the heart contracts and pushes blood through the arteries. The normal range is 60 to 80 beats per minute for an adult, 80 to 100 beats per minute for a child, and 120 to 160 beats per minute for a newborn. Your pulse should be regular, without skipped beats, and strong.

Blood Pressure

Blood pressure reflects how hard the circulating blood pushes against the arterial walls. The doctor measures this with a blood-pressure cuff, recording the millimeters of mercury on the dial when the rhythmic beating of the blood is first heard through a stethoscope placed over the brachial artery inside your arm at the elbow, and then when it disappears. The systolic pressure, or higher reading, records pressure when the heart contracts, and the diastolic, or lower reading, when it relaxes. Normal blood pressure varies with age and sex. Health-care professionals usually add 100 to the age of a male patient to determine the normal systolic pressure; thus, a 30-year-old man's normal reading should be about 130. Diastolic readings range from 65 to 90 millimeters of mercury in men, and both readings are usually 10 points lower in women. Trained athletes often have lower-than-normal blood pressure. Any systolic reading above 150, or any diastolic reading above 90, indicates elevated blood pressure. Conversely, a systolic blood pressure under 100 can indicate shock from blood loss or dehydration, except in young, healthy women, who may have a normal systolic blood pressure of 90.

Respiration

Normal adults breathe 12 to 20 times a minute, although athletes can breathe much more slowly. Normal respiration is steady, and the breaths are neither shallow nor deep.

Temperature

Average normal body temperature is 98.6°F or 37°C and is .6° higher during the second half of the month after ovulation. An elevated temperature usually means your body is fighting an infection.

OTHER COMMON TESTS

Urinalysis

Doctors test urine to detect the presence of blood, sugar, abnormal protein, or acids, or to determine whether you have an infection. To avoid contamination of your urine from menstrual blood or vaginal discharge or from skin bacteria, you should wipe your vulva area clean before urinating to provide a specimen for urinalysis. Then hold open your vaginal lips with one hand and hold the urine container with the other. Try to take the sample in the middle of your stream, avoiding the first and last portion.

Your clinician can perform an office test by dipping a stick with chemically treated paper into your urine sample to see if it changes color. Or the specimen can be sent to a lab. If the dipstick test indicates infection, a urine culture—a sample of urine—which a lab usually analyzes within 48 hours, can determine which bacterium is causing the infection, allowing for the prescription of the appropriate antibiotic. Urine tests can also detect pregnancy. If your health-care provider asks for a urine sample, find out which tests will be done; don't assume, for example, that a pregnancy test will be done unless you ask for it.

Blood Tests

The blood carries very important information about a person's physiologic state. Because each laboratory sets parameters of normalcy for each test, you should ask how the relative value of your result compares to the norm of the laboratory that reported on your blood sample.

1. A complete blood count (CBC) consists of a red blood count, a white blood count, and a differential count of white blood cells, which shows how many you have and what different types are present. An elevated white blood count indicates the presence of an infection, and it could be viral or bacterial. A CBC also includes either a hematocrit or hemoglobin. A hematocrit gives the value for the red cell portion of the blood, reveals if the hematocrit is low, and, if low, whether this is because of decreased iron stores (anemia) or a current problem, such as recent blood loss from uterine or bowel bleeding. A hemoglobin study gives the level of your hemoglobin, the iron-carrying pigment in the red blood cells, which normally ranges between 12 and 14 grams per 100 cubic centimeters of blood.

2. The doctor orders a sedimentation rate if an infection is suspected. This measures the speed at which the red cells sink through the blood if it is left standing. Several conditions make this rate increase from normal levels, including cancer and the presence of a chronic infection, such as PID. Many other conditions as varied as rheumatoid arthritis and pregnancy also make the sedimentation rate go up.

3. Because the blood carries the various hormones throughout the body, a gynecologist can determine a woman's hormonal state by testing the levels of her estrogen, progesterone, assorted androgens, gonadotropin, and the pregnancy hormone hCG.

For pregnant women, the doctor orders a blood test that records the rise in hCG to determine if the pregnancy is normal. If a woman miscarries, the hCG level falls to zero in a predictable manner. If this fails to occur, it means that residual trophoblastic or placental tissue has been left in the body, and the health-care provider must determine whether it is in the uterus or fallopian tubes and whether the trophoblastic tissue remains as a form of trophoblastic cancer. (An oncologist treats trophoblastic cancer with a dilatation and curettage [D&C], followed by chemotherapy.) (See Chapter 9.)

4. Only a few blood tests can determine if a patient has an infection. Doctors sometimes order a toxoplasmosis titer for a pregnant woman who lives with a cat to make certain she has not contracted the disease from animal feces. Toxoplasmosis can cause

fetal defects, and this is why pregnant women are advised to take great care if they must change a cat's litter box.

The test for syphilis is also routinely available to establish the presence of the infection. Other blood tests that measure antibodies, and can show that there has been exposure to gonorrhea or chlamydia, are not as reliable.

Additional blood tests measure antibodies against other diseases, such as German measles, hepatitis, and HIV to determine the exposure to these agents.

5. The only blood test used commonly to test for cancer, other than the hCG titer in trophoblastic disease, is the test for a protein in the blood called CA 125 antigen. Some tumors of the reproductive tract, and bowel cancer, cause elevation of this antigen, but it is nonspecific because it is not always present when a patient has cancer, and it can be present in other, less serious conditions and benign diseases, such as endometriomas.

Lipid Profile

A lipid profile is a blood test that measures the level of various fats (lipids) in the blood—for example, cholesterol, high-density lipoproteins (HDL), low-density lipoproteins (LDL), and triglycerides. If a woman's cholesterol is high, taking oral contraceptives may increase her risk of heart disease. Therefore, some physicians are now ordering a lipid profile for women who request a prescription for the birth control pill. (See Chapter 6.)

Pap Smear

A Pap smear is a routine test that analyzes samples of cells and secretions taken from the vagina and cervix and gives your healthcare professional a great deal of information. It should be done annually since it can detect infections and abnormal or precancerous cells that can lead to cervical cancer as well as cervical cancer itself. At the time of the pelvic examination, the doctor can study wet smears from the vagina under a microscope to identify an infectious agent. Overall, the purpose of the Pap smear is to alert the caregiver and the patient to potential problems.

A clinician usually takes a Pap smear during a pelvic exam by moving a narrow plastic or wooden spatula over the cervical surface to obtain a sample of cervical tissue and using a Q-tip or brush to remove cells from the surface of the endocervical canal. The cells are then transferred to a slide, and the sample is fixed with a chemical that preserves it. It is then sent to a laboratory for evaluation by a cytotechnologist, a specially trained technician, or a cytopathologist, a doctor who specializes in evaluating tissue changes caused by disease. Along with the cells, the doctor also sends all pertinent clinical information so that the cytopathologist can return the best possible information.

A 1988 National Cancer Institute Workshop codified the classifications for the modern practice of diagnostic cytology, producing "The 1988 Bethesda System for Reporting Cervical/Vaginal Cytological Diagnoses." This report states whether the sample was adequate to make a diagnosis, and if inadequate, why. The pathologist reads the Pap smear as "within normal limits" or "other." If "other" is selected, then the pathologist adds further descriptors to tell the referring physician what pathology exists. The report may note evidence of infection, classifying the type of infection as fungal, bacterial, protozoan, viral, or other. Additional information can reveal the body's reaction to the infection, such as inflammation and healing after an infection or a traumatic injury. The report identifies viral infections and the cellular changes they cause. For example, some vaginal warts will produce damaged areas called squamous intraepithelial lesions, precancerous cells growing among other, normal cells. The report will note these early changes that might go on to become cancer and will identify cancer of the cervix in either its early or late forms.

If the Pap smear reveals infectious agents in the vagina or cervix, the analysis of a cervical culture can find out which bacteria are present and can also recognize gonorrhea and other sexually transmitted diseases. This permits the medical caregiver to use specific antibiotics or other medications to control the infection. The Pap smear can also describe some relatively normal cervical changes.

The results of most Pap smears are normal. Sometimes the test comes back marked "insufficient specimen," which means that either not enough cells for analysis were included or that the slide was prepared in an unsatisfactory manner; if this happens, you need a repeat Pap smear. If the result indicates cervical intraepithelial neoplasia (CIN), a precancerous cell abnormality, or cervical cancer itself, the next step should be a cervical biopsy.

PROCEDURES

BIOPSY

In order to rule out possible malignancy, the doctor cuts a small piece of tissue from the part of the body where disease might be present and sends it to a lab for examination under a microscope and a definitive diagnosis by a pathologist.

Cervical Biopsy

In this procedure, the gynecologist takes a sample of all the layers of cells that line the cervix, not simply the surface cells, as in a Pap smear. This office procedure is quick and usually painless, although some women experience a short cramping sensation as the doctor cuts out the small piece of tissue.

Today, with the use of the colposcope, a physician can visualize most of the cervix. Although the colposcope cannot view the inside of the endocervical canal, which extends from the cervix at the vaginal opening into the uterus, it magnifies the cervix and its surface so that the gynecologist can see any visible abnormal areas. What the gynecologist wants to biopsy is tissue from the following categories: sections where the surface is not smooth and glistening; regions containing tiny pinholes or punctuations; areas where the surface of the tissue appears white when the gynecologist rubs off mucus with an acidic swab (usually a mixture of water and acid somewhat like vinegar); and abnormal tissue with tiny, tortuous vessels.

Conization

When a Pap smear indicates that cervical cancer might be present, the gynecologist can perform a conization of the cervix. In this procedure, the doctor makes a circular incision with a knife or laser around the cervical opening (os) and extends it at an angle up into the cervical canal to obtain a cone of tissue, including the endocervical canal above the area the colposcope can view. Laboratory examination of this tissue provides a definitive diagnosis regarding the presence of cervical cancer and also allows the doctor to determine how extensive the cancer might be.

Uterine (Endometrial) Biopsy

When it is necessary to sample the lining of the uterus, either because of an irregularity or to determine the cause of unusual uterine bleeding, the gynecologist inserts a small catheter through the cervical opening and up into the uterus. Sometimes a local anesthetic is used to numb the cervix so that the procedure is less painful, although this will not deaden feeling in the uterus. The physician then attaches the catheter to a suction device and places the tip of the catheter against the side of the uterus, establishing a vacuum and pulling a strip of the endometrium off the uterine wall; this is then sent to the pathologist for analysis. The doctor may also use a curette to obtain a sample. Uterine biopsies allow doctors to look for evidence of abnormal cellular growth. They also enable the pathologist to determine what day of the menstrual cycle it reflects, which allows fertility specialists to evaluate the adequacy of a woman's uterine lining and its responsiveness to hormones when she is having trouble conceiving.

Breast Biopsy

See Chapter 4.

X-RAY TECHNIQUES

Hysterosalpingogram

The hysterosalpingogram is one of the most common X rays used in gynecology. First the gynecologist injects an opaque substance through the cervix into the uterine cavity and out through the tubes into the abdominal cavity. As the dye fills the uterus and passes through the tubes, the radiologist takes a series of X rays of the pelvis. These visualize the interior of the uterine cavity, allowing the doctor to see if the tubes are open. Doctors also use this test to evaluate the condition of the uterine wall when abnormal uterine bleeding is present; to look for abnormally shaped uterine cavities (i.e., with a septum, with two cavities, or shaped like a "T" instead of a triangle); and as a diagnostic tool in treating infertility.

GI Series

The GI (gastrointestinal) series uses the same technique, but there the patient first swallows a radiopaque substance that passes into the stomach and small intestine. A subsequent X ray of the upper abdomen will show the dye in the stomach and outline the small bowel. To diagnose problems of the large bowel, doctors first administer an enema of a radiopaque substance (barium), which outlines the colon and allows the clear viewing of a subsequent X ray of the lower abdomen.

Pyelogram

Urologists use this test to study the kidneys. Here the doctor injects into a vein a radiopaque substance, which then passes into the bloodstream. As the dye is cleared from the blood, it concentrates in the kidneys and is excreted into the ureters and bladder. An X ray of the abdomen will then be able to show an outline of the kidneys, ureters, and bladder. Gynecologists order pyelograms when they want to determine whether uterine disease is impinging on these organ systems.

Skull Films

Doctors sometimes order X rays of the head, particularly of the pituitary gland, to evaluate an abnormality in menstrual function. However, this is rarely done today because the CAT scan and MRI are much more accurate.

Mammogram

A mammogram is an X ray of the breast that can usually detect lumps before you can feel them. Because early diagnosis is a key element in curing breast cancer, the American Cancer Society now recommends having your first mammogram between 35 and 40 years of age, with additional mammograms every year or two between ages 40 and 50, and annual mammograms thereafter. If you have a family history of breast cancer on the maternal side, or if there is any question about the findings of a routine mammogram, your doctor will recommend more frequent mammography. (See

Chapter 4 for the importance of mammography's being performed on up-to-date equipment by experienced professionals and interpreted by technicians with expertise in reading mammograms.)

Sonogram

The gynecologist's most frequently used tool for evaluating pelvic structures is ultrasound. As the name implies, ultrasound directs sound waves into the body, which send back echoes that differ depending upon their structure and physical properties and form a picture on a TV screen. This irreplaceable tool allows the practitioner to see any organ system in very complete detail. Newer techniques using a vaginal probe facilitate highly detailed studies of the pelvic area.

Computerized Axial Tomography (CAT Scan)

Using a special X-ray machine that moves the patient gradually forward, CAT scans produce a series of highly focused images that are further refined by a sophisticated computer. CAT scans are enormously useful, but they are also expensive and overused. Be sure you need one.

Magnetic Resonance Imaging (MRI)

This sophisticated new tool uses magnetic fields and radio waves to produce detailed images of internal organs. The images differ from the ones furnished by ultrasound and CAT scan because they reflect the water content of the different organs and add information about their physiological state. Doctors use MRI mostly in examining the head region, because it is capable of detecting brain tumors, although it can also reveal spinal cord lesions and irregularities in other internal organs. Because this technology has the capability of providing information about metabolic activity of the areas it images, it may one day help determine who has cancer and who does not before surgery is performed. Because patients must sometimes remain within the confining metal core of the MRI device for up to an hour while enduring loud noise as well as the close quarters, many find it very difficult to tolerate, and repeated attempts of this procedure are often necessary.

SURGERY

Although any surgery is usually a matter of concern, there is an additional element of anxiety when an operation involves any part of the sexual system. After all, our sexual identity involves all the sexual organs, and surgery on any of them may well involve our perceptions of ourselves as a whole. The media know that the newspaper, magazine, and television audience is likely to be much more interested if a prominent woman has breast or gynecological surgery than if she has an operation on her bowel. The only other operation that generates as much apprehension as breast or gynecological surgery is brain surgery. Nevertheless, reviewing the descriptions that follow will demystify the business of gynecological surgery and help you in evaluating whatever procedures you might need to consider. If you do decide to have surgery, it is wise to donate blood in advance in case you should require a blood transfusion during the procedure, as your own blood is always the safest. If this isn't possible, be aware that careful screening procedures have now greatly reduced the risks of catching some disease from the blood of donors.

ANESTHESIA

There are three types of anesthesia: local, regional, and general. Local anesthesia employs a Novocain-type drug that is injected at the surgical site and blocks pain locally for up to an hour. Allergic reactions such as hives, rashes, asthma, or changes in heart rhythm are possible but relatively rare. Doctors do not usually use local anesthesia for surgical procedures that take longer than 10 minutes.

Obstetricians often employ regional anesthesia—such as a spinal, epidural, or caudal block—to ease the pain of delivery during childbirth, and gynecologists and surgeons use it for less complicated procedures such as tubal ligation, removal of a small intrauterine fibroid, and vaginal hysterectomy. The anesthesiologist injects medication into the space surrounding the spinal cord, deadening the lower half of your body but leaving you awake, alert, and aware during the procedure. The most common side effect of this type of anesthesia is pain at the site where the needle entered the back. Less common but more problematic is a postspinal headache, which can vary from mild to severe and can last from a few hours to days, or even a week or two. Regional anesthesia can also cause a drop in blood pressure, which doctors treat by giving fluids intravenously. This is why the blood pressure is checked frequently once you receive this type of medication.

General anesthesia renders you unconscious and is the treatment of choice for major surgery. Doctors use it for major or otherwise prolonged surgical procedures and if the patient does not wish to be conscious during the surgery. The anesthesiologist, after interviewing you before the surgery, administers a sedative to calm you immediately before you reach the operating room, and there puts you to sleep with a quick-acting drug such as sodium pentothal or Diprivan, administered by injection. This is followed by ventilation anesthesia. If you are having a short procedure, such as a D&C, the anesthesiologist will place a mask over your nose and mouth so that you can receive oxygen plus inhalation anesthesia. For a longer operation, a tube will be placed through your mouth into your windpipe to ensure that you will be able to breathe easily during the surgery. You will not feel this, but you may have a slight sore throat afterward. During the surgery, the anesthesiologist will continue to administer anesthesia and oxygen.

You will be sleepy and/or groggy after general anesthesia for varying amounts of time, depending on the agent used and how long you were unconscious during surgery. You will recover more rapidly from a quick procedure, of course, such as a D&C, than from an operation that lasted five hours. Even if you rebound swiftly, do not drive or use heavy tools or machinery for the first 24 hours, because general anesthesia slows the reflexes and hampers normal coordination. You cannot eat or drink anything for eight hours prior to receiving general anesthesia, as your stomach must be totally empty. If it is not, you could vomit and inhale the acidic vomitus, which could damage your lungs.

The risk of general anesthesia is slight for young, healthy women, but it rises with age and it can be significant if you have a chronic condition, such as hypertension, respiratory illness, diabetes, heart trouble, or an allergy of which you are unaware. You should discuss your specific risk with the anesthesiologist prior to surgery, and be sure to consider it as you review all the pros and cons of elective surgery beforehand. The main risks from general anesthesia are stroke and cardiac and/or respiratory arrest. If you have any drug allergies or have had adverse reactions to a drug in the past, be sure you tell the anesthesiologist during the presurgery interview. You should also report any recent drugs you have taken, and any medical problems you have. The doctor will usually ask about the dates of your last menstrual period, but be sure to tell both the surgeon and the anesthesiologist if there is any chance that you might be pregnant so that you can have a pregnancy test to confirm or eliminate this possibility.

SURGICAL TOOLS

Scopes

Surgeons use optical aids so as to clearly see what they are doing. One favored tool is the laparoscope, used to examine the inside of the abdomen; another is the hysteroscope, which permits the surgeon to inspect the uterine cavity; and a third is the colposcope, employed to observe the cervix and vagina. Specialists doing reparative and reconstructive surgery employ microscopes that have been adapted to operating room use to enlarge the operating field and improve their ability to see tiny structures, a process called microsurgery. Thus, gynecologic surgeons now routinely reconstruct fallopian tubes that have been previously tied as a sterilizing procedure, connecting them end to end by using sutures that are smaller than the diameter of a human hair. The microscopes help surgeons identify the many different layers of tissue that need to be sewn together or that must be separated from other tissues and removed.

Pelvic surgeons have become very adept at using the range of scopes. Today, operations that previously required large enough incisions through the abdominal wall to accommodate a surgeon's hands or fingers are done with incisions measured only in centimeters, which admit the laparoscope and some operative probes. In fact, gynecologists have been visualizing the appendix and gallbladder for decades during gynecological surgery; only recently have general surgeons employed the laparoscope to remove the gallbladder, and they have turned to the gynecologist to learn how to use this equipment.

Lasers

Doctors employ lasers in their offices as well as in the operating room. A laser is an intense beam of light that focuses on tissue and burns it so that very tiny blood vessels can be cut without bleeding. Lasers have become an important part of pelvic surgery because the vessels that must be severed and closed off without bleeding are so small. If you look at the whites of your eyes and see the tiny red lines there, you will have an idea of just how minuscule these blood vessels are. Not only can a laser cut such tiny vessels, but it can seal the edge of the cut with its beam. Lasers are high-tech tools that require expensive equipment and trained personnel to use them correctly.

LAPAROSCOPIC SURGERY

Doctors use the laparoscope to visualize the abdominal cavity and to operate in the abdomen without having to open it with more than a one-half-inch incision, a capability that has made one-day surgery a reality in the treatment of a number of pelvic problems.

The clinician first introduces the laparoscope into the abdomen through a small incision in the umbilicus to diagnose the problem, which might range from an ectopic pregnancy, adhesions, or blocked fallopian tubes to fibroids and endometriosis. Doctors also use the laparoscope to detect other illnesses, including cancer, bowel disease, gallbladder disease, and appendicitis. Not only can the physician identify the pathology with the use of the laparoscope, but in many cases she or he can operate, with the help of tiny scissors, probes, suturing equipment, and either electrical or laser-driven cautery. The surgeon commonly removes small ectopic pregnancies, dissolves adhesions, treats endometriosis with lasers, and attempts to open fallopian tubes. Infertility surgeons use the laparoscope extensively when retrieving eggs and placing fertilized eggs in the fallopian tube.

Fewer complications are associated with laparoscopic surgery than with any other type of surgery. The main ones have to do with the blind insertion of two instruments into the abdomen. The first is the needle used to inject gas into the abdomen so that the abdominal wall is moved away from the bowel. The second is the laparoscopic "trocar," the sharp, pointed instrument that guides the sleeve of the laparoscope into the abdominal wall. The trocar is removed, allowing the laparoscope to be inserted through the remaining sleeve. (See Chapter 10.) Either insertion can perforate the bowel in a woman who has adhesions of the bowel that have attached to the abdominal wall. Bleeding can also be a problem if the surgeon hits or unintentionally cuts a blood vessel during the procedure. If this happens, the surgeon must open the abdomen and repair the damage.

Surgeons usually use general anesthesia for laparoscopic surgery, although they can perform tubal ligations and simple diagnostic laparoscopies under local anesthesia. If you elect local anesthesia, you should understand that the procedure can be quite uncomfortable, and that some pain is unavoidable. In addition, when the abdomen is distended with gas there is often the distressing feeling of being unable to breathe; that is why the laparoscopy is almost always done under general anesthesia. In either event, patients recover quite rapidly from laparoscopic surgery and are able to return to normal activity within a few days.

TECHNIQUES OF TRADITIONAL SURGERY

Much of pelvic surgery is still carried out in the classical way. The surgeon identifies the organ or area to be removed, repaired, or restored; frees it from surrounding structures; and then operates on it. For example, a piece of bowel might be stuck to the uterus. To free the uterus from the bowel, the surgeon puts tension on both the uterus and the bowel to identify the adhering area. Sometimes the adhering area will come loose with simple tension; if not, the surgeon must separate them with sharp dissection, using scissors, laser, or a small surgical knife called a scalpel. If the organ has to be removed, as in a hysterectomy, the surgeon clamps the blood vessels leading to the uterus to stop the flow of blood to the area, cuts the tissue, and sutures (ties) the region behind the clamp so that when the clamp is removed there will be no blood flow into the operative field. There are several ways to clamp, cut, tie, and then restore the anatomy to as normal a configuration as possible, and the surgeon chooses among them depending on the patient's individual anatomy, the degree of damage to the organ, and sometimes the degree of the surgeon's own expertise. At the end of the operation, the surgeon repairs each level of tissue that has been disturbed and closes the wound with sutures.

When surgeons restore pelvic structures, as they must do, for example, in infertility surgery, it is very important to allow only minimal bleeding and to use extremely few sutures. Sutures, no matter how tiny or how nonreactive they are, are nevertheless foreign bodies, and a patient's tissue can react to them and form adhesions, a type of scar tissue. If the surgeon must repair a pelvic structure with adhesions that have formed as a result of disease or previous surgery, the point is to remove them without causing new ones. Before the laser became available, surgeons used cautery with an electric current to accomplish this. The procedure damaged relatively large amounts of surrounding tissue; the laser is more focused and cauterizes only the tissue hit by the light beam. The burn does not spread beyond the site of the beam's focus.

MINOR PELVIC SURGERY

Minor pelvic surgery is usually performed either in the physician's office or in an outpatient facility. Medical personnel consider as minor any operation that does not require an overnight stay in the hospital, even if it takes place in a day surgery unit where general anesthesia is used and the procedure lasts six hours.

The most common minor outpatient gynecological surgery involves the vulvar area, the vagina, and the cervix. Doctors employ minor surgery to sample the endometrium, perform an abortion, remove cysts and warts, and drain infections from the vulvar area.

VULVAR CYSTS

One of the routine types of cysts that require surgical attention are those of the Bartholin's duct, located in the vestibular bulbs on either side of the vaginal opening. This cyst is caused by an obstruction of the Bartholin's duct at a site near its opening. Obstruction can be the result of an infection from gonorrhea or other infectious causes or from trauma; often the cause remains unknown. Sometimes the obstetrician cuts the duct following vaginal repair of an episiotomy, an incision that, while not always necessary, is done routinely in hospitals to ease the passage of the baby's head during childbirth. The Bartholin's glands continue to produce mucous secretions despite the obstruction; if they become infected, there can be a rapid production of pus that blocks off the numerous glandular compartments. If the duct does not become infected and does not grow or cause discomfort, then surgery is unnecessary.

When draining this type of cyst in the office, the gynecologist injects the vulvar area with a local anesthetic, then makes an incision over the surface of the swollen area and inserts a catheter inside the cyst. The catheter has a bulb on its end that the doctor then inflates, causing it to stay in place because the outer incision is smaller than the balloon. With the catheter left in place, the duct heals around the catheter, and the opening enlarges and expels the balloon. The incision is kept open so the duct will heal in that position and not close off again.

The gynecologist can perform this procedure with relative ease if the cyst is not infected. If the cyst cannot be drained effectively, the doctor can do a marsupialization of the cyst in the office, making a larger incision and sewing the inner edges of the cyst to the outer edge of the incision. This turns the cyst inside out, allowing it to drain and heal.

INTRAABDOMINAL (OVARIAN) CYSTS

Doctors usually diagnose these cysts in younger women at the time of a routine physical exam and confirm the diagnosis with ultrasound. However, if the cost becomes less prohibitive, magnetic resonance imaging (MRI) will be used more frequently for diagnosis because it evaluates water content, and cysts are usually filled with fluid. The gynecologist can drain a cyst with a needle under ultrasonic guidance, but many physicians are reluctant to do this because ultrasound and MRI are not yet sophisticated enough to guarantee that the cyst is not malignant. Unlike breast cysts, which are almost never malignant, ovarian cysts can be. Draining a malignant cyst can make matters worse, because cancerous cells may escape to other parts of the body, decreasing the chances for recovery. Therefore, doctors operate to remove most ovarian cysts that are larger than four to six centimeters and persist for more than one or two menstrual cycles.

WARTS

Genital warts are another common problem that can either irritate the vulvar area or become intrusive during intercourse. (See Chapter 11.) Doctors commonly apply a drug called podophyllin to warts. If the warts are not eliminated, or if they are extensive or are situated in areas that are too delicate to handle, such as the clitoral hood or the opening of the urethra, the gynecologist first numbs the area with local anesthesia, and then uses cryosurgery either to cauterize or freeze the wart(s). Another approach utilizes the laser, which has made outpatient treatment of recalcitrant warts, those that are small or in particularly sensitive areas, much easier and more routine than in the past.

HYMENEAL SURGERY

The entrance to the vagina usually has a hymeneal ring that has opened before birth. It is common for this ring to be only partially open or to have bands across it, so that if a girl tries to use a tampon, inserting or removing it can cause pain. When the hymen has multiple, very small openings, it is referred to as a cribriform hymen. A gynecologist can repair this condition with tiny incisions and a few sutures. Doctors usually perform this procedure in the office, using local anesthesia. If the patient is an extremely sensitive young girl, the surgery can be done in the hospital, but this involves possible psychological trauma as well as the risk of general anesthesia. The clinician should discuss all aspects of this procedure with the girl and her family—if she wants her parents to be involved.

CERVICAL SURGERY

Precancerous Tissue

If a cervical biopsy shows precancerous lesions, the doctor can cauterize the whole area of the cervix, using cold rather than heat. In this outpatient procedure, the clinician opens the vagina with a speculum, places a metal tubing in the vagina to permit good visualization of the cervix, and inserts a probe to freeze the diseased tissue and destroy it superficially while leaving the underlying tissue undamaged. Patients do not need anesthesia; most women feel only a cramp while the tissue is frozen, and a few additional cramps afterward, because the cervix does not have nerves that respond to cold. Since the vagina senses cold, great care is taken to touch only the cervix with the probe, because the doctor does not want to damage the vagina or freeze another part of the perineum. If the physician is skilled and accurate with the probe, the procedure will accomplish the freezing and destruction of all the abnormal cells. These cells are most commonly found at the endocervical junction between the cervical canal and the surface of the cervix. The patient will expel strong-smelling, slightly bloody tissue from the vagina for 10 days or more as the cervix sloughs off the dead tissue. She will also have a copious watery discharge during the healing process. Healing occurs as normal tissue from the edge of the frozen area grows back over the raw cervical region, forming a new endocervical junction.

Nabothian Cysts

These are small mucous cysts commonly found on the cervix that, if present, are easily felt when you check for an IUD string or manipulate a diaphragm. They will sometimes burst and release a small amount of blood and mucus. Nabothian cysts do not need treatment unless they become large and interfere with intercourse or cause other discomfort. If they do require drainage, the doctor can lance large ones with a needle or the tip of a scalpel, and puncture smaller ones with a needle.

Polyps

Endocervical polyps are another problem that a physician can handle easily in the office. These are outgrowths of the endocervical glands, and the gynecologist can usually remove them by grasping them with a pair of forceps or a small clamp and twisting with a modest amount of traction. Since bleeding following intercourse is a symptom of polyps, you should see your health-care provider and have a pelvic exam if you experience such bleeding. Bleeding can also signal a cervical problem, including the most serious one, cervical cancer.

MAJOR PELVIC SURGERY

Major surgery usually employs general anesthesia and involves a hospital stay of a few days or more. The advantages of hospitalization include observation by trained medical personnel, who can check for the common postoperative complications of bleeding or infection, manage postoperative care of the surgical field itself, and supervise pain medication.

As we have noted, having a relative or friend on hand as often as possible to serve as your advocate during a hospital stay is useful in terms of your keeping posted about your treatment, including testing and medication.

VULVAR SURGERY

When doctors note lesions in the vaginal and vulvar area that do not heal, they use biopsies to determine if there is a malignancy. If the malignancy is confirmed, the cancerous area needs surgical removal. The early operations developed to treat vulvar cancer were extremely disfiguring, but more recently surgeons have attempted to develop less drastic procedures and to treat early lesions with minimal excision. Women with a diagnosis of vulvar cancer should seek out a surgeon who is specially trained in gynecologic oncology. Cancer of the vulva occurs far more frequently among older women than it does in younger ones.

Bartholin's Cyst

When a Bartholin's cyst recurs and the procedure to remove it cannot be handled on an outpatient basis, the doctor will remove it in the hospital. This can be a difficult operation because the area around the Bartholin's gland is surrounded by a large number of interconnecting blood vessels. In fact, a good reason to perform this surgery in an operating room is concern about the possibility of excessive bleeding, as well as the time and skill required for the surgeon to find the major areas of infection and be certain that all foreign and contaminated material is removed. The hospital procedure is not very different from the office-based one except that the surgeon does more cutting, draining, and suturing. This surgery requires a hospital stay of a few days. Afterward, you will usually be given antibiotics and have to soak in a sitz bath to relieve soreness.

VAGINAL SURGERY

The hospital is the venue for most vaginal surgery. Some cysts on the vaginal wall require removal and drainage in an operating room because of their size and location. Surgeons frequently remove large vaginal warts in an operating room and use a laser that, because it focuses on a limited area and provides greater magnifications, allows the surgeon to see the vagina better and enables the bleeding vessels to be sutured more easily.

The most common reason for vaginal surgery is to repair the vagina after damage during a delivery. Because some women experience pain with intercourse after a repair of vaginal tears suffered during childbirth, a second surgical procedure may be needed to correct the problem. Complications in vaginal delivery can also compromise the function of the bladder, rectum, and anus so that the bladder, which normally lies on top of the vagina, or the rectum, which is typically behind it, are not in their correct anatomical positions. If the vaginal wall becomes weak, the bladder and rectum may protrude into the vagina, making it difficult to have a bowel movement or to urinate properly. In extreme cases, so much relaxation of the vagina takes place that the uterus will come out of the vagina, or herniate, leaving the cervix visible at the opening of the vagina or, possibly, allow the cervix to come out of the vagina entirely. When the uterus protrudes from the vagina, it is commonly called falling of the uterus, or prolapse. (Sometimes, doctors prescribe a pessary to prevent vaginal prolapse. If you have a pessary, you must take it out once a week to wash it. A pessary can cause vaginal ulcers; if you experience bleeding or odor, you should consult your doctor immediately about further treatment.) If the supports that cover the rectum and separate it from the vagina are destroyed, the rectum can protrude out of the vagina from the pressure of a bowel movement. If there is destruction of the rectal sphincter during delivery, a woman can be incontinent of stool and gas.

Another situation that clearly needs in-hospital correction is the presence of a fistula, which sometimes forms after childbirth and occasionally following surgery. Here, tissues from the vagina and bladder, or the vagina and rectum, grow together and form a hole connecting the two tracts. In these cases, a woman is incontinent of urine or feces, depending on whether the bladder or rectum is involved. During surgery, the gynecologist attempts to restore the structures and boundaries needed to separate the vagina from the other organs, rebuilding the perineal body that separates the vagina from the rectum so that the woman has a more functional, anatomically correct vaginal opening.

All surgery involving reconstruction of the vagina uses the same procedure. After the anesthesiologist puts the patient to sleep, the surgeon opens up the area that has been damaged, then dissects the incision up the vagina and out toward the side walls, exposing the structures of the vaginal wall. The surgeon then searches for tough, strong, fibrous tissue that can hold a suture, and stitches this tissue over the defect, rolling the flaw under the newly re-created, layered structure. The surgeon usually removes stretched, excess vaginal tissue and closes the vagina over the area of the now-corrected fistula.

When a vaginal weakness, such as a rectocele, is present, there is often some herniation of the uterus, in which case the gynecologist usually removes the uterus, a procedure called a vaginal hysterectomy. If you do not want a hysterectomy because you wish to retain your fertility, you will need a cesarean section for your next delivery, because the vaginal repair will not hold up during another vaginal birth.

UTERINE SURGERY

Dilatation and Curettage (D&C)

If your doctor does an endometrial biopsy and it fails to provide the needed information, the next step is a D&C—dilatation of the cervix and curettage of the endometrium. The hysteroscope has recently improved basic D&C technique. In the past, the surgeon's ability to remove endometrial polyps or to diagnose a submucous fibroid—one that is beneath the mucous membrane—relied on his or her ability to feel the intruding growth when the curette passed over an irregularity in the uterine wall. Now the hysteroscope makes it possible to look inside the uterus and visualize the cavity, so that the doctor can see polyps or abnormal endometrial tissue that might be precancerous or cancerous. If a polyp is present, the doctor can grasp it with a polyp forceps and remove it. If a submucous fibroid is the problem, the doctor can identify it and, frequently, can remove it with cauterization. If excessive menstrual bleeding is the difficulty and it is inadvisable to do a hysterectomy, the doctor can cauterize vascular abnormalities on the lining of the uterus. (For example, a patient in kidney failure who requires routine dialysis would be a poor candidate for major surgery.) The hysteroscope can also locate a lost IUD or a uterine septum, a cause of infertility.

Today, doctors routinely do D&Cs in the office or in an outpatient operating room setting. Your D&C will begin with anesthesia, either regional or general, depending on what you have chosen when talking with the anesthesiologist beforehand. First, the doctor will wash the vaginal area with antiseptic and drape it with sterile sheets, leaving only the vagina exposed. After performing a bimanual pelvic exam to inspect your uterus, tubes, and ovaries, the doctor will insert a speculum and clamp the cervix with a tenaculum to hold it in place. A uterine sound, a thin metal rod that shows the angle of your cervix and the depth of your uterus, is then inserted. If a tissue sample is needed, the doctor will scrape off some tissue from your cervical canal with a small curette. Using tapered rods in graduated sizes, the doctor will then open your cervical canal. Any polyps will then be removed, and samples will be taken from different areas of the uterine lining with a curette. Both specimens will be sent to the lab for microscopic examination. The doctor then removes the curette, tenaculum, and speculum.

Light bleeding or spotting is normal after a D&C, but you should call your doctor if you develop a fever, abdominal cramping and pain, heavy bleeding, fainting or dizziness, or a vaginal discharge with an odor. Bleeding can indicate accidental damage to the uterus, bladder, rectum, or a blood vessel, which requires surgical repair; a fever and strong-smelling discharge usually indicates an infection. To avoid pushing bacteria from the cervix up into the uterus, tubes, and ovaries, you should avoid intercourse, douches, and tampons or inserting anything into your vagina until the bleeding and discharge stop. You should also be sure to see the doctor for a follow-up visit to find out if you have an infection or if you otherwise need any additional treatment.

Fibroid Removal

The uterus can develop fibroids, or myomas. As their name implies, these are fibrous growths in the wall of the uterus. (See Chapter 12.) When fibroids become a problem because of their location or size, doctors usually recommend surgically removing them.

Since fibroids are sensitive to estrogen, withdrawing estrogen will reduce their size. To do this, physicians prescribe antagonists to the gonadotropin-releasing factor—GnRH analog (Lupron, nafarelin)—to stop the pituitary from signaling the ovary to produce estrogen, creating a medical menopause. Women can take GnRH analog only for short periods because they experience the side effects of menopause, such as hot flashes, and would be at greater risk for osteoporosis if they continued the drug. The treatment shrinks the fibroid and its blood supply temporarily and, if still necessary, makes the surgical removal easier for the surgeon and less risky for the patient. However, shrinking fibroids prior to surgery can have disadvantages; the gynecologist may have a harder time locating the boundaries between the shrunken fibroid and the healthy tissue around it. And reducing the size of small fibroids may cause the doctor to miss them completely during surgery, only to see them grow again when the woman stops taking the medication.

The gynecologist decides on the best method of removal based on the fibroid's size and location. Those on the uterine wall can be excised simply by isolating them and cutting them away. If they are small enough, a hysteroscope can be used to view the interior of the uterus; sometimes the fibroid can then be detached with a scissors, electric current, or laser. When a fibroid is buried deep within the uterine wall, careful surgical judgment is required, and every case needs its own individual consideration, because surgical reconstruction is as much an art as it is a science.

Myomectomy

If it is important to retain the uterus, the gynecologist performs a myomectomy, removing only the fibroid and repairing the uterus. During a hysterectomy, the doctor can clamp off the blood vessels feeding the uterus. However, fibroids have multiple blood vessels supplying them and their anatomic position is random, not pre-determined or predictable. Therefore, a great deal of bleeding often takes place during myomectomy, more so than in hysterectomy.

Fifteen to 20 percent of the time the patient will need additional surgery after myomectomy because fibroids tend to recur. Most doctors don't recommend subsequent myomectomies because of their risk and the fact that surgery causes scar tissue or adhesions that can be painful and make later surgery even more difficult. If you have no plans to become pregnant and no longer want the risk of continued uterine problems, a hysterectomy may be safer and more effective.

Hysterectomy

Hysterectomy, the surgical removal of the uterus, can be a life-saving procedure; the operation is clearly necessary for a woman who has any cancer of the reproductive tract (vagina, cervix, uterus, fallopian tubes, or ovaries), who is bleeding uncontrollably, or who is suffering from a severe infection that does not respond to other treatment. But hysterectomy is most frequently an elective pro-cedure; more commonly, it is used as therapy for fibroids, endo-metriosis, continuous irregular bleeding, excessive bleeding that becomes incapacitating, pelvic pain, and, in older women, severely painful menstrual periods (see Figure 14.1). Gynecologists also per-form vaginal hysterectomies to correct severe cases of prolapse of the uterus.

In 1988, 578,000 hysterectomies were performed in the United States. The recognition that many hysterectomies are unnecessary, along with the fact that most women want to preserve their uteri, has reduced the use of this surgery by 20 percent since the mid-1970s, although American doctors still perform more hysterecto-mies than do their counterparts in Europe. Rates are lower in the Northeast than in other regions of the country, for reasons that have not been researched. Some investigators believe that the way doctors are trained, the sheer availability of gynecologists and hos-pital beds, as well as the profitability of the procedure and the local style of medical practice all play a role. In any case, you should know that you may receive very different medical advice about whether to have a hysterectomy depending on whether you have medical insurance, where you live, and which doctor you consult.

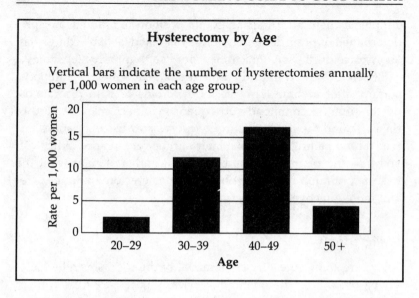

Hysterectomy by Age

Vertical bars indicate the number of hysterectomies annually per 1,000 women in each age group.

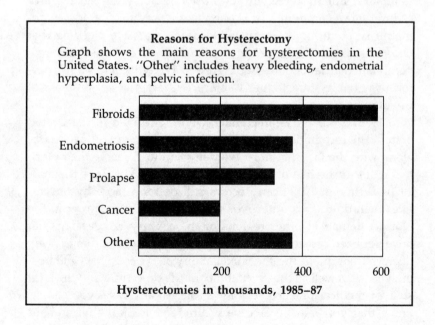

Reasons for Hysterectomy

Graph shows the main reasons for hysterectomies in the United States. "Other" includes heavy bleeding, endometrial hyperplasia, and pelvic infection.

Because of this, it is particularly important that you satisfy yourself about the necessity of the surgery before you consent to it.

Hysterectomies fall into four categories:

1. Simple (subtotal) hysterectomy removes only the uterus through the abdomen.
2. Total hysterectomy removes the uterus and cervix.
3. Hysterectomy with bilaterial salpingo-oophorectomy removes the uterus, cervix, fallopian tubes, and ovaries.
4. Radical hysterectomy, performed because of invasive cervical cancer, removes the uterus, cervix, tubes, ovaries, the upper third of the vagina, the nearby lymph nodes, and the uterine ligaments.

Vaginal Removal of the Uterus

Surgeons prefer to remove the uterus through the vagina if the patient has other vaginal problems, such as a cystocele, where the urinary bladder protrudes through the vaginal wall, or a rectocele, a similar inversion of the rectum, because they can correct these abnormalities at the same time. The other advantages over the abdominal method are that the hospital stays and recovery periods are shorter, complications fewer, and there is no visible scar. About a quarter of the hysterectomies performed on women under 65, and 40 percent of those over 65, are vaginal.

During the vaginal procedure, you will be in the same position as you are during a pelvic exam, with feet in stirrups and legs apart. After anesthesia has taken effect and your thighs and vagina have been cleansed, the gynecologist will hold open the vaginal walls with instruments while making an incision in your vagina where its walls meet the cervix and then cutting through connective tissue and the abdominal lining (peritoneum) into the abdominal cavity. Clamping the cervix so that it can be pulled down, the gynecologist then locates, ties off, and cuts the ligaments and blood vessels that attach the uterus to other structures in the pelvis, removing the uterus and cervix through the vagina. After repairing each layer that has been cut, the surgeon closes the incision.

Abdominal Removal of the Uterus

Gynecologists use the abdominal procedure, also called a laparotomy, a term used to denote any abdominal procedure, when large fibroids, adhesions from previous surgery, or an unusually small pelvis make removal of the uterus through the vagina difficult or impossible. If other organs, such as the ovaries and tubes, must also be removed, most gynecologists prefer the abdominal approach, using either a vertical or horizontal incision in the abdominal wall.

Here the surgeon cuts through connective tissue and the peritoneum, separates the abdominal muscles, and holds the incision open with instruments so that the operating fields can be seen. After checking adjacent structures for abnormalities, the doctor clamps the ligaments and blood vessels leading to the uterus and other structures (ovaries, tubes) that will be excised, frees and removes them, and then stitches each layer of tissue closed.

Should Healthy Ovaries Be Removed?

Whether or not to remove healthy ovaries when excising the uterus remains a medical controversy. The advantage, of course, is eliminating the risk of ovarian cancer. The disadvantage is the loss of the estrogen and androgens that the ovaries secrete even beyond menopause, which protect against heart disease and osteoporosis and enhance libido. Young women certainly should retain their healthy ovaries. Menopausal women must weigh the potential danger of ovarian cancer against the value of not disturbing normal physiological function. You will have to decide for yourself, of course, balancing your age, risk factors, and the level of your general concern about the possibility of your developing ovarian cancer. In doing so, remember to review your family history to determine if close relatives have had cancer of the ovary; remember, too, that if you have used oral contraceptives for one year, your risk of this disease drops by 50 percent. Several follow-up studies of women who have retained their ovaries after hysterectomy show a very low rate of subsequent ovarian cancer, only 0.1 percent of 10,638 women in seven studies done between 1963 and 1977.

Complications of Hysterectomy

The most common complications of hysterectomy are infection at the site of the incision and bleeding during the operation; 25 to 50 percent of patients experience some complication, and 10 percent need a blood transfusion. Some gynecologists give antibiotics routinely when they operate, which has markedly reduced post-operative infections. Hysterectomy also presents an increased risk of blood clots traveling from a pelvic or leg vein to the lung (pulmonary embolism), which can be life-threatening. There is always a heightened risk from general anesthesia. And occasionally the gynecologist can inadvertently damage other organs (bladder, ureter, bowel) during the surgery, which must be repaired. Overall, the mortality rate is 6.6 deaths for every 100,000 hysterectomies.

One long-range complication from any type of abdominal surgery involves the formation of adhesions, the bands of thin tissue that sometimes develop between abdominal structures and cause a great deal of pain, often requiring another operation to remove them. Another issue is the loss of prostacyclin, a hormone the uterus secretes that dilates blood vessels and helps to keep blood platelets from sticking together, which may be a factor in preventing coronary heart disease. Some epidemiological studies suggest that premenopausal hysterectomy increases the risk of coronary heart disease for the rest of the premenopausal years, even if the healthy ovaries are left in place to continue producing protective estrogen. But other areas of the body produce prostacyclin as well, and more research is clearly needed before this risk is established.

Does Hysterectomy Affect Sex Life?

Some women feel that sex is different following a hysterectomy, while others do not. Some doctors ascribe this to the fact that certain sensory nerves are cut during the surgery, and that women consequently may miss the feeling of the penis touching the cervix and the uterus contracting during orgasm. Others point out that all the pelvic floor muscles are still there to contract during orgasm, and that the only nerves cut are those to the uterus itself. Women for whom uterine contractions were a major factor in orgasm will therefore notice a difference in orgasm after hysterectomy. A 1981 review of more than a thousand hysterectomy patients found that 50 percent of the women reported no change in the level of their desire, 9 percent said their desire had declined, and 9 percent said it had increased. Clearly, further research is needed here as well.

Psychological Reactions to Hysterectomy

The psychological reactions women have to hysterectomy also vary. Many become depressed after the surgery, and for a woman who wanted to begin or continue childbearing, the experience can be devastating. Others are relieved and enjoy freedom from pain, bleeding, the discomfort of uterine prolapse, or whatever other symptoms led them to choose the procedure. How women react depends on many factors, including the general state of their mental health, their self-esteem, and the support they receive from their partners and friends. Investigators agree that women who are thoroughly familiar with the reasons for the surgery and have made their own decision about having it are less likely to experience adverse psychological reactions.

OVARIAN SURGERY

Cysts

Doctors suspect ovarian pathology when they can feel an enlarged ovary, or when a patient complains of pain. Since ovaries normally enlarge during mid-cycle, your doctor probably will want to follow a cyst for a month or more. If it does not disappear, or if it exceeds four to six centimeters in size, the gynecologist will turn to other diagnostic techniques to determine the nature of the mass. The doctor may order a sonogram, which will show whether the problem is a single cyst or multiple masses and whether it is solid or filled with liquid. By following the mass, the doctor knows whether or not it is growing. A CA 125 blood test can help determine if the mass might be malignant, although CA 125 may be elevated in benign ovarian cysts. An X ray can tell if the cyst has calcium deposits. (If it has, your doctor will usually recommend immediate removal.) In young women this can indicate a dermoid cyst, derived from an egg that tried to divide on its own and form a fetus. A dermoid cyst has disorganized tissue, and the calcium deposits are usually malformed fetal teeth. It does not go away on its own, and if it ruptures, the fatty material in it causes major irritation to the abdominal cavity.

During surgery, the gynecologist "shells" a benign cyst out of the ovary and stitches the ovary closed, trying to reconstruct the normal ovarian anatomy. Malignant ovarian tumors require wide removal, including the fallopian tubes and the uterus, followed by radiation and/or chemotherapy.

Endometriomas

An endometrioma, which is endometrial tissue that has formed a mass by bleeding into itself, sometimes becomes embedded in the ovary and is often difficult to excise. Endometriomas frequently have caused destruction of ovarian tissue with major distortions and pain. Infertility surgeons are trained to operate on these cysts and to restore the ovary to its best possible state. Sometimes the destruction of the ovary is so extensive, however, that it is impossible to save it. In very severe cases of endometriosis, the surgeon must remove both ovaries. In the past, the uterus was also removed during this operation, since the woman could not become pregnant but could develop later uterine pathology. With the availability of in vitro fertilization and the ability to maintain hormone levels artificially, doctors now leave the uterus in women who still want to attempt a pregnancy with a previously frozen embryo or a donor embryo.

The most common complication of ovarian surgery is the formation of adhesions around the ovary, which may result in infertility. If you have your ovaries removed before menopause, you should consider estrogen replacement therapy to avoid increasing your risk of osteoporosis and heart disease.

SURGERY ON THE FALLOPIAN TUBES

Sterilization by Tubal Ligation

While much of the surgery performed on the fallopian tube is to restore function and enable a woman to have a child (see Chapter 10), a common reason for surgery on the fallopian tubes is sterilization. If you are considering a tubal ligation (closing of the tubes), you should understand that this procedure is permanent in its effects. While it is true that pregnancies occur—albeit rarely—after tubal ligation, and that the tubes can sometimes be restored, unless you are absolutely certain that you do not want to become pregnant, you should not choose sterilization. Conversely, if you *are* sure, tubal ligation is a relatively safe and easy procedure with an extremely small failure rate, as low as one in 2,000 procedures using laparoscopic sterilization.

While only one basic technique is involved in tubal ligation, the tying off, or occlusion of, the fallopian tubes, the location of the incision and the method of occlusion can differ. Your gynecologist may use a one-inch horizontal incision just below the navel, or a one-quarter- to one-half-centimeter incision just above the pubic hairline. The doctor may either cauterize the tubes (burning and sealing them); make a loop of the tube, tie it with suture thread, and cut the loop away; or use clips or elastic rings to close each tube.

A typical tubal ligation procedure starts with general anesthesia, although local and regional anesthesia may also be a possibility. After the anesthesia has taken effect, the gynecologist inserts a needle through the umbilicus and pumps air into the abdomen to distend it so that the organs of the abdomen are separated from each other, enabling the doctor to see well and move instruments around in the abdomen without hitting the bowel. The doctor then places the laparoscope directly into the abdomen through a small incision just below the navel, identifies the fallopian tubes, grasps them, and ties them off, using cautery, silastic clips, or bands. A speculum may be placed in the vagina so that the doctor can clamp the cervix and move the uterus and tubes into an advantageous position. The clips, rings, or cautery can be inserted either through a channel in the laparoscope or separately through a tiny incision above the pubic hairline. The decision to use one incision or two depends on the equipment available and the patient's anatomy. After tying the tubes, the gynecologist inspects them to make sure no bleeding is present, removes the instruments, closes the incision with one or two stitches, and covers it with a Band-Aid—which is why this procedure is sometimes referred to as Band-Aid surgery.

If your gynecologist does not have access to a laparoscope, he or she will perform a mini-laparotomy. This procedure involves making a small incision (one to two inches long) just above the pubic area, opening the abdomen, identifying the tubes, and then tying them off. This incision was common before the laparoscope greatly simplified tubal ligation.

An obstetrician can perform a tubal ligation immediately after birth or within the first 48 hours after delivery. If you have an epidural block for your delivery, the doctor may be able to tie off your tubes without additional anesthesia as soon as the baby is born; if you wait a day, then you will need another anesthetic, which can be general or regional. The advantage of postpartum sterilization is that the uterus is enlarged and lies high in the abdomen, and the surgeon can reach the tubes with a one- to two-inch incision just under the navel, tie them off, and close the incision. This procedure does not normally extend your obstetrical hospital stay. The disadvantage of postpartum sterilization is major: The failure rate is as high as one in 50 procedures. This is because the increased blood supply that exists right after delivery makes it more likely that the tubes will heal and their channels will reopen. This is far less likely when the tubes are tied at least six weeks after delivery. Then the increased blood supply of pregnancy will have returned to normal.

Complications

Tubal ligations are usually quick, and patients suffer very little pain afterward; most women go home the same day. One hazard is a future pregnancy in the closed-off fallopian tube (an ectopic pregnancy), a danger because the tube can rupture. This can occur at any time after a tubal ligation but is more likely in the first few years after the procedure. If you experience sudden, intense pain, irregular bleeding, faintness, or dizziness, which can indicate internal bleeding, call your doctor at once. (See Chapters 9 and 10.)

Other complications of tubal ligation include problems from anesthesia, a rare development; a surgeon's unintentional damage to internal organs; or infection and bleeding. The danger signals that should alert you to call your surgeon are fever; significant pain, requiring more medication than the doctor has prescribed; bleeding from your incision that does not stop with a pressure dressing; red or tender skin around the incision; feeling faint; or experiencing breathing problems.

The fallopian tube has its own diseases, most of which stem from its ability to close off and form a structure that does not open into the peritoneal cavity. If the infection causes blockage, the tube may form a septic abscess or a large hydrosalpinx, a collection of watery fluid. Pelvic inflammatory disease (PID) can cause tubal blockage, as can infection from a miscarriage, abortion, or IUD. Whatever the cause, infected fallopian tubes are a major problem. Doctors usually treat them with long-term, high-dose antibiotics, and this often requires hospital admission so that the medications can be given intravenously. If the abscess does not resolve or if the tubes become massive or painful, they must be drained. The clinician usually does this through an abdominal incision. If the infection or abscess has become massive, the surgeon may have to remove one or both tubes. These infections can be life-threatening; the surgery prevents the loss of life.

MALE STERILIZATION: VASECTOMY

You and your partner may opt for male sterilization as a *permanent* method of birth control. There are good reasons to choose this alternative. Failure rates are low (one in 1,000 procedures), the surgery takes only 20 minutes in a doctor's office, there is little pain and discomfort, recovery usually occurs within 24 to 48 hours, and complications are fewer than for tubal ligation. There is no evidence that vasectomy changes hormone levels, sex drive, or has any long-term negative effect on a man's health.

The procedure starts with cleaning, shaving, and surgically draping the scrotum area. Some surgeons give a mild sedative before doing this. The doctor locates each of the tubes that carries sperm from testes to penis (the vas deferens), injects a local anesthetic into the scrotum, and, after it takes effect, makes one central incision or two incisions, one above each vas deferens. The incision is small, one half to one inch. The surgeon then lifts the first vas deferens through the incision, removes a one-half- to one-inch section of it, and ties or cauterizes the ends to seal them; the same is done with the second vas deferens. The incision is then closed with one or two stitches. If the doctor does not use absorbable sutures, the stitches must come out in about four days.

Physicians recommend that a man wear jockey shorts or an athletic support after surgery to relieve the ache that sometimes accompanies vasectomy, that someone drive him home afterward, and that he rest for a day or two after surgery. He should keep the incision area dry for a day or so and avoid strenuous activity and lifting for about a week. A couple can resume intercourse once he feels comfortable, but he becomes sterile only after all sperm have exited both vasa deferentia; therefore, he must use another type of birth control until his sperm count is zero. This takes three to six months.

Complications

The rate of problems after vasectomy is low. Blood clots occur in one or two men out of 100, in which case the surgeon usually has to reopen the incision and remove them. Infection happens at about the same low rate, and it can usually be controlled with antibiotics. Occasionally, an abscess develops, which must be drained. Swelling, if it occurs, usually subsides within a week; an ice pack, wearing a support, and rest are the best treatments. A nonprescription medication is usually sufficient for pain relief. Rarely, a lump of inflamed tissue called a granuloma forms because of sperm leaking from the cut end of the tube; while this usually requires treatment only if it becomes infected, it can cause the tube to grow again with consequent vasectomy failure, so the surgeon should be consulted.

CANCER SURGERY

If the gynecologist diagnoses cervical, endocervical, or uterine cancer, the next step will be to try to determine the extent of the disease. A simple hysterectomy is the treatment of choice for small, noninvasive cancers. Once the cancer has spread from the local site, the gynecologist will probably refer you to a gynecologic oncologist, a cancer specialist. You may need radiation therapy and then surgery. Whatever the therapy, it should be individualized for your disease. You should have a thorough discussion with your physician about the choices, risks, and benefits of any proposed treatment. (See Chapter 13.)

Remember that unless you are faced with a life-threatening situation that requires immediate action, you have time to evaluate all the choices open to you once treatment is proposed. You can do this by getting additional medical opinions and learning as much as possible about the relative benefits and risks of the drugs, tests, or surgical procedures you are considering. Often, carefully monitoring a medical condition or following a course of medication or other noninvasive therapy can produce results that make surgery unnecessary. No matter what you decide, fully informing yourself about the options you have is the best way to make yourself a full partner in your health care.

15

Menopause and Beyond

Florence Haseltine, M.D.

Aging means an end to the childbearing years, but for an increasing number of women it also means liberation: the luxury of putting oneself first and the opportunity of considering options that were inconceivable during the years of nurturing and otherwise supporting a family. For the woman who retains her health and energy, these years can be a thoroughly fulfilling period of life. Dr. Sadja Greenwood has coined the acronym PMZ to describe this positive side of aging: postmenopausal zest. Whether older women continue their family responsibilities by caring for aging parents and/or grandchildren, or whether they enter or reenter the work force and start new careers, the rewards of this period of life can be substantial. Given the tremendous leap in life expectancy that has taken place in recent years, as well as the fact that women over 50 make up a burgeoning portion of our population, the medical community needs to turn far more research attention to menopause and the years beyond than it has done in the past.

The definition of menopause is quite clear: the end of menstruation for at least six months due to a cessation in the function of the ovaries. Menopause, therefore, reflects the aging of the female reproductive system. The resulting infertility and loss of ovarian hormones are the two most immediate and obvious consequences of menopause.

Menopause is a normal life event, but it is also a time of biological change that inevitably alters some of the metabolic functions that regulate the body and interact with the aging process. Women usually experience menopause between the ages of 45 and 55. A woman's pattern is often the same as her mother's and sisters', but it may also differ. Smoking, for example, is linked to the onset of early menopause because it causes lower estrogen levels, probably because smoking affects the ovary.

Women do not lose their libido at menopause. Although the ovulating process stops, the ovaries continue to produce small amounts of male hormones that preserve sexual response, and women can continue to have satisfying sex lives for many years. In fact, many postmenopausal women report that the freedom from concern about pregnancy and, later, the freedom from using birth control permits them to experience levels of sexual pleasure they may not have previously allowed themselves.

You should continue to use a barrier method of birth control until your periods have stopped for at least six months, as some women can, and occasionally do, become pregnant this late in life. Of course, if you are taking a birth control pill, you will continue to have periods. Be sure to consult your doctor about how long to keep on using oral contraceptives.

The onset of menopause manifests itself in diverse ways, and it is normal for its qualities to vary from woman to woman. The most obvious of these features is that the menstrual cycle becomes irregular and then ceases completely, a process that can happen suddenly or take place over several years. Bleeding patterns may change as well: sometimes the flow becomes lighter and lasts for fewer days than in the past, or it may become much heavier, sometimes to the point of flooding.

HORMONAL CHANGES AND THEIR EFFECTS

A marked phenomenon in menopause is the change that takes place in the gonadotropins, those substances that affect the ovaries, such as the luteinizing hormone (LH) and the follicle-stimulating hormone (FSH). Before puberty, the levels of LH and FSH are low. They rise during puberty, first at night, and then during the fertile period at mid-cycle, when they climb precipitously, or spike. At menopause, this pattern changes again. Both of these hormones increase, and the rate between them changes. FSH rises more than LH does in relation to the levels that existed during childhood.

This change in women's hormonal status does not happen overnight, but occurs over a long period of time, starting when we are in our late 30s and continuing through the 40s and 50s. From age 35 to 55, women experience a tremendous change in ovarian function. Initially, the gonadotropin hormone levels do not seem to alter, but ovarian function does. Fertility studies have shown that while the ovary continues to produce follicles, they are far less capable of initiating and maintaining a pregnancy. When work on in vitro fertilization began, investigators found it was very difficult to collect eggs from the ovary that would fertilize and implant. (See Chapter 10.) When women reach their late 40s and early 50s and the ovaries stop producing follicles, a marked rise takes place in the levels of the luteinizing hormone and the follicle-stimulating hormone from the pituitary. At the same time, the ovaries begin to decrease their production of estrogen. But women are not left totally and abruptly without estrogen. The ovaries continue to make small quantities of it for about 10 years after menopause. Meanwhile, in response to ovarian slowdown, the adrenal glands take over and produce androstenedione, which converts to estrone, another type of estrogen. The body's fatty tissues also produce estrogen.

The changes in these hormone levels and ratios may affect several systems. One is the ratio of estradiol to estrone. Different estrogens have varying effects on blood lipids and on estrogen-sensitive tissue. There also appears to be a relative increase in the amount of androgen compared to estrogen, which may show up as acne or as a receding hairline. And of course, the ovary stops manufacturing progesterone while the secretion of prolactin, the hormone that stimulates milk production, falls. While these hormonal changes are notable, most of them are secondary to the decrease in estrogen.

SOME CHARACTERISTICS OF MENOPAUSE

HOT FLASHES

About 70 to 75 percent of women experience hot flashes, also called flushes, while others remain entirely free of this common menopausal experience. If present, the flushes can be from occasional to frequent and from mild to severe. Some women find them quite uncomfortable, particularly if they take the form of profuse sweating that appears suddenly. A noticeable hot flash can happen as often as once an hour, and women who experience them repeatedly and with great intensity find it helpful to avoid wearing synthetic fabrics, to wear lighter clothes, particularly cotton, and to dress in layers of light clothing that can be removed quickly if needed. Some women are able to identify certain triggers that bring on hot flashes, such as stress, caffeine, alcohol, hot or spicy foods, and hot drinks; by avoiding these, they are able to decrease the intensity and frequency of the flashes. A remedy as simple as drinking ice water can sometimes be very helpful.

Hot flashes are not imaginary; those women who experience them usually have elevated pulse rates and elevated levels of luteinizing hormone (LH) before the flash occurs. A part of the hypothalamus called the arcuate nucleus contains a signaling mechanism that permits the regular delivery of the gonadotropin-releasing hormone (GnRH), and this makes interior body heat come to the body's surface; it occurs simultaneously with hot flashes. GnRH signals the pituitary gland to release LH and FSH, but researchers have not yet established the precise mechanism that causes hot flashes. Although all postmenopausal women have occasional elevated levels of GnRH, why some women experience flushes and others don't is still a mystery.

As noted, many women are aware of when a hot flash is imminent, and maintaining an accurate daily record of how often and with what intensity they occur can help to predict and thus sometimes to control their occurrences. In addition, certain sensors can provide an objective predictor of flashes. One sensor measures finger temperature. When the blood vessels open (dilate), the finger temperature rises, a phenomenon that can help predict when a flash is coming and measure its intensity.

SLEEP DISTURBANCES

Hot flashes that take place at night interrupt sleep, sometimes causing insomnia and a subsequent lack of the kind of light sleep that takes place when dreaming occurs. Dreaming is an important part of normal sleep, and without it individuals may become tense and irritable, thus exhibiting the kind of behavior that has become so highly stereotyped as a common symptom of menopause. Researchers are now finding that sleep disturbances are an important cause of accidents at work and disruption in family life. Partners also often lose sleep as a result of these disturbances—when an overheated woman throws off the bedcovers, for example, or when the sheets become wet during the night from her intense sweating.

VAGINAL CHANGES

With ovarian failure, the vaginal lining thins because the vagina is very sensitive to the lowered level of estrogen that takes place at this time. This thinning can cause pain and bleeding during intercourse, and can seriously impair a couple's normal sex life. Even for women who don't experience such pain and/or bleeding, more time may be needed for arousal because the vagina, cervix, and uterus all become smaller at menopause and the degree of labial swelling that normally accompanies sexual excitement is reduced. Consequently, lovemaking may have to be more leisurely. It is important for you to be able to tell your partner if your sexual responsiveness changes. Since male sexuality also slows with age, you may find your partner very receptive to this information and happy to experiment with changes in sexual style. Be sensitive to the fact that your confiding these new needs may also threaten a man, particularly if he feels that his usual behavior no longer arouses you. This is a time when it is important for you and your partner to talk about making sexual adjustments in order to preserve and enhance your sex life.

Women with good muscle tone have an advantage in easily continuing a pleasurable sex life, so that Kegel exercises, which improve vaginal muscle strength, are particularly important at this time. (See Chapter 5.)

OTHER CHARACTERISTICS

Menopause has been associated with other qualities of the aging process, such as the wrinkling and drying out of the skin caused by low estrogen levels. In some women, the atrophy of the vagina can produce bladder symptoms, such as burning, increased frequency of urination, or unintended loss of urine. If the atrophy is brought on by estrogen depletion, estrogen therapy can help markedly.

Interestingly, while boys' voices drop at around the age of 13, women's voices lower at around age 50. Because of this subtle difference that occurs after menopause, opera singers usually have to stop singing soprano roles at this age because of the alteration in their voices.

Women can also experience heart palpitations, headaches, and breast tenderness during menopause. And certain other physiological changes take place, including a decrease in bone density. If severe, this can lead to osteoporosis, or to alterations in the cardiovascular system that require medical evaluation. All of these changes are a normal response to menopause.

ESTROGEN AS THERAPY

Estrogen was first identified in the late 1920s. By the mid-1950s, in an effort to treat some of the unwanted symptoms of menopause, doctors were prescribing estrogen in increasing doses for more and more menopausal women, even though studies about its cumulative effects had not been undertaken. This early treatment was called unopposed estrogen therapy, meaning that the estrogen was administered without progestin, the synthetic form of the hormone progesterone. Then, in the early 1970s, a series of research reports indicated that the rising number of estrogen prescriptions appeared to be causing an increase in cancer of the endometrium, the lining of the uterus. These findings led to a dramatic drop in the use of estrogen therapy.

It seems that the heavy estrogen doses doctors prescribed during the 1960s produced a histological picture that resembled cancer in many of the women who used them. But these women did not appear to face the same long-range risk of dying as did those who got endometrial cancer but did not receive estrogen-replacement therapy (ERT). The increase in endometrial cancers that was reported in the 1970s was based on observing tissues that *looked like* cancer but may not have been cancer. Where the tumors *were* cancerous, they were minimally malignant, and these patients usually had a favorable outcome.

After researchers evaluated a great deal of epidemiologic data, the result of this controversy has been to focus on the problems of the relationship between unopposed estrogen and the endometrium. These epidemiologic studies revealed that untreated women, compared with those receiving ERT, experienced an increase in diagnosed endometrial carcinoma. The data also demonstrated a protective effect of estrogen and progestin agents— that is, the epidemiologists noted that women on lower estrogen doses did not seem as vulnerable to endometrial cancer as those who took higher doses, while those who received high doses of estrogen and who also took progesterone did not get cancer. These findings led to the current ERT regimen of lower estrogen doses taken with progesterone. Progesterone was added to the estrogen regimen to down-regulate (balance) the estrogen. The reduced cancer rate was more likely due to the reduction in estrogen doses than to the addition of progesterone, but good long-range studies have yet to be conducted to evaluate the benefits and risks of combined therapy. Since the 1970s, most responsible doctors have tried to find a balance between the relative advantages and disadvantages of ERT and to monitor its use carefully.

Women who have their ovaries removed because of infection or disease before they are 50 experience a very abrupt hormonal loss, severe hot flashes, and other menopausal symptoms. Some sort of estrogen therapy is indicated, but doctors still do not agree on the length of treatment. Most doctors believe the therapy should continue at least until the age of 50, but others prescribe ERT until age 55 or 60. Although menopause before the age of 45 is rare, women with early menopause probably should consider ERT, because they face a markedly increased risk of osteoporosis and heart disease. Be sure to read "How Safe Is Estrogen Therapy?" later in this chapter before you consider estrogen therapy.

ESTROGEN VAGINAL CREAMS

One type of ERT employs a vaginal cream containing estrogen. The original idea here was that, without being ingested, the estrogen would not be absorbed into the bloodstream and carried throughout the body, but would affect only the vagina; thus, a woman would not get endometrial cancer as a result. However, a landmark experiment in the late 1970s demonstrated that estrogen still enters the circulation if administered vaginally, though at a lower dosage than by other methods of administration. The vagina does absorb the estrogen in vaginal cream, which can then affect the endometrium. The reason doctors did not note endometrial cancer in women who used vaginal cream may be because its relatively small estrogen dose compared to that in oral estrogen did not overstimulate the endometrium. Furthermore, although very little effect was noted initially on the FSH, which stays in the body for a long time, a slight decrease in the LH appeared rather quickly. While estrogen vaginal creams can indeed reduce the number and intensity of hot flashes or sometimes can eliminate them entirely, depending on the dose, doctors prescribe it mostly for its effects on the vagina and urethra.

ORAL ESTROGEN

There are two kinds of oral estrogen-replacement therapy: one using estrogen alone and one that adds progestin to estrogen use. Estrogen-only therapies employ several different estrogen compounds, differentiated chiefly by where they come from; some are extracted from horse urine, others are synthetic. These have varied life spans in the blood, and each has slightly different effects on the endometrium. Gynecologists add progestin to estrogen because they assume that, in addition to protecting the endometrium from both cancer and precancerous abnormalities like adenomatous hyperplasia, it may reduce the incidence of breast cancer. ERT regimens use only the progestin Provera, which is different from progestins used in oral contraceptives. However, more research is needed to prove or disprove the assumptions on the role hormones play in various cancers. For now, the typical pattern in the treatment of menopausal symptoms is to take estrogen only for the first 25 days, take progestin concomitantly for the last 10 to 14 days of the estrogen cycle, and have 5 days without medication. Many doctors prescribe estrogen every day and add progestin for the first 10 to 14 days, providing continual therapy. Whichever course your doctor prescribes, it is a good idea to mark your calendar daily so that you can keep track of when to take each medication.

TRANSDERMAL PATCH

A third and more recent type of estrogen administration is through the skin, using a patch that dispenses estrogen over a period of time, referred to as transdermal delivery. However, estrogen given this way may fail to affect blood lipids favorably. Therefore, for women using the patch, doctors should probably add progestin at least every three months to protect against endometrial cancer, and many physicians prescribe it monthly.

HOW EFFECTIVE IS ESTROGEN THERAPY?

There is no question that ERT reduces symptoms. Within a few hours of estrogen administration, the elevated LH and FSH levels drop rapidly, with FSH decreasing more slowly, indicating that estrogen exposure can have an immediate effect on the levels of these hormones. Symptoms such as hot flashes do not lessen significantly until approximately one week after therapy begins; after that, estrogen reduces nocturnal flashes and the insomnia they cause in some women. Unfortunately, oral estrogen occasionally causes nausea and elevated blood pressure. If you experience these, you may try either a vaginal estrogen cream or a skin patch.

Researchers have investigated a number of replacement regimes, using estrogen alone or with progestin, recording the LH/FSH ratio as well as the woman's own subjective measurement of her hot flashes. From these studies, it seems clear that exposure of the central nervous system to estrogen preconditions the brain so that researchers see very specific responses when they withdraw estrogen. For example, women's hot flashes became worse when they stopped taking estrogen, exceeding the norm that existed before therapy began. This rebound effect is a very interesting phenomenon. It implies that another set point exists when women stop taking estrogen abruptly, and that estrogen exposure and withdrawal reversibly alters the action of the hypothalamus, the part of the brain responsible for signaling the pituitary to make FSH and LH, which cause the ovaries to produce estrogen. Women not exposed to estrogen do not show this effect. In other words, hot flashes are the body's response to estrogen withdrawal once a person has experienced it and are not related to age.

HOW SAFE IS ESTROGEN THERAPY?

At present, estrogen is the only drug doctors have with which to treat menopausal symptoms, a fact that clearly reflects the dearth of research that has been conducted in the whole area of women's health. A major effort is needed to find and test other nonhormonal medications that can change the course of estrogen deficiency. In the meantime, physicians and researchers must carefully examine their ideas about estrogen use. If they are to use hormones wisely and safely, they must understand how the body metabolizes and absorbs estrogens and progestins. The metabolic pathways of the different estrogenic and progestational drugs need extensive study, as do the crucial questions of how the mode of administration and the dose affect high-density lipoproteins (HDL), low-density lipoproteins (LDL), the breasts, the brain, and the endometrium. Once physicians know pathways and dosage effects, they should be able to prescribe more accurately with greater benefit and less harm to patients. For example, if we had a compound that could lubricate vaginal tissue or reduce hot flashes without having an impact on the breast, it could be prescribed for women with a family history of breast cancer, or for those who now have breast cancer. At present, these women are unable to use medication at menopause because of worries that estrogen may increase their risk of breast cancer.

The method of administration of any hormone is also important. For example, when the ovary converts androgens from the adrenal gland to estrogens, they enter the bloodstream directly. But if a woman takes estrogens orally, they proceed to the stomach and liver and may raise the level of liver enzymes. Some estrogens affect HDL and LDL levels if taken by mouth but do not appear to influence these levels if they are given vaginally or transdermally. It has not been established whether this is a dosage or a pathway effect. Some of these reactions may also relate to the history of medication use—that is, how much and for how long a woman has been taking a hormone or any other drug.

Doctors have been dropping the doses of oral estrogen they prescribe, but they are now raising the estrogen dosage administered by the transdermal patch delivery system. Because of the previous concern that arose from treating women with high levels of estrogen replacement, the transdermal patch was first employed with a very low dose, which physicians now find they must raise for it to be effective.

The tendency in the last few years has been for women to forgo estrogen-replacement therapy because the earlier association between ERT and cancer outweighed other considerations, such as the possible benefit of ERT in preventing cardiovascular disease and osteoporosis. But the decision whether or not to use estrogen replacement therapy has become somewhat easier with the publication in September 1991 of the largest and longest study of the hormone's postmenopausal benefits. This ten-year research effort, which followed almost 49,000 nurses who were 30 to 65 years old and had no history of cancer or heart disease when the study began, found that the women who were taking estrogen had half the number of heart attacks as those who were not taking the hormone. Heart disease is the greatest killer of older women; the risk of dying from it for women between 50 and 94 is 31 percent, while the chance of dying from breast or uterine cancer for the same age group is only 2.8 percent and .7 of 1 percent respectively.

The study is persuasive but not conclusive, and the National Institutes of Health is planning a double-blind clinical trial to eliminate doubt. However, results will not be available for ten years. At present, fewer than 10 percent of postmenopausal women take estrogen. Many women who want to consider ERT have responsibly sought further information regarding its potential benefits, side effects, and the risks involved, but because the state of medical knowledge is so inadequate, fully informed consent has not been possible. For example, the rate of breast cancer is rising in this country, and the reasons are not clear. While current ERT medications, primarily Premarin and Provera, do not seem to be a major contributing factor, the breast cancer question is far from answered. Some studies have found estrogen to be protective against breast cancer; others have not documented any difference in rates of breast cancer between estrogen users and nonusers; and a few have indicated an increased risk. But as more of our population reaches menopause, and as recommendations for hormonal replacement therapy change, we must learn not only how these drugs affect the breast but what long-term effects they may have on the body in general. Until then, and until physicians educate themselves as fully as possible about how estrogen works, its use should be considered with caution.

CONTRAINDICATIONS TO HORMONE THERAPY

While most areas are gray, some guidelines are clear:

You should not use hormones if you have or ever have had blood clots. This includes pulmonary embolism (a clot in the lungs) and phlebitis (a clot in the leg). You should avoid hormones if you have had a stroke; cancer of the breast, uterus, or ovary; or any abnormal vaginal bleeding. However, some oncologists do recommend ERT to some patients with early-stage uterine cancer who have been free of recurrence of the disease for five years. Because it is the liver that breaks down estrogen, you should not use hormones if you suffer from impaired liver function.

You should be especially careful about using hormones if you have heart or kidney disease, diabetes, epilepsy, or asthma.

You should be wary of using estrogen if you have breast disease, fibroid tumors of the uterus, or have received abnormal results from a mammogram. Since estrogen increases the risk of gallbladder disease, you should be cautious about taking it if you have this problem. If you have high blood pressure or diabetes, your doctor should prescribe hormones only with care and follow you closely, in case the estrogen causes a rise in your blood pressure or a change in the way your body handles sugar.

INDICATIONS FOR HORMONE THERAPY

Who, then, might benefit from hormonal therapy? If you experience either a natural or surgical premature menopause, you probably should take hormones, because you are at greater risk of severe postmenopausal symptoms and osteoporosis. If you are at high risk for osteoporosis or have been tested and found to have low bone density, you should probably start a course of ERT. If your menopausal symptoms are severe, hormonal therapy is the only therapy available that will give you relief.

For the vast area between these two poles, you must balance the risks with the benefits. Either decision—to take hormones or to avoid them—is perfectly reasonable, of course. After asking your clinician all the questions you have about ERT, you will decide for yourself, as always, what is best for you.

OSTEOPOROSIS

Ten to 15 years after the onset of menopause, more than 25 percent of women have developed osteoporosis because of the loss of bone tissue. In its most extreme form, it can cause the "hump" and bent-over posture that sometimes result from collapsed vertebrae in the back; it can also cause significant back and neck pain.

Between 2 and 5 million Americans seek medical help each year for some problem linked to osteoporosis, and upwards of 15 million have osteoporosis to some degree. Although all the body's bones are affected by this condition, fractures of the spine, the wrist, and the hip are typical. Of these, hip fracture is the most devastating; 75 percent of those with a fractured hip must give up their independence, and between 10 and 20 percent die of complications, mostly pneumonia, because of the anesthesia needed during surgery and the lack of mobility afterward.

CAUSES

The risk of developing osteoporosis increases with age, is eight times greater in women than in men, and is more prevalent in whites than in African Americans. The cause of this disease appears to reside in the mechanisms underlying the normal loss of bone mass that follows menopause in women and occurs in all of us with advancing age. Alterations in hormones regulating bone growth and reabsorption, a number of hormonal changes such as a lack of estrogen, and a sedentary life-style all contribute to its development.

Osteoporosis is a leading cause of disability in the elderly. Women with this disorder are often severely handicapped. In this disease, the trabeculae that normally support the bone structure of the vertebrae become thin and deteriorate, causing fractures. Unfortunately, once these trabecular structures are destroyed, they cannot be rebuilt.

RISK FACTORS

Caucasian women who are fair, slender, small, and of northern European background are at greater risk for osteoporosis. Having close relatives (mother or sisters) with osteoporosis increases your chances of developing the disease. A high-protein diet may be a contributing factor because it increases the amount of calcium excreted in the urine; an inadequate lifetime calcium intake, as well as not getting enough sunlight, also raise your risk. Using certain medications can also put you in jeopardy, among them antacids containing aluminum, thyroid pills, steroids, Dilantin, and heparin. Medical problems that elevate your chances of osteoporosis include premature menopause, the absence of menstruation, anorexia nervosa, the presence of abnormal sex chromosomes, diabetes, some types of kidney disease, and hyperthyroidism.

TESTING

Certain tests can report on the status of your bones. Single-photon absorptiometry measures bone density in the arm or heel, which, if low, indicates a greater chance of fractures. This procedure is relatively simple and can be done as an office procedure by any specialist who has the machine. Dual-photon absorptiometry measures bone density of the spine, and can therefore predict vertebral fractures and the development of a hump. But the equipment is much more complex and the test more expensive than the single-photo variety. Both these procedures take only a few minutes.

CAT scans can obtain an exact picture of a cross section of bone. But this procedure is more costly than either form of absorptiometry, takes longer, and exposes the patient to radiation.

Testing can predict risk. Prospective studies show that women with the lowest bone mass in the radius bone of the forearm and the calcaneus (heel bone) have a higher risk of all kinds of fractures in the ribs, the metacarpal bones of the hand, and the forearms. A recent large prospective inquiry, the Study of Osteoporotic Fractures, investigated women over 65 years of age to determine whether those with lower bone density in the radius and calcaneus might also have a higher incidence of hip fracture. The investigators measured bone mineral density in these two bones at the beginning of the study, and every four months for 20 months, using single-photon absorptiometry. Among the 9,703 Caucasian women in the study, they found 53 hip fractures. The study showed that the lower the bone density, the higher the risk of hip fracture, and that both sites predicted the women's risk for this type of fracture equally well. The risk of hip fracture in this population doubled for each 10-year increase in age.

If you have any risk factors for osteoporosis, if you have had a fracture from a mild stimulus, or if your height has decreased, you should consider being tested, because estrogen-replacement therapy can be most effective in reducing bone loss when it is started early.

PREVENTING OSTEOPOROSIS

It is wise to make your home as accident-proof as possible. Eliminate any conditions that lead to slipping and falling, such as scatter rugs, loose carpeting, extension cords or other loose wiring, insufficient stairway railings, highly polished floors, and poor lighting. Since medications that cause dizziness or poor coordination increase the risk of falling, and because more hip fractures occur among patients who take certain sleeping pills, antianxiety drugs, and tranquilizers, it is a good idea to review all your medications with your doctor to see if they multiply your risk of falls and fractures.

Exercise and proper diet, including an adequate lifetime calcium intake, can help to prevent bone loss and keep bones strong. Because our bodies need vitamin D to absorb calcium and other minerals, ask your doctor about derivatives of vitamin D that may also be an effective preventive treatment for osteoporosis. (See Chapter 6.)

LIVING WITH OSTEOPOROSIS

A series of evaluations from Scandinavia that studied the mineral content of the bones in the hand (metacarpals) in patients who did not receive estrogen therapy found that the bones' mineral content dropped steadily. At the point that bone density had decreased severely in these women, the investigators were able to predict when fractures would occur. On the other hand, they found that the women who were on ERT lost bone at a much lesser rate.

Researchers have established that, at menopause, a steady loss of mineral content in the bone takes place over a 36-month period. This is not enough loss to produce fractures, and even at this point, some rebuilding of the bone can be obtained with the use of ERT because the trabecular bone architecture has not been destroyed, just thinned. In fact, women begin to lose bone during the pre-menopausal period because bone loss is a normal part of the aging process. But lack of estrogen can exacerbate the problem. For maximum protection against osteoporosis, it is best to consider starting estrogen-replacement therapy within three years of menopause. The usual dose is 0.625 milligrams of conjugated estrogen, which is sufficient to reduce bone loss as well as hot flashes. How to determine the exact amount that works for each woman has not yet been established, but doctors favor the 0.625 dose since this amount shows no association with a higher rate of endometrial cancer. Progesterone alone also protects against bone loss and hot flashes.

Remember that the medical community is in disagreement about how long ERT can be safely and effectively continued, as well as whether lower doses can suffice with aging. Intermittent treatment is apparently less beneficial than continuous treatment, however, because bone loss starts again as soon as the estrogen is discontinued.

As in all aspects of women's health, further research is needed in treating osteoporosis. Etidronate, an oral compound, has been found safe and effective in treating osteoporosis by slowing bone reabsorption, but it is very expensive and has not yet been approved by the FDA for this purpose.

EXERCISE

Regular exercise can specifically benefit menopausal women because it stimulates cells that build bones. Weight-bearing exercise that puts stress on your long bones is most effective. Walking, jogging, bicycling, jumping rope, and using various exercise machines can all improve the condition of your bones, though jogging and jumping rope might cause injury to bones and joints by the pounding they entail. Swimming, while an excellent overall conditioner, is not useful in strengthening bones.

A variety of studies has shown that weight-bearing exercise, started at any age, increases the calcium content of bones and their resistance to fracture. One study found that a group of women in their 80s living in a nursing home who did chair exercises for 30 minutes three times a week for three years increased their bone density by 2.29 percent, while among a similar group of inactive women, bone loss averaged 3.28 percent. Another study, of men and women in their 70s conducted at the Michigan School of Public Health, found that two 40-minute exercise sessions weekly brought a number of health improvements after three months, among them increases in flexibility, balance, and the ability to move quickly and steadily, which lessens the risk of accidents. These older people also experienced reduced blood pressure, relief from arthritis pain, and a more upbeat mood.

If you have not been active, you should see your doctor before starting any strenuous activity, to make sure that you are in proper health to embark on a regular exercise program. Once you receive this clearance, it is a good idea to begin slowly, gradually increasing the length and number of exercise sessions as your overall fitness improves.

CARDIOVASCULAR DISEASE

Aside from the caution and care you should exercise in general in considering the use of ERT, the more specific approach is to consider the balance between the possible increased risk of breast and endometrial cancers that it poses versus the slowing of bone loss and decreased chance of osteoporosis that it achieves. In addition, estrogen replacement may also influence cardiovascular disease, and treating cardiovascular disease is one of the main reasons physicians give for using ERT. Nevertheless, the effect of estrogen on heart disease and the mechanism of its action is not clear, and there is no evidence that it is actually protective. At the same time, cardiovascular disease is the most likely disease a 50-year-old woman will die from over the five to 15 years after menopause.

Although most women are more frightened of breast cancer and osteoporosis, they actually face double the risk of developing cardiovascular disease than they do of developing any form of cancer, and a tenfold increase of cardiovascular disease over breast cancer alone. This does not mean that the other diseases are not serious; it simply indicates how thoughtlessly health authorities have been avoiding the major health issue that the threat of heart disease represents to older women.

The relationship between menopause and cardiovascular disease is not explicit, although there is some evidence that normal ovarian function protects the cardiovascular system. Until women reach the menopausal years, their rate of heart disease does not rise at the same rate as it does for men. In the 40- to 48-year-old age group, for example, men face a five times greater risk of heart disease than do women. The ratio of women developing cardiovascular disease does not approach that of men until they are between 65 and 69, at which point 22.1 of every 1,000 women get the disease, compared to 26.7 of every 1,000 men.

What evidence we have on this topic has not totally resolved the issue. Data from the Framingham study, which includes women who are pre- and postmenopausal and compares the rates at which they get cardiovascular disease, shows that there is a twofold increase as women enter menopause up to about age 55. Age is clearly the main risk factor here, because a woman's risk of heart disease increases as she ages, whether or not she is menstruating or has ovarian function.

The HANES (Health and Nutrition Examination Survey) study, which relates the factors of smoking, high blood pressure, diabetes, elevated cholesterol, and weight to cardiovascular disease at five-year age intervals, compared two similar groups, one using estrogen and one not using it. For women who had an early menopause—that is, before age 45—those who took estrogen reduced their risk of cardiovascular disease by 10 to 40 percent. Unfortunately, the study failed to look at the much larger population of women who had a normal menopause, and consequently we have no indication of whether estrogen therapy benefits them or not.

As in so many other areas of general health, most of the information on cardiovascular disease comes from studies of men. Although investigators have tried to extrapolate the data to women, it is not necessarily totally applicable. For example, in men, the ratio of high-density lipoproteins (HDL) to low-density lipoproteins (LDL) is important: the higher the HDL, the lower the risk of cardiovascular disease, while the higher the LDL, the higher the risk of cardiovascular disease. The same may be true for women; serum cholesterol seems to be associated with an elevated risk of cardiovascular disease, and in women who have passed menopause, it is mainly the LDL that rises, not the HDL. Thus, one concern about treatment with estrogens and progestational agents is how they affect fats. Studies show that some forms of estrogen decrease the level of LDL and slightly increase the level of HDL; some of the progestational agents seem to have the opposite effect on HDL and LDL, and this is one of the concerns with the therapy as it is now used.

As our population ages, the benefits of achieving good health and the practices for maintaining and perpetuating it in later life are being investigated, expanded on, and adopted by greater and greater numbers of people. As enlightened consumers of health-care services, women have been in the forefront of pressing the medical community for needed services and humanizing medical practice.

Our society is slowly learning that the health-care issues of later life deserve the same scrutiny and evaluation as those of youth and midlife. The future study of aging, especially for women, seems promising indeed.

Appendix

TERATOGEN INFORMATION SERVICES*

KEY

Calls accepted from:

P = Public
H = Health-Care Providers

Type of service:

T = Telephone Service
C = Clinical Service

U.S.A.

1. Arizona Teratogen Information Service
   Department of Pediatrics
   University of Arizona Health Sciences Center
   2504 East Elm
   Tucson, AZ 85716
   Eugene Hoyme, M.D., Lynn Hauck, M.A., Dee Quinn, M.S.
   1-800-362-0101 (AZ only); (602) 626-6016 [P,H,T,C]
   1-800-544-7543 (New Mexico only) [H,T]

*Compiled by MA Teratogen Information Service (updated 5/91)

2. Teratogen Counseling Information Service
   Arkansas Genetics Program
   University of Arkansas for Medical Sciences
   4301 West Markham, Slot 518
   Little Rock, AR 72205
   Chris Cunniff, M.D., Donald R. Mattison, M.D.
   Elizabeth Alderson, R.N.P., LaJuana Morrison, R.N.
   (501) 686-5994 [H,T]

3. California Teratogen Registry
   Department of Pediatrics H814B, UCSD Medical Center
   University of California
   225 Dickinson Street
   San Diego, CA 92103
   Kenneth L. Jones, M.D., Kathleen Johnson, B.S.
   1-800-532-3749 (CA only); (619) 294-6084 [P,H,T]

4. Colorado/Wyoming Teratogen Information and Education
   Service
   Children's Hospital, Division of Genetics
   1056 East 19th Avenue
   Denver, CO 80218-1088
   David Manchester, M.D., Karen Prescott, M.S.,
   Cathy Marquez
   1-800-332-3073 or 2082 (CO only); 1-800-442-2701 (WY only);
   (303) 861-6395 [P,H,T,C]

5. Connecticut Pregnancy Exposure Information Service
   Division of Human Genetics, Department of Pediatrics
   University of Connecticut Health Center
   263 Farmington Ave.
   Farmington, CT 06032
   Sally Rosengren, M.D., Glenda Dings Spivey, M.S.
   1-800-325-5391 (CT only); (203) 679-1502 [P,H,T,C]

6. Teratogen Information Service
   Department of Pediatrics, Division of Genetics
   Box J-296 JHMHSC, University of Florida
   Gainesville, FL 32610-0296

Charles A. Williams, M.D., Donna Poynor, M.A.
(904) 392-3050 [P,H,T,C]

7. Teratogen Information Service
    University of Miami School of Medicine
    Mailman Center, P.O. Box 016820
    Miami, FL 33101
    Herbert A. Lubs, M.D., Virginia H. Carver, Ph.D.
    Yezmin Perrilla, M.S., Anna C. Carpenter, M.P.H.
    (305) 547-6464 [H,T,C]

8. Teratogen Information Service
    Department of Pediatrics, College of Medicine
    University of South Florida
    12901 Bruce B. Downs Boulevard, Box 15-G
    Tampa, FL 33612-4799
    Suzanne R. Sage, R.N., M.S., Boris G. Kousseff, M.D.
    James K. Hartsfield, Jr., D.M.D., M.S., M.M.Sc.
    (813) 974-2262 [P,H,T,C]

9. Centers for Disease Control
    Birth Defects and Genetic Diseases Branch, Koger 2033 (F-37)
    1600 Clifton Road
    Atlanta, GA 30333
    Jose Cordero, M.D., M.P.H., Muin Khoury, M.D., Ph.D.
    (404) 488-4717 [P,H,T]

10. Illinois Teratogen Information Service
    Northwestern Memorial Hospital, Suite 1564, Prentice
    Pavilion
    333 East Superior Ave.
    Chicago, IL 60611
    Eugene Pergament, M.D., Ph.D.,
    Maureen Smith-Deichmann, M.S.
    1-800-252-4847 (IL only); (312) 908-7441 [P,H,T,C]

11. Iowa Teratogen Information Service
    Department of Pediatrics/Medical Genetics
    University of Iowa, Hospitals and Clinics
    Iowa City, IA 52242

James Hanson, M.D., Roger A. Williamson, M.D.
Ann Muilenburg, R.N., Christine Headley, R.N.
(319) 356-2674 [H,T,C]

12. Prenatal Diagnosis & Genetics Clinic
HCA Wesley Medical Center
550 North Hillside
Wichita, KS 67214
(316) 688-2360

13. Food and Drug Administration
HFD 733
Rockville, MD 20857
(301) 443-2306

14. Massachusetts Teratogen Information Service
National Birth Defects Center, Franciscan Children's Hospital
30 Warren Street
Boston, MA 02135
Murray Feingold, M.D., Jane O'Brien, M.D.,
Susan Rosenwasser, M.Ed., Katryn Miller, M.Ed.,
Robin Maltz, M.P.H., Karen Treat, M.S.
1-800-322-5014 (MA only); (617) 787-4957 [P,H,T,C]

15. Genis (Genetics and Environmental Information Service)
Washington University School of Medicine
OB/GYN—Genetics Department
216 South King's Highway, First Floor
St. Louis, MO 63110
Heidi Beaver, M.P.H., Cindy Johnson, M.S.,
Laura Turlington, M.S., James Crane, M.D.
(314) 454-8172 [P,H,T,C]

16. Nebraska Teratogen Project
MRI, University of Nebraska Medical Center
600 South 42nd Street
Omaha, NE 68198-5430
Beth Conover, R.N., M.S., Bruce Buehler, M.D.
(402) 559-5071 [H,T,C]

17. New Jersey Pregnancy Risk Information Service
    Department of Pediatrics and Genetics
    School of Osteopathic Medicine
    University of Medicine and Dentistry of New Jersey
    401 Haddon Avenue
    Camden, NJ 08103
    Michael McCormack, Ph.D., Carol Zuber, M.S.
    (609) 757-7869; 1-800-441-0025 (NJ only) [P,H,T,C]

18. Western New York Teratogen Information Service
    1200 East & West Place, Building 16
    West Seneca, NY 14224
    Luther K. Robinson, M.D., Jan Robinson, P.N.P.,
    Carolyn Farrell, M.S.
    (716) 833-9359; 1-800-869-9606 (western NY only) [P,H,T,C]

19. Perinatal Environmental and Drug Exposure Consultation
    Service (PEDECS)
    Department OB/GYN, University of Rochester Medical Center
    601 Elmwood Ave.
    Rochester, NY 14642
    Richard K. Miller, Ph.D.
    (716) 275-3638 [H,C]

20. Pregnancy Healthline
    Genetics Section, Seventh Floor, Spruce Building
    Pennsylvania Hospital, Eighth and Spruce Streets
    Philadelphia, PA 19107-6192
    Alan E. Donnenfeld, M.D.
    Ronald J. Librizzi, D.O., Leslie Vought, M.S.
    (215) 829-5437 [P,H,T,C]

21. Pregnancy Safety Hotline
    Department of Medical Genetics, Western Pennsylvania
    Hospital
    4800 Friendship Avenue
    Pittsburgh, PA 15224
    Karen A. Filkins, M.D., Christiann Jackson, M.D.
    Catherine Ritter, M.S., Michael Kerr, M.D.,

Kathy Bournikos, M.S.
(412) 687-SAFE [P,H,T,C]

22. Reproductive Genetics, Magee-Women's Hospital
Forbes and Halket Street
Pittsburgh, PA 15213
Sandra G. Marchese, M.S., Dee Pegram, M.Ed.
(412) 647-4168 [P,H,T,C]

23. South Dakota Teratogen and Birth Defects Information Project
Birth Defects Genetics Center
University of South Dakota Medical School
414 East Clark Street
Vermillion, SD 57069
Patricia Ann Skorey, M.N.S., Carol Walton, M.S.
1-800-962-1642 (SD only), (605) 677-5623 [P,H,T,C]

24. Teratogen Information Service
Pediatric Subspecialty Building
T. C. Thompson Children's Hospital
910 Blackford Street
Chattanooga, TN 37403
Richard M. Roberts, Ph.D., M.D.,
Joie Davis, R.N., C.P.N.P, M.S.N.
(615) 778-6112 [P,H,T,C]

25. UTCHS Medical Genetics
Department of Pediatrics
711 Jefferson, Room 523
Memphis, TN 38163
(901) 528-6595 [C only]

26. Genetic Screening and Counseling Service
Texas State Department of Mental Health and Mental
Retardation
3600 McKinney
P.O. Box 2467
Denton, TX 76202-2467
Charles Combs, M.Ed., Rick Macias, M.D.,

Joseph Sears, M.D., Lori Wolfe
(817) 383-3561 [P,H,T,C]

27. Pregnancy Riskline (Utah, Montana, Nevada)
Utah State Department of Health
44 Medical Drive
Salt Lake City, UT 84113
John Carey, M.D., Marsha Leen-Mitchell, B.S.,
Lynn Martinez, B.S.
1-800-822-BABY (UT, excluding Salt Lake City); (801) 583-2229
(Salt Lake City area); 1-800-521-2229 (MT and NV) [P,H,T,C]

28. Vermont Pregnancy Risk Information Service
Vermont Regional Genetics Center
96 Colchester Avenue
Burlington, VT 05401
Alan E. Guttmacher, M.D., Elizabeth F. Allen, Ph.D.
1-800-531-9800 (VT only); (802) 658-4310 [P,H,T,C]

29. Washington State Poison Control Network
Children's Hospital
4800 Sand Point Way N.E.
Seattle, WA 98105
William Robertson, M.D., Timothy Fuller, R.Ph.,
Steven Bobbink, R.Ph.
1-800-732-6985 (WA only); (206) 526-2121 [P,H,T]

30. Central Laboratory for Human Embryology
Department of Pediatrics RD20, School of Medicine
University of Washington
Seattle, WA 98195
Thomas Shepard, M.D.
(206) 543-3373 [P,H,T,C]

31. Wisconsin Teratogen Project
Waisman Center, Room 347, University of Wisconsin
1500 Highland Avenue
Madison, WI 53705-2280
Renata Laxova, M.D., Jody Hahn, M.S.
1-800-362-3020 (WI only); (608) 262-4719 [P,H,T,C]

32. Eastern Wisconsin Teratogen Service
Medical Genetics Institute, S.C.
4555 West Schroeder Drive, Suite 180
Brown Deer, WI 53223
Rafel Elejalde, M.D., Maria M. de Elejalde, R.N.
(414) 357-6555 [P,H,T,C]

33. Teratogen Information Program (TIP)
Birth Defects Center
Children's Hospital of Wisconsin
9000 West Wisconsin Ave.
P.O. Box 1997
Milwaukee, WI 53201
(414) 266-2900

34. Great Lakes Genetics
2323 North Mayfair Road, Suite 410
Wauwatosa, WI 53226
(414) 475-7223

CANADA

35. Motherisk
Hospital for Sick Children
555 University Avenue
Toronto M5G 1X8, Ontario, Canada
Gideon Koren, M.D., Natalie Horlatsh, B.Sc.
Sheelagh Martin, R.N., Anne Pastuszak
(416) 598-6780 [P,H,T,C]

36. Info-Grossesse: The Pregnancy Healthline
[closed because of lack of funds]
Department of Epidemiology, McGill University
1020 Pine Avenue West
Montreal H3A 1A2, Quebec, Canada
Abby Lippman, Ph.D., Marie LeDuc, R.N., B.A.
F.C. Frasere, M.D., Ph.D., M. Vekemans, M.D., Ph.D.

37.   Safe-Start Teratogen Project, Room 1E-1
      Chedoke-McMaster Hospitals
      Box 2000, Station A
      1200 Main St. West
      Hamilton L8N 3Z5, Ontario, Canada
      Elizabeth Chow-Tung, Pharm.D.
      (416) 521-2100 x6788 [H,T,C]

38.   Ottawa Motherisk
      Regional Poison Center
      Children's Hospital of Eastern Ontario
      401 Smyth Road
      Ottawa K1H 8L1, Ontario, Canada
      Michelle Brill-Edwards, M.D.
      (613) 737-2320 [P,H,T,C]

39.   Teratogen Information Service
      Department of Medical Genetics
      University Hospital—Shaughnessy Site
      4500 Oak Street
      Vancouver V6H 3N1, British Columbia, Canada
      Jan Friedman, M.D., Ph.D., Wendy Hird, M.Sc.
      Heidi Hogg, M.Sc.
      (604) 875-2157 [P,H,C]

40.   Fetal Risk Assessment from Maternal Exposure
      (FRAME) Program
      Division of Clinical Pharmacology
      Children's Hospital of Western Ontario
      800 Commissioner's Road East
      London N6C 2V5, Ontario, Canada
      Michael Rieder, M.D., F.R.C.P.C., Ph.D.
      (519) 685-8140 [P,H,T,C]

FRANCE

41.   Centre Régional d'Information sur les Tératogènes
      Institut Européen des Génomutations
      86, Rue Edmond Locard

F69005 Lyon, France
Elisabeth Robert, M.D.
(33) 78-25-82-10

42. Centre de Renseignements sur les Agents Tératogènes
(CRAT)
CHU St. Antoine Laboratoire d'Embryologie
184, Rue du Faubourg
75102 Paris, France
Dr. Elisabeth Elefant, Charles Roux, Marie Boyer, M.D.
(1) 43-41-26-22; (1) 43-41-71-00 poste 1462

GERMANY

43. Beratungsstelle für Embryotokiuologie
Pulsstr. 3
D1000 Berlin 19, Germany
49-30-3023022

ISRAEL

44. Teratogen Information Service, Laboratory of Teratology
Hebrew University, Hadassah Medical School, PO Box 1172
Jerusalem, Israel
Asher Ornoy, M.D., Judy Arnon, Ph.D.
02-428430/5

45. Beilinson Teratogen Information Center
Beilinson Medical Center
Petah Tikva 49100, Israel
03-937747312

ITALY

46. Red Telephone: Pregnancy Counseling Service
Osepale San Paolo, Clinica Ostetrica
Via A. Di Rudini 8

Milan, Italy 20142
Sabina Dal Verme
02-8184286

47.   Telefono Rosso
      Servizio di Epidemiologia e Clinica dei Difetti Congeniti
      Instituto di Clinica Pediatrica
      Universita Cattolica del Sacro Coure
      Largo Gemelli 8
      Rome 00168, Italy
      Pierpaolo Mastroiacovo, M.D.
      0039-06-3372779/3381344

THE NETHERLANDS

48.   Teratology Information Service
      Department of Teratology
      National Institute of Public Health and Environmental
      Hygiene
      P.O. Box 1, 3720 BA Bilthoven
      The Netherlands
      Paul Peters, Ph.D., D.V.M., J.M. Garbis-Berkvens, B.Sc.
      31-30-742017/742944

SWITZERLAND

49.   Swiss Teratogen Information System
      Institut d'Histologie et d'Embryologie
      Université de Lausanne, Rue du Brignon 9
      1005 Lausanne, Switzerland
      Thomas Pexeider, M.D., A. Bueret, M.D., D. Bloch, M.D.
      41-21-492-952/41-21-313-2952

UNITED KINGDOM

50.   Teratology Information Service of the National Poisons
      Information Service

Department of Pharmacology and Toxicology
U.M.D.S., Guys Hospital Medical School,
University of London
St. Thomas St.
London SE1 9RT, U.K.
Frank M. Sullivan, B.Sc., Patricia R. McElhatton, Ph.D.
44-71-955-4240

Index